Restless Legs Syndrome and Sleep Related Movement Disorders

Editor

DENISE SHARON

SLEEP MEDICINE CLINICS

www.sleep.theclinics.com

Consulting Editor
TEOFILO LEE-CHIONG Jr

September 2015 • Volume 10 • Number 3

ELSEVIER

1600 John F. Kennedy Boulevard • Suite 1800 • Philadelphia, Pennsylvania, 19103-2899

http://www.theclinics.com

SLEEP MEDICINE CLINICS Volume 10, Number 3
September 2015, ISSN 1556-407X, ISBN-13: 978-0-323-39585-4

Editor: Patrick Manley
Developmental Editor: Donald Mumford

Sleep Medicine Clinics (ISSN 1556-407X) is published quarterly by Elsevier Inc., 360 Park Avenue South, New York, NY 10010-1710. Months of issue are March, June, September and December. Business and Editorial Offices: 1600 John F. Kennedy Blvd., Ste. 1800, Philadelphia, PA 19103-2899. Customer Service Office: 3251 Riverport Lane, Maryland Heights, MO 63043. Periodicals postage paid at New York, NY and additional mailing offices. Subscription prices are $195.00 per year (US individuals), $95.00 (US residents), $406.00 (US institutions), $230.00 (Canadian individuals), $235.00 (international individuals), $135.00 (Canadian and international residents) and $452.00 (Canadian and international institutions). Foreign air speed delivery is included in all *Clinics* subscription prices. All prices are subject to change without notice. **POSTMASTER:** Send change of address to *Sleep Medicine Clinics*, Elsevier Health Sciences Division, Subscription Customer Service, 3251 Riverport Lane, Maryland Heights, MO 63043. Customer Service: **Tel: 1-800-654-2452 (U.S. and Canada); 314-447-8871 (outside U.S. and Canada). Fax: 314-447-8029. E-mail: journalscustomerservice-usa@elsevier.com (for print support); journalsonline support-usa@elsevier.com (for online support).**

Reprints. For copies of 100 or more of articles in this publication, please contact the Commercial Reprints Department, Elsevier Inc., 360 Park Avenue South, New York, NY 10010-1710. Tel.: 212-633-3874; Fax: 212-633-3820; E-mail: reprints@elsevier.com.

Sleep Medicine Clinics is covered in *MEDLINE/PubMed (Index Medicus)*.

PROGRAM OBJECTIVE
The goal of *Sleep Clinics of North America* is to keep practicing physicians up to date with current clinical practice by providing timely articles reviewing the state of the art in patient care.

TARGET AUDIENCE
All practicing physicians and other healthcare professionals.

LEARNING OBJECTIVES
Upon completion of this activity, participants will be able to:
1. Review the epidemiology and diagnosis of the Restless Leg Syndrome/Willis-Ekbom Disease (RLS/WED).
2. Discuss the comorbidity of RLS/WED with other issues such as psychiatric disorders and growing pains.
3. Recognize the roles of both pharmacologic and non-pharmacologic treatments in the management of RLS/WED.

ACCREDITATION
The Elsevier Office of Continuing Medical Education (EOCME) is accredited by the Accreditation Council for Continuing Medical Education (ACCME) to provide continuing medical education for physicians.

The EOCME designates this enduring material for a maximum of 15 *AMA PRA Category 1 Credit*(s)™. Physicians should claim only the credit commensurate with the extent of their participation in the activity.

All other health care professionals requesting continuing education credit for this enduring material will be issued a certificate of participation.

DISCLOSURE OF CONFLICTS OF INTEREST
The EOCME assesses conflict of interest with its instructors, faculty, planners, and other individuals who are in a position to control the content of CME activities. All relevant conflicts of interest that are identified are thoroughly vetted by EOCME for fair balance, scientific objectivity, and patient care recommendations. EOCME is committed to providing its learners with CME activities that promote improvements or quality in healthcare and not a specific proprietary business or a commercial interest.

The planning committee, staff, authors and editors listed below have identified no financial relationships or relationships to products or devices they or their spouse/life partner have with commercial interest related to the content of this CME activity:
Nadir Askenasy, MD, PhD; Jean-Jacques Askenasy, MD, PhD; Philip M. Becker, MD; Terry M. Brown, DO; Maria Clotilde Carra, DMD, PhD; Giacomo Chiaro, MD; Sudhansu Chokroverty, MD, FRCP; Norma G. Cuellar, PhD, RN, FAAN; Thomas J. Dye, MD; Raffaele Ferri, MD; Michela Figorilli, MD; Bernard Fleury, MD; Anjali Fortna; Stephany Fulda, PhD; Cathy Goldstein, MD; Nelly Huynh, PhD; Brian B. Koo, MD; Susan Mackie, MD; Mauro Manconi, MD, PhD; Patrick Manley; Mahalakshmi Narayanan; Chiara Prosperetti, MD; Federica Provini, MD, PhD; Monica Puligheddu, MD; Erin Scheckenbach; Denise Sharon, MD, PhD, FAASM; Narong Simakajornboon, MD; Marietta P. Stanton, PhD, RN, FAAN; Mary Suzanne Stevens, MD, MS; Naoko Tachibana, MD, PhD; Lynn Marie Trotti, MD, MSc; Debra Whisenant, PhD, MSPH, RN; Rochelle S. Zak, MD.

The planning committee, staff, authors and editors listed below have identified financial relationships or relationships to products or devices they or their spouse/life partner have with commercial interest related to the content of this CME activity:
Richard P. Allen, PhD, FAASM is a consultant/advisor for Luitpold Pharmaceuticals, Inc.
Diego García-Borreguero, MD, PhD is on the speakers bureau for UCB, Inc. and Otsuka Holdings Co., Ltd., a consultant/advisor for Merck & Co., Inc.; Jazz Pharmaceuticals plc; and Ferrer, and receives research support from XenoPort, Inc.
Gilles Lavigne, DMD, PhD, FRCD is a Canada Research Chair.
Teofilo Lee-Chiong Jr, MD has stock ownership, a research grant, and an employment affiliation with Koninklijke Philips N.V., is a consultant/advisor for CareCore National and Elsevier B.V.; and has royalties/patents with Elsevier B.V.; Lippincott; John Wiley & Sons, Inc.; Oxford University Press; and CreateSpace, a DBA of On-Demand Publishing, LLC.
David B. Rye, MD, PhD is a consultant/advisor for UCB, Inc.; XenoPort, Inc.; and Jazz Pharmaceuticals plc.
Arthur S. Walters, MD is a consultant/advisor for, with research support from, UCB, Inc. and Mundipharma International.
John W. Winkelman, MD, PhD is a consultant/advisor for UCB, Inc.; XenoPort, Inc.; INSYS Therapeutics, Inc.; Merck & Co., Inc.; and Flex Pharma, Inc., and has research support from UCB, Inc.; XenoPort, Inc.; Purdue Pharma L.P.; and Neurometrix, Inc.

UNAPPROVED/OFF-LABEL USE DISCLOSURE
The EOCME requires CME faculty to disclose to the participants:
1. When products or procedures being discussed are off-label, unlabelled, experimental, and/or investigational (not US Food and Drug Administration [FDA] approved); and
2. Any limitations on the information presented, such as data that are preliminary or that represent ongoing research, interim analyses, and/or unsupported opinions. Faculty may discuss information about pharmaceutical agents that is outside of FDA-approved labelling. This information is intended solely for CME and is not intended to promote off-label use of these medications. If you have any questions, contact the medical affairs department of the manufacturer for the most recent prescribing information.

TO ENROLL

To enroll in the Sleep Medicines Clinic Continuing Medical Education program, call customer service at 1-800-654-2452 or sign up online at http://www.theclinics.com/home/cme. The CME program is available to subscribers for an additional annual fee of USD $140.

METHOD OF PARTICIPATION

In order to claim credit, participants must complete the following:

1. Complete enrolment as indicated above.
2. Read the activity.
3. Complete the CME Test and Evaluation. Participants must achieve a score of 70% on the test. All CME Tests and Evaluations must be completed online.

CME INQUIRIES/SPECIAL NEEDS

For all CME inquiries or special needs, please contact elsevierCME@elsevier.com.

SLEEP MEDICINE CLINICS

THE CLINICS ARE AVAILABLE ONLINE!
Access your subscription at:
www.theclinics.com

Contributors

CONSULTING EDITOR

TEOFILO LEE-CHIONG Jr, MD
Professor of Medicine, National Jewish Health;
Professor of Medicine, School of Medicine,
University of Colorado Denver, Denver,
Colorado; Chief Medical Liaison, Philips
Respironics, Pennsylvania

EDITOR

DENISE SHARON, MD, PhD, FAASM
Assistant Professor of Medicine, Tulane
University School of Medicine, New Orleans,
Louisiana; Clinical Director, Advanced Sleep
Center, Metairie, Louisiana

AUTHORS

RICHARD P. ALLEN, PhD, FAASM
Associate Professor, Department of
Neurology, Johns Hopkins University,
Baltimore, Maryland

JEAN-JACQUES ASKENASY, MD, PhD
Department of Neurology, Sackler Medical
School, Tel-Aviv University, Tel Aviv, Israel

NADIR ASKENASY, MD, PhD
Frankel Laboratory, Petach Tikva, Israel

PHILIP M. BECKER, MD
President, Sleep Medicine Associates of
Texas; Clinical Professor, Department of
Psychiatry, University of Texas Southwestern
Medical Center, Dallas, Texas

TERRY M. BROWN, DO
Medical Director, Sleep Medicine Associates,
LLC, Sleep Disorders Center, St. Joseph
Memorial Hospital, Murphysboro, Illinois

MARIA CLOTILDE CARRA, DMD, PhD
Assistant Professor, Department of
Periodontology, Service of Odontology,

Rothschild Hospital, Assistance Publique -
Hopitaux de Paris, Université Paris 7 – Denis
Diderot, Unité de formation et recherche of
Odontology, Paris, France

GIACOMO CHIARO, MD
Department of Biomedical and Neuromotor
Sciences, Bellaria Hospital, University of
Bologna, Bologna, Italy

SUDHANSU CHOKROVERTY, MD, FRCP
Director of Sleep Medicine Research; Co-Chair
Emeritus; Professor of Neuroscience,
Department of Neurology, JFK Neuroscience
Institute, Edison, New Jersey; Professor,
Department of Neuroscience, Seton Hall
University, South Orange, New Jersey

NORMA G. CUELLAR, PhD, RN, FAAN
Full Professor, Capstone College of Nursing,
University of Alabama, Tuscaloosa, Alabama

THOMAS J. DYE, MD
Assistant Professor of Pediatrics, Cincinnati
Children's Hospital Medical Center, Cincinnati,
Ohio

RAFFAELE FERRI, MD
Senior Staff Specialist and Head, Department
of Neurology I.C., Sleep Research Centre, Oasi
Institute for Research on Mental Retardation
and Brain Aging (IRCCS), Troina, Italy

MICHELA FIGORILLI, MD
Specialist Collaborator, Neurophysiology Unit,
Sleep Disorder Center, University of Cagliari,
Monserrato, Cagliari, Italy

BERNARD FLEURY, MD
Sleep Medicine and Respiratory Function Unit,
Saint Antoine Hospital, Assistance Publique -
Hopitaux de Paris, Paris, France

STEPHANY FULDA, PhD
Sleep and Epilepsy Center, Neurocenter of
Southern Switzerland, Civic Hospital (EOC) of
Lugano, Lugano, Switzerland

DIEGO GARCÍA-BORREGUERO, MD, PhD
Director, Sleep Research Institute, Madrid,
Spain

CATHY GOLDSTEIN, MD
Assistant Professor, Department of Neurology,
University of Michigan Sleep Disorders Center,
Ann Arbor, Michigan

NELLY HUYNH, PhD
Faculty of Dental Medicine, Université de
Montréal, Montreal, Quebec, Canada

BRIAN B. KOO, MD
Department of Neurology, Yale University
School of Medicine, New Haven, Connecticut;
Department of Neurology, West Haven VAMC,
Connecticut Veterans Affairs Healthcare
System, West Haven, Connecticut

GILLES LAVIGNE, DMD, PhD, FRCD
Dean, Faculty of Dental Medicine, Université
de Montréal, Montreal, Quebec, Canada

SUSAN MACKIE, MD
Instructor in Medicine, Department of Internal
Medicine, Brigham and Women's Hospital,
Harvard Medical School, Boston,
Massachusetts

MAURO MANCONI, MD, PhD
Sleep Center, Neurocenter of Southern
Switzerland, Civic Hospital of Lugano, Lugano,
Switzerland

CHIARA PROSPERETTI, MD
Sleep Center, Neurocenter of Southern
Switzerland, Civic Hospital of Lugano, Lugano,
Switzerland

FEDERICA PROVINI, MD, PhD
Department of Biomedical and Neuromotor
Sciences, Bellaria Hospital, University of
Bologna; IRCCS Institute of Neurological
Sciences of Bologna, Bologna, Italy

MONICA PULIGHEDDU, MD
Assistant Professor, Neurophysiology Unit,
Sleep Disorder Center, University of Cagliari,
Monserrato, Cagliari, Italy

DAVID B. RYE, MD, PhD
Professor, Program in Sleep, Department of
Neurology, Emory University School of
Medicine, Atlanta, Georgia

DENISE SHARON, MD, PhD, FAASM
Assistant Professor of Medicine, Tulane
University School of Medicine, New Orleans,
Louisiana; Clinical Director, Advanced Sleep
Center, Metairie, Louisiana

NARONG SIMAKAJORNBOON, MD
Professor and Director, Sleep Disorders
Center, Cincinnati Children's Hospital Medical
Center, Cincinnati, Ohio

MARIETTA P. STANTON, PhD, RN, FAAN
Full Professor, Capstone College of Nursing,
University of Alabama, Tuscaloosa, Alabama

MARY SUZANNE STEVENS, MD, MS
Clinical Assistant Professor, Department of
Neurology, University of Kansas, Kansas City,
Kansas

NAOKO TACHIBANA, MD, PhD
Center for Sleep-related Disorders, Kansai
Electric Power Hospital, Fukushima, Osaka,
Japan

LYNN MARIE TROTTI, MD, MSc
Assistant Professor, Department of Neurology
and Sleep Center, Emory University School of
Medicine, Atlanta, Georgia

ARTHUR S. WALTERS, MD
Professor, Department of Neurology,
Vanderbilt University, Nashville,
Tennessee

DEBRA WHISENANT, PhD, MSPH, RN
Assistant Professor, Capstone College of
Nursing, University of Alabama, Tuscaloosa,
Alabama

JOHN W. WINKELMAN, MD, PhD
Chief, Sleep Disorders Clinical Research
Program, Departments of Psychiatry and

Neurology, Massachusetts General Hospital,
Harvard Medical School, Boston,
Massachusetts

ROCHELLE S. ZAK, MD
Sleep Disorders Center, University of California
San Francisco, San Francisco, California

Contents

> There are more than 50 epidemiologic studies measuring the prevalence of restless legs syndrome/Willis-Ekbom disease (RLS/WED) across 5 of the 6 inhabited continents (not Australia), most conducted in North America and Europe. Sufficient studies have been conducted in Asia, North America, and Europe to make inferences on RLS/WED prevalence by region. RLS/WED prevalence is thought to be highest in North America and Europe and lower in Asia. These differences across regions may be explained by cultural, environmental, and genetic factors. Future investigation is needed to determine to what extent these factors affect expression of RLS/WED according to world region.

> Restless leg syndrome/Willis-Ekbom disease has brain iron deficiency that produces excessive dopamine and known genetic risks, some of which contribute to the brain iron deficiency. Dopamine treatments work temporarily but may eventually produce further postsynaptic down-regulation and worse restless leg syndrome. This article includes sections focused on pathophysiologic findings from each of these areas: genetics, cortical-spinal excitability, and iron and dopamine.

> Neuroimaging studies are of crucial relevance in defining the pathophysiology of restless legs syndrome (RLS). MRI studies showed no structural brain lesions and confirmed a central iron deficiency. Structural and functional studies showed an involvement of the thalamus, sensorimotor cortical areas, and cerebellum in RLS and assessed neurotransmission abnormalities in the dopaminergic and opiate systems. Finally, glutamatergic hyperactivity has been proposed as a cause of disrupted and shortened sleep in RLS. Differences among the results of the studies make it difficult to draw any definitive conclusions, thus, suggesting the need for future research.

Restless legs syndrome (RLS) is a common sensorimotor trait defined by symptoms that interfere with sleep onset and maintenance in a clinically meaningful way. Non-volitional myoclonus while awake and asleep is a sign of the disorder and an informative endophenotype. The genetic contributions to RLS/periodic leg movements are substantial, are among the most robust defined to date for a common disease, and account for much of the variance in disease expressivity. The disorder is polygenic, as revealed by recent genome-wide association studies. Experimental studies are revealing mechanistic details of how these common variants might influence RLS expressivity.

Restless leg syndrome, or Willis-Ekbom disease, is a neurosensorimotor disorder with significant impact that is diagnosed through 5 clinical criteria. Adherence to 5 criteria and a thorough physical examination are often sufficient for diagnosis. Associated features prove helpful in young children or the cognitively impaired. Polysomnography is not routinely required unless the patient has other sleep-related symptoms. The finding of periodic leg movements in sleep only suggests, instead of confirms, the diagnosis. It is important to arrive at appropriate diagnosis because the prevalence is in the millions and treatment significantly improves sleep quality and daytime function.

Periodic leg movements during sleep (PLMS) are a highly active research topic and accumulating recent evidence has led to reevaluation of key aspects on the role of PLMS in restless legs syndrome (RLS). This article summarizes the recent developments in 3 areas: the relationship of PLMS to cortical arousals in patients with RLS, the differential effect of dopaminergic and non-dopaminergic treatment on PLMS, and the possible emergence of PLMS as a sleep-related cardiovascular risk factor.

Restless legs syndrome (RLS) mimics cannot always be differentiated from RLS/Willis-Ekbom disease (WED) based only on the 4 essential criteria; hence, a fifth criterion has recently been established. RLS comorbidities may provide us important clues for understanding the neurobiology of RLS/WED. Iron-dopamine connection, hypoxia pathway activation, and dopamine-opioid interaction are important pathophysiological mechanisms in RLS; this knowledge is derived from our understanding of RLS associations with a variety of medical, neurologic, and other conditions. Clinicians must formulate an RLS differential diagnosis based on history and physical examination, but laboratory tests may sometimes be needed to arrive at a correct diagnosis.

Restless legs syndrome (RLS) is a sensorimotor disorder that can cause significant discomfort, impaired quality of life, poor mood, and disturbed sleep. Because the disorder is chronic and associated with multiple comorbidities, RLS can be seen in an inpatient or perioperative setting. Certain characteristics of the hospitalized or surgical context can exacerbate or unmask RLS. Importantly, RLS and the associated discomfort and insomnia can prolong hospital stay and negatively impact outcomes. RLS medications should be continued during the hospital admission when possible. Avoidance of excessive phlebotomy and medications known to trigger RLS is helpful. Patients should increase activity when acceptable.

Recent studies have shown that restless legs syndrome (RLS) and periodic limb movement disorder (PLMD) are common in the pediatric population. The diagnostic criteria for Pediatric RLS have recently been updated to simplify and integrate with newly revised adult RLS criteria. Management of RLS and PLMD involves pharmacologic and nonpharmacologic interventions. Children with low iron storage are likely to benefit from iron therapy. Although there is limited information on pharmacologic therapy, there are emerging literatures showing the effectiveness of dopaminergic medications in the management of RLS and PLMD in children. This article covers clinical evaluation of RLS and PLMD in children and the relationship with growing pains.

Restless legs syndrome (RLS)/Willis-Ekbom disease is 3-fold more prevalent in pregnant than in non-pregnant women. Symptoms are particularly strong and frequent during the third trimester of pregnancy and disappear around delivery. A preexisting form of RLS tends to worsen during pregnancy. Women who experience RLS during pregnancy have a higher risk of symptoms in further pregnancies and of developing a primary form of RLS later in life, than women free of symptoms during pregnancy. This article reviews the literature for pregnancy-related RLS, with particular attention to its epidemiology, course, possible mechanisms, management, and the impact of symptoms.

There is great interest in the study of sleep in healthy and cognitively impaired elderly. Sleep disorders have been related to quality of aging. Sleep-related movements are a frequent correlate of disordered sleep and daytime sleepiness; restless legs syndrome/Willis–Ekbom disease (RLS/WED), in particular, is often unrecognized in the elderly. This review explores RLS/WED in the elderly population which may be subdivided into 3 groups: healthy, dependent, and frail. The RLS/WED could be a predictor for lower physical function; its burden on quality of life and health care-related costs, in the elderly, should be an important clinical and public health concern.

Restless Leg Syndrome in Neurologic and Medical Disorders 343

Nadir Askenasy and Jean-Jacques Askenasy

Leg quiescence homeostasis is a model that ensures quiet sleep through concerted activities of several neurotransmitters in key centers of the nervous system. Restless legs syndrome (RLS) is a functional perturbation of this model, which produces striatal motor activity along activation of the thalamocortical circuits responsible for the conscious urge and discomfort. This model explains the association of restless leg syndrome with a wide variety of associated pathologies emphasizing that perturbed function and imbalance may occur under different steady states of neurotransmitter levels. Likewise, this concept links various central and peripheral etiologies and integrates the augmenting and transient effects of therapeutic neuromodulators.

Restless Legs Syndrome and Psychiatric Disorders 351

Susan Mackie and John W. Winkelman

There are strong epidemiologic ties between restless legs syndrome (RLS) and a wide array of psychiatric conditions. Although the mechanism of this association is not fully understood, there are likely bidirectional cause-and-effect relationships. Appreciation of psychiatric comorbidity is an essential component of the treatment of RLS. Clinicians should be prepared to facilitate appropriate psychiatric treatment and consider the complex interactions between psychiatric medications, RLS medications, and the clinical course of both illnesses.

Living with Restless Legs Syndrome/Willis-Ekbom Disease 359

Naoko Tachibana

Restless legs syndrome/Willis-Ekbom disease (RLS/WED) is commonly seen in patients with end-stage renal disease (ESRD), but this condition has not been properly recognized. The prevalence of RLS/WED in ESRD shows the ethnic variation (7%–68%), with the similar tendency of primary RLS/WED. Although RLS/WED in ESRD is defined in secondary RLS/WED, the factors of ESRD that are involved in the genesis of RLS/WED remain unknown. Even after renal transplantation, RLS/WED symptoms do not completely disappear, and genetic predisposition to RLS/WED may play an important role in causing RLS/WED. Long-term intervention for RLS/WED and ESRD will be necessary.

Restless Legs Syndrome/Willis-Ekbom Disease Morbidity: Burden, Quality of Life, Cardiovascular Aspects, and Sleep 369

Mary Suzanne Stevens

Restless legs syndrome (RLS)/Willis-Ekbom disease (WED) has a significant negative effect on quality of life. The decreased quality of life is similar to that of other chronic diseases, such as diabetes type 2, depression, and osteoarthritis. RLS/WED disrupts sleep length, sleep quality, and daytime alertness. Sleep disruption can contribute to depression. RLS/WED has been associated with cardiovascular disease and high blood pressure, possibly because of increased sympathetic tone caused by periodic limb movements of sleep. RLS/WED is underdiagnosed, leading to chronic sleep disruption and daytime consequences. Patients with RLS/WED have decreased productivity at work, which potentially has far-reaching economic consequences.

Sleep bruxism (SB) is a common sleep-related jaw motor disorder observed in 8% of the adult population. SB diagnosis is based on history of tooth grinding and clenching and is confirmed by the polysomnographic recording of the electromyographic activity of jaw muscles during sleep. SB may be associated with orofacial pain, headaches, and sleep-disordered breathing. Managing SB cannot be done without a comprehensive clinical and, when indicated, polysomnographic differential diagnosis of other comorbidities, which need to be taken into account to select the best treatment approach.

Various medications and behavioral treatments for sleep-related leg cramps have been tried, but the quality of the evidence is low. Quinine seems to be effective, but dangerous. β-Agonists may be one of the more common causes of secondary leg cramps. Statins may not be implicated in leg cramps as much as has been believed. Potassium-sparing diuretics may have a higher incidence of sleep-related leg cramps than potassium-depleting diuretics. Plantar flexion of the feet may elicit most sleep-related leg cramps. More research into behavioral treatments is needed. A standardized sleep-related leg cramp questionnaire would be useful to expand research.

A scoping review is an approach to identify or map the extent of key concepts and main sources and types of evidence available on a topic. Hypnic jerks are considered a parasomnia categorized as a sleepwake transition disorder. Although hypnic jerks are considered a benign sleep/movement disorder, some of the latest research indicates that they may be a clinical characteristic for other sleep disorders that affect health care outcomes. This article conducts a scoping review of the literature to determine the extent, range, and nature of the research activity related to hypnic jerks and identifies research gaps in the existing literature.

Preface

Restless Legs Syndrome and Sleep Related Movement Disorders

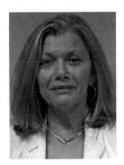

Denise Sharon, MD, PhD, FAASM
Editor

This issue of *Sleep Medicine Clinics* highlights the current understanding of Restless Legs Syndrome/Willis-Ekbom Disease (RLS/WED), sleep bruxism, leg cramps, and hypnic jerks—all part of sleep-related movement disorders. These pathologic entities are characterized by simple, usually stereotyped movements that interfere with the ability to achieve or maintain sleep. As such, their diagnosis and management may fall between the cracks of specialized medicine. Frequently, patients transition between primary care, neurology or movement specialists, and sleep medicine and pain specialists. These transitions prolong the time elapsed between the initial symptoms and the diagnosis, sometimes up to 12 years, as mentioned in the article by Simakajornboon, Dye, and Walters on RLS/WED and growing pains in children and adolescents.

RLS is included with sleep-related movement disorders but might be also considered as an exception to this category. RLS is not diagnosed during sleep, but it can affect sleep. The patient typically engages in walking or nonstereotyped movements to ease the urge to move the legs, arms, or other body parts. The name itself has been an issue of debate lately.

Karl-Axel Ekbom coined the expression of restless legs in his doctoral thesis in 1945 when he described the movement disorder as we know it today. However, arms or other body parts may present with similar symptoms. Therefore, even though the symptoms typically start in the legs, it is not all

about the legs. There was also a sense among RLS patients that their symptoms are trivialized because legs are supposed to move anyway. In addition, this disorder became a subject of jokes, questioning its medical validity and setting it as an example of disease mongering and revenue source for the pharmaceutical companies. Since RLS is a common condition in the United States and other western countries as reported by Koo in his assessment of RLS epidemiology around the globe, many patients felt degraded and uncomfortable when attempting to describe their symptoms. Some continued to suffer in silence, often to the point of being unable to work or fulfill their social obligations. The proposed name change to Willis-Ekbom disease (WED) was meant to honor Sir Thomas Willis, who provided the first medical description of RLS in the seventeenth century, and Karl-Axel Ekbom, for his work in the last century.

The transition from syndrome to disease was prompted by recent, important pathophysiologic and genetic findings. Richard Allen presents a primer to the pathophysiology of RLS/WED. Provini and Chiaro discuss the role of neuroimaging in understanding RLS/WED, and Rye discusses the common genetic variants affecting RLS/WED expressivity. A disease is characterized by a set of distinguishing signs and symptoms that impair normal functioning, as shown by Becker in an article on the diagnosis and assessment of RLS/WED. Periodic limb movements (PLMs) are frequently part of the RLS/WED phenotype, and

Sleep Med Clin 10 (2015) xvii–xviii
http://dx.doi.org/10.1016/j.jsmc.2015.07.001

sleep.theclinics.com

Fulda explores the relationship between RLS and PLMs. Currently, there are no specific diagnostic tests in use to properly diagnose RLS/WED in clinical practice. Chokroverty underlines the importance of considering the differential diagnoses, the mimics, and the comorbidities when assessing an RLS/WED patient.

Several articles in this issue are devoted to the management and treatment of RLS/WED. The limited research available on nonpharmacologic options is detailed in my review on the topic. Manvir Bhatia presents an interesting insight into the world of yoga. The dopaminergic options are summarized in Zak's review, while Garcia-Borreguero presents the problematics associated with dopaminergic treatment. Finally, Trotti reviews the quality measures for the diagnosis and management of the RLS/WED patient.

Living with RLS/WED poses a number of challenges that affect patients in specific conditions, including hospitalizations and perioperative situations. Goldstein discusses how these conditions can trigger or worsen RLS/WED and provides suggestions for managing these situations. Children and adolescents often get undiagnosed, misdiagnosed, and mislabeled, potentially affecting their well-being and development. In addition, as Simakajornboon, Dye, and Walters point out, better differentiation is needed between entities such as RLS, periodic limb movement disorder, and growing pains in this population. Another segment population that can have significant difficulty living with RLS/WED are pregnant women. As Prosperetti and Manconi point out in their article, RLS/WED frequently occurs in this population, and the pharmacologic options are very limited. RLS/WED tends to worsen with age and often manifests in the second half of life, posing significant difficulties in the diagnosis and management due to the potential frailty and cognitive impairment of the patient, as reported by Figorilli, Puligheddu, and Ferri.

As a chronic disease, RLS/WED has been associated with many other disorders that can exacerbate the symptoms. Conversely, the treatment of these disorders can trigger or worsen RLS/WED symptoms. In this issue, we chose to concentrate on three groups of co-morbidities. Askenasy and Askenasy review the neurologic and medical comorbidities. Winkelman and Mackie review the psychiatric disorders and their specific association with RLS/WED. Tachibana focuses on the common association of RLS/WED and end-stage renal disease, as this comorbidity can further worsen the quality of life of these patients. RLS/WED significantly impacts patients and their lives. However, as Stevens points out in her assessment of RLS/WED morbidity and burden, it can impact work productivity and affect society as a whole.

Even though some of the sleep-related movement disorders are common, their representation in evidence-based studies is scarce. Among these are sleep bruxism, leg cramps, and hypnic jerks. Carra, Huynh, Fleury, and Lavigne review sleep bruxism, and its recently published definition and grading criteria are presented.

Finally, leg cramps and hypnic jerks are very common occurrences, although less common as a sleep disorder. In his review of leg cramps, Brown makes a strong case for further research to better understand the nature of this disorder. Cuellar presents an extensive literature review on hypnic jerks and points to existing gaps in our understanding of this condition.

This issue of *Sleep Medicine Clinics* provides us with an opportunity to present a series of articles by an international group of well-published scientists and clinicians on RLS/WED and sleep-related movement disorders. This issue is too narrow in scope to cover all aspects, some of which are still poorly understood. Its purpose is to increase awareness of this field and to engage the reader to seek further information and a better understanding regarding sleep-related movement disorders, all in an attempt to bridge the gaps in our knowledge and comprehension.

Denise Sharon, MD, PhD, FAASM
Tulane University School of Medicine
1430 Tulane Avenue
New Orleans, LA 70112, USA

Advanced Sleep Center
2905 Kingman Street
Metairie, LA 70006, USA

E-mail address:
denisesharon@cox.net

Epidemiology of Restless Legs Syndrome/Willis-Ekbom Disease

Epidemiology of Restless Legs
Syndrome/Willis-Ekbom
Disease

Restless Leg Syndrome Across the Globe
Epidemiology of the Restless Legs Syndrome/Willis-Ekbom Disease

Brian B. Koo, MD[a,b,*]

KEYWORDS

- Restless legs syndrome • RLS • Epidemiology • World • Willis-Ekbom disease

KEY POINTS

- There are more than 50 epidemiologic studies measuring restless legs syndrome (RLS)/Willis-Ekbom disease (WED) prevalence across 5 of the 6 inhabited continents (not Australia), most conducted in North America and Europe.
- There is historical precedent for the large number of studies that have been conducted in Europe, especially in Scandinavia.
- Limitations when comparing prevalence across these studies are related to use of various ascertainment methods and differing RLS/WED criteria.
- Sufficient studies have been conducted in Asia, North America, and Europe to make inferences on RLS/WED prevalence by region.
- RLS/WED prevalence is thought to be highest in North America and Europe with most estimates ranging from 5.5% to 11.6% and lower in Asia with most estimates ranging from 1.0% to 7.5%.
- These differences across regions may be explained by cultural, environmental, and genetic factors.
- Future investigation is needed to determine to what extent each of these different factors affects expression of RLS/WED according to world region.

BACKGROUND

The restless legs syndrome, recently renamed Willis-Ekbom Disease (RLS/WED), is a neurologic condition that consists of an inexorable urge to move the legs in the evening and nighttime, when rest is most desired. The first widely accepted historical account of RLS/WED originated from London, England, in 1685 and was described by Sir Thomas Willis, after whom the first half of the disorder is named.[1] The first truly convincing published account of RLS may have actually come before these writings in the ancient Chinese book of *Neike Zhaiyao* (Internal summary), written by Xue Ji in 1529.[2] It was not until several centuries later in the 1940s that RLS/WED was described and studied in detail in Upsala, Sweden, by Karl Ekbom, after whom the latter half of the disorder is named.[3] In modern times, investigation of RLS/WED has primarily been conducted in North America and Europe. It is clear from this history of description and research that RLS/WED is a condition that affects persons around the world

B.B. Koo has no disclosures to report.
[a] Department of Neurology, Yale University School of Medicine, 15 York Street, New Haven, CT 06510, USA;
[b] Department of Neurology, West Haven VAMC, Connecticut Veterans Affairs Healthcare System, 950 Campbell Avenue, West Haven, CT 06516, USA
* Department of Neurology, West Haven VAMC, 950 Campbell Avenue, West Haven, CT 06516.
E-mail address: koobri@gmail.com

with diverse ethnic, cultural, and genetic backgrounds.

RLS/WED is common, and the epidemiology, namely, prevalence, of this disorder has been studied in persons living on 5 of the 6 inhabited continents (not Australia).[4-8] This article outlines the world epidemiology of RLS/WED. To do this, different epidemiologic studies of RLS/WED carried out in community populations are reviewed by continent. Following this epidemiologic summary, genetic variation in RLS and how this may affect global RLS expression are discussed. Studies that have specifically focused on the question of ethnic variability in RLS are reviewed. Finally, the many factors other than genetic, ethnic, and geographic that could affect RLS prevalence are discussed. Briefly, these factors include differing RLS/WED definitions used over the years, varying methodology used to diagnose RLS/WED, and cultural aspects of disease perception.

RESTLESS LEGS SYNDROME/WILLIS-EKBOM DISEASE CRITERIA

Properly designed epidemiologic studies that aimed to determine the prevalence of RLS/WED used the accepted diagnostic criteria at the time of the study. RLS/WED diagnostic criteria have undergone different revisions over the years, and thus, before moving on to describe different epidemiologic studies of RLS/WED, it is important to provide an overview of some of these changes. RLS/WED was first officially defined by the International RLS Study Group in 1995, including 4 minimal criteria for diagnosis: (1) a desire to move the extremities, often associated with parasthesias/dysesthesias; (2) motor restlessness; (3) worsening of symptoms at rest with at least temporary relief by activity; and (4) worsening of symptoms in the evening or night.[9] In 2003, these criteria were revised with some changes in wording; the criterion of motor restlessness was removed, and the previous criterion (3) was separated into 2 criteria so that the final criteria included (1) an urge to move the legs, usually accompanied by uncomfortable sensations in the legs, (2) the urge to move or unpleasant sensations begin or worsen during periods of rest or inactivity, (3) the urge to move or unpleasant sensations are partially or completely relieved by movement, and (4) worsening of symptoms in the evening or night.[10]

Again in 2014, RLS/WED criteria were amended. The 4 criteria outlined in 2003 were kept, but a fifth criterion of differential diagnosis was added. In addition, specifiers were added to delineate clinically significant RLS/WED and to classify RLS/WED as chronic-persistent or intermittent.[11]

It should also be noted that RLS/WED diagnostic criteria were published by 3 different organizations: the American Academy of Sleep Medicine, the American Psychiatric Association, and the International Restless Legs Syndrome Study Group (IRLSSG); luckily the criteria were similar for all groups.[11-13]

All of these studies, discussed in this monograph, were conducted before the release of the various 2014 criteria and used criteria that were current at the time each study was conducted. Each of the studies is described in **Table 1**, including location, year of publication, ages included, numbers, criteria used, number of questions used, prevalence, and important notes.

AFRICA

There have been only 2 studies that have examined the prevalence of RLS/WED in regions of Africa. These studies were conducted in Tanzania, a 2010 study in a rural area and a 2014 study in an urban area.[5,14] Both studies modeled questions based on the four 2007 IRLSSG criteria and translated these questions into Kiswahili and then back to English to ensure accuracy. Prevalence estimates were low, partly because of the 2-phase screening approach: first questionnaire screening and, if positive, then an interview and examination by a neurologist. In the 2010 study, only 10 of 7654 persons screened positive and only 1 person was thought to have RLS by physician interview, yielding a screening RLS/WED prevalence of 0.11% and actual prevalence of 0.013%. In the 2014 study, only 156 of 28,606 persons screened positive for RLS/WED and there were only 10 confirmed cases of RLS/WED, which yielded a screening prevalence of 0.55% and an actual RLS/WED prevalence of 0.037%.

ASIA

Studies to determine RLS prevalence in Asia have been conducted in South Korea, Taiwan, Japan, Singapore, China, Saudi Arabia, and India. Most studies to measure RLS prevalence were carried out in South Korea. There was a wide range of RLS prevalence in different South Korean studies, varying from 0.9% to 12.1%.[6,15-18] This wide prevalence variation likely is attributable to the ranging stringency in criteria used to define RLS/WED. For example, in the study finding 12.1% prevalence, RLS/WED was considered if there was an affirmative answer to only 1 question: "Have you ever experienced an urge to move your legs or unpleasant sensations like creepy-crawling feelings in your legs before sleep?",[17] whereas studies that

Table 1
Epidemiologic studies measuring RLS/WED prevalence

	Authors (Year of Publication)	Location	Ages	N (Total, Men)	Criteria	Question	Prevalence (%)	Comments
Africa	Winkler et al,[5] 2010	Tanzania	≥14	(7654, 3825)	IRLSSG 2007	3	0.03	Face-to-face interview. Those who answered at least 1 RLS question positively (n = 10) were reinterviewed by a neurologist
	Burtscher et al,[14] 2014	Tanzania	≥14	(35,008)	IRLSSG 2007	4	0.47	Face-to-face interview. Those who answered at least 1 RLS question positively (n = 248) were reinterviewed by a neurologist
Asia	Kim et al,[17] 2005	South Korea	40–69	(9939, 4711)	None	1	12.1	Face-to-face interview. "Have you ever experienced an urge to move your legs or unpleasant sensations, creepy-crawling feelings in your legs before sleep?"
	Cho et al,[15] 2008	South Korea	20–69	(5000, 2470)	IRLSSG 2003	4	7.5	Telephone interview, Johns Hopkins RLS diagnostic interview. Positive to 4 IRLSSG criteria; once a month or 20 lifetime episodes
	Cho et al,[6] 2009	South Korea	18–64	(6509, 2581)	IRLSSG 2003	4	0.9	Face-to-face interview. Positive to 4 IRLSSG criteria
	Park et al,[18] 2010	South Korea	40–69	(1000 women)	IRLSSG 2003	4	6.5	Questionnaire. Positive to 4 IRLSSG criteria
	Kim et al,[16] 2012	South Korea	≥65	(1990, 901)	IRLSSG 2003	4	9.5	Questionnaire. Positive to 4 IRLSSG criteria
	Kageyama et al,[23] 2000	Japan	≥20	(4612, 1012)	None	1	~5–10	Self-administered questionnaire; single question: "Have you ever experienced sleep disturbance due to a creeping sensation or hot feeling in your legs?" (Yes/No/Sometimes)

(continued on next page)

Table 1
(continued)

Authors (Year of Publication)	Location	Ages	N (Total, Men)	Criteria	Question	Prevalence (%)	Comments
Yokoyama et al,[24] 2008	Japan	≥70	(1769, 769)	None	1	11.4	Home interviews, single question: "Is your sleep interrupted by a creeping sensation or hot flushes in your legs after you go to bed at night?" RLS: sometimes, often, always
Nomura et al,[22] 2008	Daisen, Japan	≥20	(2812, 1223)	IRLSSG 2003	4	1.8	Telephone interview. 4 questions assessing RLS. If 2 positive answers, then interview neurologist
Tsuboi et al,[25] 2009	Ajimu, Japan	≥65	(1251, 439)	IRLSSG 1995	4	1.0	1. Written questionnaire. 4 IRLSSG criteria (1995) 2. Verify answers telephone interview 3. Face-to-face interview
Chen et al,[27] 2010	Taiwan	15–70	(4011, 1634)	IRLSSG 2003	4	1.6	Telephone interview. Positive to 4 IRLSSG criteria. Symptoms were assessed for the past month
Li et al,[28] 2012	Wangtai, China	≥16	(2101, 1061)	IRLSSG 2003	4	7.2	Questionnaire. Positive to 4 IRLSSG criteria
Ma et al,[29] 2012	Shanghai, China	≥50	(2609, 895)	IRLSSG 2003	4	0.7	1. Written questionnaire. 4 IRLSSG criteria (2003) 2. Verify answers telephone interview neurologist 3. Face-to-face interview
Rangarajan and D'Souza,[26] 2007	Bangalore, India	18–90	(1266, 699)	IRLSSG 2003	4	2.2	Face-to-face interview, positive to 4 IRLSSG criteria

Region	Study	Location	Age	(N, cases)	Criteria		Prevalence %	Method
Europe	Sevim et al,[31] 2004	Mersin, Turkey	≥18	(3234, 1571)	IRLSSG 1995	4	3.2	Face-to-face interview, positive to 4 IRLSSG criteria
	Erer et al,[32] 2009	Orhangazi, Bursa, Turkey	40–95	(1124, 550)	IRLSSG 2003	4	9.7	Face-to-face interview. One screening question. Participants answering positive interviewed by movement disorder specialist using IRLSSG
	Tasdemir et al,[33] 2010	Kandira, Turkey	≥18	(2111, 1007)	IRLSSG 2003	4	3.4	Face-to-face interview. Positive to 4 IRLSSG criteria
	Hadjigeorgiou et al,[34] 2007	Larissa, Greece	≥18	(3033, 1419)	IRLSSG 2003	4	3.9	Face-to-face interview. Positive to 4 IRLSSG criteria
	Ohayon and Roth,[35] 2002	UK, Germany, Italy, Portugal, Spain	15–100	(18,980; 9241)	International Classification of Sleep Disorders (ICSD)	3	5.5	Telephone interview, ICSD criteria 1. Unpleasant sensation in the legs at night 2. Disagreeable sensations of creeping in the calves, often with general aches/pains in legs 3. The discomfort is relieved by movement
	Allen et al,[4] 2005	France Germany Italy Spain United Kingdom	≥18	(1884) (1929) (1768) (1896) (1950)	IRLSSG 2003	4	10.8 4.1 6.7 4.9 8.6	Face-to-face and telephone interview, Positive to 4 IRLSSG criteria
	Hogl et al,[36] 2005	Bruneck, Italy	50–89	(701, 335)	IRLSSG 1995	4	10.6	Face-to-face interview. Positive to 4 IRLSSG criteria
	Vogl et al,[37] 2006	S Tyrol, Italy	≥18	(530)	IRLSSG 2003	4	8.9	1. Questionnaire, Positive to 4 IRLSSG criteria 2. Movement disorder specialist history
	Celle et al,[38] 2010	St-Etienne, France	≥18	(667, 271)	IRLSSG 2003	4	24.2	Questionnaire 1. Unpleasant sensation in legs 2. Urge to move 3. Relief by movement 4. Worsening in evening or night 5. Symptoms greater than once per week in last 6 mo

(continued on next page)

Table 1 (*continued*)

Authors (Year of Publication)	Location	Ages	N (Total, Men)	Criteria	Question	Prevalence (%)	Comments
Tison et al,[39] 2005	France	≥18	(10,263; 4762)	IRLSSG 1995	4	8.5	Face-to-face interview. Positive to 4 IRLSSG criteria
Rothdach et al,[40] 2000	Augsburg, Germany	65–83	(369, 196)	IRLSSG 1995	3	9.8	Face-to-face interview, 3 questions based on IRLSSG
Berger et al,[41] 2004	Pomerania, Germany	20–79	(4310, 2018)	IRLSSG 1995	3	10.5	Face-to-face interview. Positive response to 3 questions based on IRLSSG criteria
Happe et al,[42] 2008	Dortmund, Germany	25–75	(1312, 618)	IRLSSG 2003	3	8.8	Face-to-face interview. Positive to 3 questions based on 4 IRLSSG criteria or previous RLS diagnosis
Rijsman et al,[43] 2004	Krimpen, Netherlands	≥50	(1485, 789)	None	1	7.1	Questionnaire: One question: "Is your sleep disturbed by leg movements?" "Never, Sometimes, Often, Always"; RLS often or always
Pekmezovic et al,[44] 2013	Sombor, Serbia	≥18	(2112)	IRLSSG 2003	4	5.1	Face-to-face interview. Positive to 4 IRLSSG criteria
Benediktsdottir et al,[45] 2010	Reykjavik, Iceland Uppsala, Sweden	≥40	(769) (601)	IRLSSG 2003	3	18.3 11.5	Face-to-face interview. Positive to 4 IRLSSG criteria
Juuti et al,[46] 2010	Oulu, Finland	57	(995, 439)	IRLSSG 2003	1	18.0	Have you ever suffered from restless legs? By restless legs, we mean unpleasant feelings in the legs at rest, especially when going to bed, which urge you to move your legs or walk
Bjorvatn et al,[47] 2005	Denmark Norway	≥18	(1005) (1000)	IRLSSG 2003	4	8.8 14.3	Telephone interview, Positive to 4 IRLSSG criteria
Ulfberg et al,[48] 2001	Dalarna, Sweden	18–64	(2608 men)	IRLSSG 1995	4	5.8	Questionnaire. Positive to 4 IRLSSG criteria
Ulfberg et al,[49] 2001	Dalarna, Sweden	18–64	(140 women)	IRLSSG 1995	4	11.4	Questionnaire. Positive to 4 IRLSSG criteria
Ulfberg et al,[8] 2007	Sweden	18–90	(1000, 490)	IRLSSG 2003	4	4.9	Telephone interview. Positive to 4 IRLSSG criteria
Broman et al,[50] 2008	Uppsala, Sweden	20–59	(1335, 586)	IRLSSG 2003	3	18.8	Questionnaire, 3 questions IRLSSG criteria
Wesstrom et al,[51] 2008	Sweden	18–64	(3516 women)	IRLSSG 2003	5	15.7	Questionnaire. Positive to 5 questions based on 4 IRLSSG criteria

S America	Persi et al,[7] 2009	Buenos Aires, Argentina	≥18	(471, 187)	IRLSSG 2003	3	20.2	Questionnaire: "Do you have unpleasant sensations in your legs combined with an URGE or need to move your legs?' If yes, 2 subset questions: "Do these symptoms occur mainly or only at REST and they IMPROVE with movement?" and "Are these symptoms WORSE in the evening or night than in the morning?" Positive to all 3
	Miranda et al,[60] 2001	Santiago, Chile	≥18	(100, 31)	IRLSSG 1995	4	13.0	Face-to-face interview. Positive to 4 IRLSSG criteria
	Castillo et al,[61] 2006	Quito, Ecuador	25–85	(500, 190)	IRLSSG 2003	4	2.0	Indigenous population. Telephone interviews. 4 RLS questions. Needed 4 positive answers to have RLS
	Castillo et al,[62] 2014	Quito, Ecuador	≥40	(665, 279)	IRLSSG 2003	4	6.0	Mostly indigenous population. Questionnaire with 4 IRLSSG questions. Those who screened positive were interviewed by neurologist/sleep specialist. Positive to 4 IRLSSG criteria
	Eckeli et al,[63] 2011	Cassia dos Coqueiros (CQ), Brazil	≥18	(1081, 650)	IRLSSG 2003	4	6.4	CQ has 2706 inhabitants, mostly immigrants from Italy and Portugal. 2 phases: Face-to-face interview by neurologist/sleep physician and repeat face-to-face interview by same neurologist/sleep physician. Positive to 4 IRLSSG criteria

(continued on next page)

Table 1
(continued)

Authors (Year of Publication)	Location	Ages	N (Total, Men)	Criteria	Question	Prevalence (%)	Comments
N America Lavigne and Montplaisir,[64] 1994	Canada	≥18	(2019, 996)	None	2	15.0	Face-to-face interview, 2 questions: 1. At bedtime, does restlessness in your legs very often, often, occasionally, or never delay your falling asleep? 2. When you wake up during the night, do you very often, often, occasionally, or never feel unpleasant sensation in your leg muscles that require you to move your legs/walk to be more comfortable?
Froese et al,[65] 2008	British Columbia, Canada	≥18	(430, 185)	IRLSSG 2003	4	17.7	Indigenous population. Face-to-face interview. Positive to 4 IRLSSG criteria
Phillips et al,[66] 2000	Kentucky, USA	≥18	(1803)	None	1	9.4	Telephone interview, single question: "Do you have unpleasant feelings in your legs (eg, creepy-crawly or tingly feelings) when you lie down at night that make you feel restless and keep you from getting a good night's sleep?" Had to occur ≥5 times/mo
Phillips et al,[67] 2006	United States	≥18	(1506, 731)	IRLSSG 2003	2	9.7	Telephone interview. 2005 National Sleep Foundation Poll, 2 questions based on IRLSSG criteria. "In the past year, according to your own experience or what others tell you, how often did you have unpleasant feelings in your legs like creepy, crawly, or tingly feelings at night with an urge to move when you lie down to sleep?" Answering "every night/almost every night" or "a few nights a week" were asked: "Would you say these feelings in your legs are worse, about the same as, or better at night or in the evening compared with other times of day?"
Lee et al,[68] 2006	Baltimore, MD, USA	≥18	(1028)	IRLSSG 2003	7	4.2	Face-to-face interview. 7-item RLS questionnaire based on 4 minimal IRLSSG criteria

Author	Location	Age	Sample (cases, controls)	Criteria	Questions	Prevalence	Comments
Winkelman et al,[69] 2006	Wisconsin, USA	30–60	(2821, 1335)	None	4	15.8	Multilevel questionnaire. "How often, when you are sitting or lying down, do you have any of the following feelings in your legs?" Two symptoms of RLS, "repeated urge to move your legs" and "strange and uncomfortable feelings in the legs," Answer: never, less than once per month, monthly, weekly and daily/nightly If reported either symptom more than never, asked if symptoms "get better when you get up and start walking" and "disrupt your sleep"; RLS if both leg symptoms at least monthly, and symptoms be both relieved by movement and produce sleep disruption
Allen et al,[4] 2005	United States	≥18	(5964)	IRLSSG 2003	4	7.6	Face-to-face and telephone interview. Positive to 4 IRLSSG criteria
Winkelman et al,[70] 2008	United States	≥18	(3433, 1559)	IRLSSG 2003	4	5.1	Self-administered questionnaire. Positive to 4 IRLSSG criteria
Gao et al,[71] 2009	United States	M >56	(65,554)	IRLSSG 2003	3	4.1	Questionnaire: "Do you have unpleasant leg sensations (like crawling, paresthesia, or pain) combined with motor restlessness and an urge to move?" If yes then: 1. "Do these symptoms occur only at rest and does moving improve them?" and 2. "Are these symptoms worse in the evening/night compared with the morning?" Positive for all 3 for RLS
		W, 38–55	(23,119)	IRLSSG 2003	3	6.4	
Ram et al,[72] 2010	Unites States	≥16	(6139, 2965)	Unknown	NA	0.4	Face-to-face interview by trained research assistant; but no details given
Sawanyawisuth et al,[73] 2013	San Diego, CA, USA	≥18	Hispanic (1754, 772) White (1913, 973)	IRLSSG 2003	4	14.4 / 18.3	Telephone interview. Positive to all 4 RLS questions
Allen et al,[74] 2011	United States	Unknown	(61,792)	IRLSSG 2003	4	7.3	Computer questionnaire. Positive to all 4 RLS questions

The table is organized by continent and within each continent by region. The "Author" column provides first author and (year of publication). "Location" refers to country, city, or region. "Criteria" outlines which definitions were used to determine RLS/WED. "Questions" refers to the number of questions used when screening for RLS/WED. "Prevalence" is the prevalence of RLS/WED determined in the study. The "Comments" section provides notes on study methodology.

found lower prevalence used at least 4 questions that reflected the 2003 four necessary IRLSSG criteria.[15,16] In addition, there could be cultural factors related to a higher threshold to report subjective complaints in persons of Korean descent. A major multinational study estimated the prevalence of major depressive disorder, another disease diagnosed based on subjective complaints, as very low in South Korea (2.3%) compared with Western countries (16.4%), even though South Korea typically falls below Western countries on measurements of happiness.[19,20] A comparative analysis, finding lower major depression prevalence in South Korea compared with the United States, concluded that this difference may have resulted, at least in part, by a higher threshold for reporting subjective complaints among Koreans.[21]

There have been 4 studies that aimed to measure RLS/WED prevalence in Japan, and again, there was a wide range of prevalence, between 1.0% and 11.0%.[22-25] Studies finding a high RLS prevalence (10.0%–11.4%) used only 1 question to determine RLS/WED,[22,25] whereas studies finding lower prevalence (1.0%–1.6%) required that persons with RLS/WED answer 4 questions affirmatively.[23,24] In these latter studies, subjects judged to have RLS/WED by screening questionnaire were interviewed, either over telephone or in person by a neurologist.

RLS/WED prevalence was similarly low in studies conducted in Bangalore, India, and Taiwan.[26,27] In the Indian study, a questionnaire based on the four 2003 IRLSSG criteria identified that 2.1% of 1266 community-dwelling residents of Bangalore, India, suffered from RLS/WED.[26] The Taiwanese study required 4 positive responses to 4 questions modeled after the 2003 IRLSSG criteria and found that among 4011 Taiwanese residents, 1.6% had RLS/WED.[27]

"The patient has trouble sleeping at night and a feeling of soreness and hotness in the legs. In addition, the leg muscles could have spasms, leading to frequent leg movements which are from left to right or from right to left, until the patient falls asleep from exhaustion." This description of what sounds like RLS/WED was published in the ancient Chinese book of Neike Zhaiyao (Internal summary) in 1529 AD. Although descriptions of RLS may have been first published in China, epidemiologic studies of RLS/WED were not published until 2012. Two studies that yielded widely discrepant estimates of RLS/WED prevalence, 0.7% and 7.2%, were published in 2012.[28,29] The former study, which found 0.7% prevalence, used a 3-phase questionnaire-interview method in which the final interview was conducted by a physician

over the telephone, whereas the latter study used only 1 questionnaire; this methodological difference likely accounts for the discrepant findings. Apart from RLS/WED epidemiology, there is increasing interest among traditional Chinese medicine practitioners to treat RLS/WED. According to Chinese medicine principles, RLS/WED is a symptom caused by inadequate blood circulation in the legs, often associated with deficiency in the liver or kidneys. Chinese herbs used to treat RLS/WED aim to supplement Qi or life force and blood, by activating blood circulation, calming the liver to stop wind, and invigorating the kidney to eliminate dampness. There are more than 176 herbal preparations used to treat RLS/WED, and active clinical trials are ongoing to find the optimal combination of these preparations to treat RLS/WED.[30]

EUROPE

Most epidemiologic studies to estimate RLS/WED prevalence have been done in different countries of Europe. There are 16 European countries in which community-based studies have been carried out to determine RLS prevalence in 23 different studies.[4,8,31-51] Nearly all studies used IRLSSG criteria, some the 1995 and others the 2003 criteria, depending on when the study was done. As seen in Asian studies, prevalence tended to be high when few questions were used to determine RLS.[43,46] Many studies used face-to-face interviews to accrue information, but some relied on self-report questionnaire. These differences in methodology likely account for some variation in prevalence across countries (this issue of how methodology results in prevalence variation is discussed in subsequent sections).

There may still be other determinants of variation in RLS/WED prevalence across different regions, including linguistic and cultural factors. The term restless legs was coined in 1945 by Karl-Axel Ekbom in his doctoral thesis, entitled Restless Legs.[52] The English term restless legs was introduced by Ekbom, but many of his Swedish patients would use the direct Swedish translation of restless legs, rastlösa benat. There are derivations of this in other languages as well, including ruhelose-beine in German, gambe senza riposo in Italian, and piernas inquietas in Spanish. Indeed, linguistic and cultural factors are known to affect reporting of somatic and psychiatric symptoms.[53] Because RLS/WED diagnosis is based on reported and subjective somatic symptomatology, differences in culture may result in a variable threshold to report symptoms (even when directly asked) and thus differences in prevalence estimates.

Considering the European land mass, the presence of multiple countries over a broad area with latitudinal diversity allows for a determination of whether or not RLS/WED expression may vary with latitude. There is some rationale to think that it may. In an animal model of RLS/WED, alpha-melanocyte stimulating hormone (α-MSH) introduced into the rat cerebral ventricles produced an RLS-like phenotype, consisting of increased locomotive behavior, prolonged sleep latency, and increased hind limb movements in sleep.[54] The main peripheral skin receptor of α-MSH is the melanocortin-1 receptor (MC1R). Single nucleotide polymorphisms (SNPs) of the MC1R gene are associated with a fair skin phenotype, and these SNPs are overrepresented in areas of high latitude where their presence has been favored by low ultraviolet burden to maintain the ultraviolet-induced synthesis of vitamin D.[55,56]

In general, low RLS prevalence is seen in southern countries: Greece, Turkey, Spain, Portugal, and Italy[4,31–36]; high prevalence is seen in northern countries: Norway, Sweden, Iceland, and Finland[8,45–51]; and moderate prevalence is seen in central countries: England, Serbia, Germany, northern Italy, Netherlands, France, and Denmark.[4,35,37–44,47] **Fig. 1** shows a map of Europe, where prevalence is reported per 1000 persons and has been standardized so that prevalence of men and women were averaged (if reported separately), as in a previous publication.[57] When considering the correlation between prevalence of RLS/WED and country/city latitude, the correlation found in this prior study was r = 0.77 (95% confidence interval, 0.15, 0.96; P = .02).

The correlation of RLS/WED prevalence and latitude suggests that there may be an association between the expression of RLS symptoms and exposure to ultraviolet radiation. If this were the case, one would expect that symptom severity in RLS/WED would be seasonal. One study used Internet search query data for the term restless legs as a surrogate for RLS/WED symptoms and found a seasonal effect in northern and southern hemispheres that coincided with the greatest volume of searches in the summer.[58] Searches for restless legs were most frequent in June and July for northern hemispheric countries (United States, Canada, United Kingdom) and in January for southern hemispheric countries (Australia); both periods coincide with summer and are periods of greatest ultraviolet exposure. There may also be an association between RLS/WED and vitamin D. A Finnish study showed that serum levels of 25-hydroxyvitamin D were significantly lower in women with idiopathic RLS/WED than in age-matched female controls.[59]

THE AMERICAS

In South America, there have been 5 studies estimating RLS/WED prevalence in 4 countries, Argentina, Chile, Ecuador, and Brazil.[7,60–63] The prevalence has ranged broadly from 2.0% in Ecuador to 20.2% in Argentina. Conducting studies in this continent may address the question of whether RLS/WED is more prevalent in Caucasian, largely European populations (in this case immigrant) or in persons indigenous to South America. Although there were only 5 studies conducted in South America, the 3 studies of largely immigrant populations in Argentina, Chile, and Brazil found a higher prevalence of RLS/WED (20.2%, 13.0%, and 6.4%, respectively) compared with the studies of populations indigenous to Ecuador (6.0% and 2.0%).

In North America, studies have been conducted in both Canada and the United States. There have been 2 studies completed in Canada, estimating RLS/WED prevalence.[64,65] The first study was published in 1994, before the IRLSSG was formed, and thus, questions to determine RLS/WED were not standardized. The questions asked in a face-to-face interview included (1) "At bedtime, does restlessness in your legs very often, often, occasionally, or never delay your falling asleep?" and (2) "When you wake up during the night, do you very often, often, occasionally, or never feel unpleasant sensation in your leg muscles that require you to move your legs/walk to be more comfortable?" Prevalence in this study was found to be 15.0%.[64] The other study included indigenous groups in British Columbia, finding that 17.7% had RLS/WED.[65]

To date, there have been 10 epidemiologic studies that have estimated RLS/WED prevalence in the United States, broadly or in regions/states.[4,66–74] Unlike most other regions of the world, the United States is largely an immigrant population, and when conducting epidemiologic studies, this allows for interesting inferences regarding the potential role of genetics, ethnicity, environment, and culture on the expression of disease. RLS/WED prevalence ranged among studies from 0.4% to 18.3%. Again, differing methodology likely accounts for much of this variance, including the number of questions used to determine RLS/WED and the criteria used.

One study conducted in a biracial population in East Baltimore aimed to determine if the prevalence of RLS/WED was lower in African Americans than in Caucasian Americans as had been previously suggested.[75] The prevalence of RLS/WED was similar in African Americans (4.7%) and Caucasian Americans (3.8%). A 7-item questionnaire was used to determine RLS/WED symptoms,

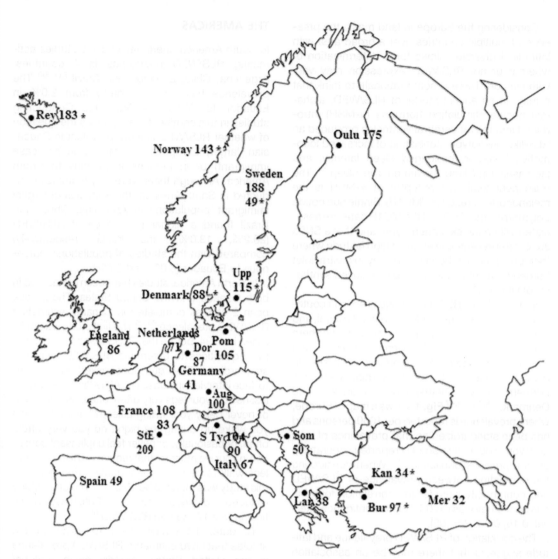

Fig. 1. Map of Europe. RLS prevalence by country or region in Europe. Shown is RLS prevalence per 1000 persons by country or city. Prevalence is standardized as the average of the RLS prevalence in men and women, as if the 1000 persons were composed of 500 men and 500 women. RLS prevalence is highest in regions with greatest northern latitude: Sweden, Finland, Norway, and Iceland; intermediate in regions with central latitude: Netherlands, Germany, England, France, Serbia, and Italy; and lowest in regions with lowest latitude: Spain, Greece, and Turkey. Aug, Augsburg, Germany; Bur, Bursa, Turkey; Dor, Dortmung, Germany; Kan, Kandira, Turkey; Lar, Larissa, Greece; Mer, Mersin, Turkey; Pom, Pomerania, Germany; Rey, Reykjavok, Iceland; S Ty, South Tyrolia, Italy; Som, Sombor, Serbia; StE, Saint Etienne, France; Upp, Uppsala, Sweden.

likely accounting for comparatively low RLS/WED prevalence. This higher prevalence of RLS/WED in persons of African descent than in European descent is not consistent with the very low RLS/WED prevalence found in Tanzania.[5,14] This result suggests that there are other factors influencing the expression of RLS/WED. These factors might include environment, culture, or medical comorbidity.

Notable among the RLS/WED epidemiologic studies done in the United States are 2 studies conducted in 2 large sleep-specific epidemiologic cohorts, the Wisconsin Study and the Sleep Heart Health Study cohorts.[69,70] The prevalence of RLS/WED determined in these studies was divergent, 15.8% in the Wisconsin cohort and 5.1% in the Sleep Heart Health Study cohort. These divergent estimates may have reflected the disparate screening questions used in the studies, 4 questions consistent with IRLSSG criteria in the Sleep Heart Health Study and 4 questions that were partially consistent with IRLSSG criteria in the

Wisconsin cohort (see **Table 1**). In addition to estimating RLS/WED prevalence, these studies aimed to determine if there was an association between RLS/WED and cardiovascular disease. In both studies, there was an observed 2- to 2.5-fold increased odds of prevalent cardiovascular disease in persons with frequent RLS/WED. Cardiovascular disease was defined as coronary bypass surgery, coronary angioplasty, insertion of a pacemaker, or self-report of myocardial infarction or coronary heart disease in the Wisconsin study and doctor-diagnosed angina, myocardial infarction, or coronary revascularization procedures in the Sleep Heart Health Study. These 2 studies were a major starting point for many other studies that analyzed this issue of cardiovascular risk in RLS/WED.[76–78]

One of the above-mentioned studies analyzed RLS/WED in the Nurses' Health Study.[77] Investigators in this same group in a different study combined data from the Nurses' Health Study II and Health Professionals Follow-up Study to estimate RLS/WED prevalence and determine if there was an association with obesity.[71] Probable RLS/WED was determined in 4.1% of men and 6.4% of women. In those with a body mass index of more than 30 compared with those with less than 23, the odds of having RLS/WED was 42% higher. Although this study had a large number of subjects, 88,693, RLS/WED prevalence was not presented by race/ethnicity.

Determining RLS/WED prevalence in different racial/ethnic groups was the focus of a study conducted in San Diego County.[73] In this large study, there were 1754 Hispanics of Mexican descent and 1913 non-Hispanic whites. Using telephone interview and asking 4 questions consistent with 2003 IRLSSG criteria, RLS/WED prevalence was 14.4% in Hispanics of Mexican descent and 18.3% in non-Hispanic whites. In Mexican Hispanics, acculturation was measured using the Short Acculturation Scale for Hispanics.[79] Mexican Hispanics with high acculturation compared with those with low acculturation had a significantly higher prevalence of RLS/WED (17.4% vs 12.8%; $P = .008$), and acculturation was an independent predictor of RLS/WED in the Mexican Hispanic group.

METHODOLOGY IN DETERMINING RESTLESS LEGS SYNDROME/WILLIS-EKBOM DISEASE PREVALENCE

One of the main issues when comparing RLS/WED prevalences in different geographic regions that have come from differing studies is the inconstant methodology used among studies. In 2014, the IRLSSG and the American Academy of Sleep Medicine revised the diagnostic criteria for RLS/WED to include clauses that rule out that symptoms arise from any one of many common RLS mimics (eg, nocturnal leg cramps, peripheral neuropathy) and that require clinical significance.[11,12] Most RLS/WED epidemiologic studies reported in this monograph were conducted before these criteria emerged and thus used 2003 IRLSSG criteria. The presence of 4 necessary criteria outlined by the IRLSSG in 2003 made it logical for investigators to use 4 questions when screening for RLS/WED; however, not all studies used IRLSSG criteria, which added variability between studies. Across studies, inconstant definitions of RLS/WED are further complicated by differences in how information is ascertained, specifically whether questionnaire or interview was used. Interview by an experienced practitioner is the gold standard for the diagnosis of RLS/WED, but in large population studies, this may not be possible. Alternatives are interview by trained research staff or use of validated questionnaires. Validated tools to diagnose RLS/WED include the Hening telephone diagnostic interview and the Cambridge-Hopkins diagnostic questionnaire for RLS[80,81]; unfortunately, only a minority of studies used these tools when determining RLS/WED.[68,74]

A study conducted by Allen and colleagues[74] demonstrates the impact of using tools such as the Cambridge-Hopkins diagnostic questionnaire for RLS to exclude RLS mimics. In this study, among 61,792 community-dwelling individuals, 4484 (7.3%) fulfilled all 4 IRLSSG criteria on an online survey. Of a random 1440 sample from the 4484 positively screened RLS/WED subjects, 37.2% were found to have an RLS mimic or secondary RLS based on medical history. Methodology and definitions used can profoundly affect prevalence estimations of RLS/WED, which are determined according to the self-report of subjective patient symptoms.

RESTLESS LEGS SYNDROME/WILLIS-EKBOM DISEASE GENETICS AND WORLD PREVALENCE

In 2007, two landmark studies of genome-wide association in RLS/WED were published.[82,83] One study found that in Icelandic and US samples, there was a significant genome-wide association between RLS/WED with periodic limb movements during sleep and a common intronic variant of the BTBD9 gene on chromosome 6p21.2 (odds ratio, 1.8; $P = 2 \times 10^{-9}$).[82] The Icelandic and US samples must have been genetically diverse. Information regarding race/ethnicity in the US sample that might allow further inferences on genetic diversity was not supplied. The second study found in German and French-Canadian populations significant associations between RLS and intronic variants in the MEIS1 gene, BTBD9 gene, and MAP2K5/LBXCOR1 genes on chromosomes 2p, 6p, and 15q, respectively.[83] This latter study contained people of European descent. This same group identified in German, Austrian, Czech, and Canadian populations association between RLS/WED and variants on yet another gene, PTPRD on chromosome 9p23-24.[84] In a separate study of Korean population, in a dominant model of inheritance, there was significant association between RLS/WED in variants of the BTBD9 gene but not PTPRD, MEIS1, or MAP2K5/LBXCOR1 genes.[85] This Korean study suggests that there is a genetic basis for the many Asian-based studies that had previously demonstrated a lower RLS/WED prevalence when compared with North American or European-based studies.[6,27] There is real need to perform additional genetic analysis of gene variants previously identified to associate with RLS/WED in populations that have not been studied before, including African, Latin-American, and Middle-Eastern populations.

SUMMARY

There are more than 50 epidemiologic studies measuring RLS/WED prevalence across 5 of the 6 inhabited continents (not Australia). There is historical precedent for the large number of studies that have been conducted in Europe, especially in Scandinavia. Limitations when comparing prevalence across these studies are related to use of various ascertainment methods and differing RLS/WED criteria. Nevertheless, there are cultural, environmental, and genetic factors that also contribute to the varied expression of RLS/WED according to world region.

REFERENCES

1. Willis T. The London practice of physic. London: Bassett and Crooke; 1685.
2. Ji X. Neike zhaiyao (Internal summary). 1529 AD. From modern reproduction. Nanjing (China): Jiang Su Scientific and Technology Publishing House; 1985.
3. Ekbom K. Asthenia crurum paraesthetica ('Irritable legs'). Acta Med Scand 1944;118:197–209.
4. Allen RP, Walters AS, Montplaisir J, et al. Restless legs syndrome prevalence and impact: REST general population study. Arch Intern Med 2005;165: 1286–92.
5. Winkler AS, Trendafilova A, Meindl M, et al. Restless legs syndrome in a population of northern Tanzania: a community-based study. Mov Disord 2010;25: 596–601.
6. Cho SJ, Hong JP, Hahm BJ, et al. Restless legs syndrome in a community sample of Korean adults: prevalence, impact on quality of life, and association with DSM-IV psychiatric disorders. Sleep 2009;32: 1069–76.
7. Persi GG, Etcheverry JL, Vecchi C, et al. Prevalence of restless legs syndrome: a community-based study from Argentina. Parkinsonism Relat Disord 2009;15:461–5.
8. Ulfberg J, Bjorvatn B, Leissner L, et al. Comorbidity in restless legs syndrome among a sample of Swedish adults. Sleep Med 2007;8:768–72.
9. Walters AS. Toward a better definition of the restless legs syndrome. The International Restless Legs Syndrome Study Group. Mov Disord 1995;10:634–42.
10. Allen RP, Picchietti D, Hening WA, et al. Restless legs syndrome: diagnostic criteria, special considerations, and epidemiology. A report from the restless legs syndrome diagnosis and epidemiology workshop at the National Institutes of Health. Sleep Med 2003;4:101–19.
11. Allen RP, Picchietti DL, Garcia-Borreguero D, et al. Restless legs syndrome/Willis-Ekbom disease diagnostic criteria: updated International Restless Legs Syndrome Study Group (IRLSSG) consensus criteria – history, rationale, description, and significance. Sleep Med 2014;15:860–73.
12. American Academy of Sleep Medicine. International classification of sleep disorders. 3rd edition. Darien (IL): American Academy of Sleep Medicine; 2014.
13. American Psychiatric Association. Diagnostic and statistical manual of mental disorders: DSM-5. Washington, DC: American Psychiatric Association.; 2013.
14. Burtscher C, Baxmann A, Kassubek J, et al. Prevalence of restless legs syndrome in an urban population of eastern Africa (Tanzania). J Neurol Sci 2014; 346:121–7.
15. Cho YW, Shin WC, Yun CH, et al. Epidemiology of restless legs syndrome in Korean adults. Sleep 2008;31:219–23.
16. Kim WH, Kim BS, Kim SK, et al. Restless legs syndrome in older people: a community-based study on its prevalence and association with major depressive disorder in older Korean adults. Int J Geriatr Psychiatry 2012;27:565–72.
17. Kim J, Choi C, Shin K, et al. Prevalence of restless legs syndrome and associated factors in the Korean adult population: the Korean Health and Genome Study. Psychiatry Clin Neurosci 2005;59:350–3.
18. Park YM, Lee HJ, Kang SG, et al. Prevalence of idiopathic and secondary restless legs syndrome in Korean Women. Gen Hosp Psychiatry 2010;32:164–8.
19. Weissman MM, Bland RC, Canino GJ, et al. Cross-national epidemiology of major depression and bipolar disorder. JAMA 1996;276:293–9.

20. Helliwell J, Layard R, Sachs J. World happiness report 2013. New York: UN Sustainable Development Solutions Network; 2013.

21. Chang SM, Hahm BJ, Lee JY, et al. Cross-national difference in the prevalence of depression caused by the diagnostic threshold. J Affect Disord 2008; 106:159–67.

22. Nomura T, Inoue Y, Kusumi M, et al. Prevalence of restless legs syndrome in a rural community in Japan. Mov Disord 2008;23:2363–9.

23. Kageyama T, Kabuto M, Nitta H, et al. Prevalences of periodic limb movement-like and restless legs-like symptoms among Japanese adults. Psychiatry Clin Neurosci 2000;54:296–8.

24. Yokoyama E, Saito Y, Kaneita Y, et al. Association between subjective well-being and sleep among the elderly in Japan. Sleep Med 2008;9:157–64.

25. Tsuboi Y, Imamura A, Sugimura M, et al. Prevalence of restless legs syndrome in a Japanese elderly population. Parkinsonism Relat Disord 2009;15: 598–601.

26. Rangarajan S, D'Souza GA. Restless legs syndrome in an Indian urban population. Sleep Med 2007;9:88–93.

27. Chen NH, Chuang LP, Yang CT, et al. The prevalence of restless legs syndrome in Taiwanese adults. Psychiatry Clin Neurosci 2010;64:170–8.

28. Li LH, Chen HB, Zhang LP, et al. A community-based investigation on restless legs syndrome in a town in China. Sleep Med 2012;13:342–5.

29. Ma JF, Xin XY, Liang L, et al. Restless legs syndrome in Chinese elderly people of an urban suburb in Shanghai: a community-based survey. Parkinsonism Relat Disord 2012;18:294–8.

30. Yan X, Wang WD, Walters AS, et al. Traditional Chinese medicine herbal preparations in restless legs syndrome (RLS) treatment: a review and probable first description of RLS in 1529. Sleep Med Rev 2012;16:509–18.

31. Sevim S, Dogu O, Kaleagasi H, et al. Correlation of anxiety and depression symptoms in patients with restless legs syndrome: a population based survey. J Neurol Neurosurg Psychiatry 2004;75:226–30.

32. Erer S, Karli N, Zarifoglu M, et al. The prevalence and clinical features of restless legs syndrome: a door to door population study in Orhangazi, Bursa in Turkey. Neurol India 2009;57:729–33.

33. Tasdemir M, Erdogan H, Boru UT, et al. Epidemiology of restless legs syndrome in Turkish adults on the western Black Sea coast of Turkey: a door-to-door study in a rural area. Sleep Med 2010;11: 82–6.

34. Hadjigeorgiou GM, Stefanidis I, Dardiotis E, et al. Low RLS prevalence and awareness in central Greece: an epidemiological survey. Eur J Neurol 2007;14:1275–80.

35. Ohayon MM, Roth T. Prevalence of restless legs syndrome and periodic limb movement disorder in the general population. J Psychosom Res 2002;53: 547–54.

36. Hogl B, Kiechl S, Willeit J, et al. Restless legs syndrome: a community-based study of prevalence, severity, and risk factors. Neurology 2005;64: 1920–4.

37. Vogl FD, Pichler I, Adel S, et al. Restless legs syndrome: epidemiological and clinicogenetic study in a South Tyrolean population isolate. Mov Disord 2006;21:1189–95.

38. Celle S, Roche F, Kerleroux J, et al. Prevalence and clinical correlates of restless legs syndrome in an elderly French population: the synapse study. J Gerontol A Biol Sci Med Sci 2010;65:167–73.

39. Tison F, Crochard A, Leger D, et al. Epidemiology of restless legs syndrome in French adults: a nationwide survey: the INSTANT Study. Neurology 2005; 65:239–46.

40. Rothdach AJ, Trenkwalder C, Haberstock J, et al. Prevalence and risk factors of RLS in an elderly population: the MEMO study. Memory and Morbidity in Augsburg Elderly. Neurology 2000;54:1064–8.

41. Berger K, Luedemann J, Trenkwalder C, et al. Sex and the risk of restless legs syndrome in the general population. Arch Intern Med 2004;164:196–202.

42. Happe S, Vennemann M, Evers S, et al. Treatment wish of individuals with known and unknown restless legs syndrome in the community. J Neurol 2008;255: 1365–71.

43. Rijsman R, Neven AK, Graffelman W, et al. Epidemiology of restless legs in The Netherlands. Eur J Neurol 2004;11:607–11.

44. Pekmezovic T, Jovic J, Svetel M, et al. Prevalence of restless legs syndrome among adult population in a Serbian district: a community-based study. Eur J Epidemiol 2013;28:927–30.

45. Benediktsdottir B, Janson C, Lindberg E, et al. Prevalence of restless legs syndrome among adults in Iceland and Sweden: lung function, comorbidity, ferritin, biomarkers and quality of life. Sleep Med 2010;11:1043–8.

46. Juuti AK, Laara E, Rajala U, et al. Prevalence and associated factors of restless legs in a 57-year-old urban population in northern Finland. Acta Neurol Scand 2010;122:63–9.

47. Bjorvatn B, Leissner L, Ulfberg J, et al. Prevalence, severity and risk factors of restless legs syndrome in the general adult population in two Scandinavian countries. Sleep Med 2005;6:307–12.

48. Ulfberg J, Nystrom B, Carter N, et al. Prevalence of restless legs syndrome among men aged 18 to 64 years: an association with somatic disease and neuropsychiatric symptoms. Mov Disord 2001;16: 1159–63.

49. Ulfberg J, Nystrom B, Carter N, et al. Restless legs syndrome among working-aged women. Eur Neurol 2001;46:17–9.

50. Broman JE, Mallon L, Hetta J. Restless legs syndrome and its relationship with insomnia symptoms and daytime distress: epidemiological survey in Sweden. Psychiatry Clin Neurosci 2008;62:472–5.

51. Wesstrom J, Nilsson S, Sundstrom-Poromaa I, et al. Restless legs syndrome among women: prevalence, co-morbidity and possible relationship to menopause. Climacteric 2008;11:422–8.

52. Ekbom K-A. Restless legs. Acta Med Scand 1945; 158(suppl):1–123.

53. Simon GE, VonKorff M, Piccinelli M, et al. An international study of the relation between somatic symptoms and depression. N Engl J Med 1999;341:1329–35.

54. Koo BB, Feng P, Dostal J, et al. Alpha-melanocyte stimulating hormone and adrenocorticotropic hormone: an alternative approach when thinking about restless legs syndrome? Mov Disord 2008;23:1234–42.

55. Abdel-Malek Z, Suzuki I, Tada A, et al. The melanocortin-1 receptor and human pigmentation. Ann N Y Acad Sci 1999;885:117–33.

56. Jablonski NG, Chaplin G. The evolution of human skin coloration. J Hum Evol 2000;39:57–106.

57. Koo BB. Restless legs syndrome: relationship between prevalence and latitude. Sleep Breath 2012; 16:1237–45.

58. Ingram DG, Plante DT. Seasonal trends in restless legs symptomatology: evidence from internet search query data. Sleep Med 2013;14:1364–8.

59. Balaban H, Yildiz OK, Cil G, et al. Serum 25-hydroxyvitamin D levels in restless legs syndrome patients. Sleep Med 2012;13:953–7.

60. Miranda M, Araya F, Castillo JL, et al. Restless legs syndrome: a clinical study in adult general population and in uremic patients. Rev Med Chil 2001; 129:179–86.

61. Castillo PR, Kaplan J, Lin SC, et al. Prevalence of restless legs syndrome among native South Americans residing in coastal and mountainous areas. Mayo Clin Proc 2006;81:1345–7.

62. Castillo PR, Mera RM, Fredrickson PA, et al. Psychological distress in patients with restless legs syndrome (Willis-Ekbom disease): a population-based door-to-door survey in rural Ecuador. BMC Res Notes 2014;7:911.

63. Eckeli AL, Gitai LL, Dach F, et al. Prevalence of restless legs syndrome in the rural town of Cassia dos Coqueiros in Brazil. Sleep Med 2011;12:762–7.

64. Lavigne GJ, Montplaisir JY. Restless legs syndrome and sleep bruxism: prevalence and association among Canadians. Sleep 1994;17:739–43.

65. Froese CL, Butt A, Mulgrew A, et al. Depression and sleep-related symptoms in an adult, indigenous, North American population. J Clin Sleep Med 2008;4:356–61.

66. Phillips B, Young T, Finn L, et al. Epidemiology of restless legs symptoms in adults. Arch Intern Med 2000;160:2137–41.

67. Phillips B, Hening W, Britz P, et al. Prevalence and correlates of restless legs syndrome: results from the 2005 National Sleep Foundation Poll. Chest 2006;129:76–80.

68. Lee HB, Hening WA, Allen RP, et al. Race and restless legs syndrome symptoms in an adult community sample in east Baltimore. Sleep Med 2006;7:642–5.

69. Winkelman JW, Finn L, Young T. Prevalence and correlates of restless legs syndrome symptoms in the Wisconsin Sleep Cohort. Sleep Med 2006;7: 545–52.

70. Winkelman JW, Shahar E, Sharief I, et al. Association of restless legs syndrome and cardiovascular disease in the Sleep Heart Health Study. Neurology 2008;70:35–42.

71. Gao X, Schwarzschild MA, Wang H, et al. Obesity and restless legs syndrome in men and women. Neurology 2009;72:1255–61.

72. Ram S, Seirawan H, Kumar SK, et al. Prevalence and impact of sleep disorders and sleep habits in the United States. Sleep Breath 2010;14:63–70.

73. Sawanyawisuth K, Palinkas LA, Ancoli-Israel S, et al. Ethnic differences in the prevalence and predictors of restless legs syndrome between Hispanics of Mexican descent and non-Hispanic Whites in San Diego county: a population-based study. J Clin Sleep Med 2013;9:47–53.

74. Allen RP, Bharmal M, Calloway M. Prevalence and disease burden of primary restless legs syndrome: results of a general population survey in the United States. Mov Disord 2011;26:114–20.

75. Kutner NG, Bliwise DL. Restless legs complaint in African-American and Caucasian hemodialysis patients. Sleep Med 2002;3:497–500.

76. Winter AC, Schurks M, Glynn RJ, et al. Restless legs syndrome and risk of incident cardiovascular disease in women and men: prospective cohort study. BMJ Open 2012;2:e000866.

77. Li Y, Walters AS, Chiuve SE, et al. Prospective study of restless legs syndrome and coronary heart disease among women. Circulation 2012; 126:1689–94.

78. Szentkiralyi A, Volzke H, Hoffmann W, et al. Multimorbidity and the risk of restless legs syndrome in 2 prospective cohort studies. Neurology 2014;82:2026–33.

79. Marin G, Sabogal F, Marin BV, et al. Development of a short acculturation scale for hispanics. Hisp J Behav Sci 1987;9:183–205.

80. Hening WA, Allen RP, Washburn M, et al. Validation of the Hopkins telephone diagnostic interview for restless legs syndrome. Sleep Med 2008;9: 283–9.

81. Allen RP, Burchell BJ, MacDonald B, et al. Validation of the self-completed Cambridge-Hopkins questionnaire (CH-RLSq) for ascertainment of restless legs syndrome (RLS) in a population survey. Sleep Med 2009;10:1097–100.

82. Stefansson H, Rye DB, Hicks A, et al. A genetic risk factor for periodic limb movements in sleep. N Engl J Med 2007;357:639–47.

83. Winkelmann J, Schormair B, Lichtner P, et al. Genome-wide association study of restless legs syndrome identifies common variants in three genomic regions. Nat Genet 2007;39:1000–6.

84. Schormair B, Kemlink D, Roeske D, et al. PTPRD (protein tyrosine phosphatase receptor type delta) is associated with restless legs syndrome. Nat Genet 2008;40:946–8.

85. Kim MK, Cho YW, Shin WC, et al. Association of restless legs syndrome variants in Korean patients with restless legs syndrome. Sleep 2013;36:1787–91.

Pathophysiology of Restless Legs Syndrome/Willis-Ekbom Disease

Pathophysiology of Restless
Legs Syndrome/Willis-Ekbom
Disease

Restless Leg Syndrome/ Willis-Ekbom Disease Pathophysiology

Richard P. Allen, PhD

KEYWORDS

• Iron • Dopamine • RLS/WED • PLMS • RLS augmentation

KEY POINTS

- Iron management is impaired in restless leg syndrome/Willis-Ekbom disease, leading to brain iron deficiency.
- Brain iron deficiency acting partly through hypoxic pathway activation produces increased presynaptic and synaptic dopamine. This produces postsynaptic down-regulation that overcorrects for the normal evening and nocturnal decrease in dopamine-producing restless leg syndrome/Willis-Ekbom disease symptoms. Increasing dopamine activation in the evening and night corrects this problem reducing restless leg syndrome symptoms.
- Eventual continued increased dopamine stimulation with long-term dopamine treatment leads to further postsynaptic desensitization and gradual worsening of restless leg syndrome/Willis-Ekbom disease, especially at the higher doses and possibly more for shorter-acting medications.
- Brain iron deficiency also reduces myelin, possibly accounting for brain white matter decreases in restless leg syndrome/Willis-Ekbom disease.
- Hypoxia (eg, with chronic obstructive pulmonary disease) activates hypoxic pathways leading to dopamine increases and restless leg syndrome/Willis-Ekbom disease independent of iron status.

INTRODUCTION

Three major clinical features of restless leg syndrome/Willis-Ekbom disease (RLS/WED) unique for common neurologic disorders enabled somewhat surprising pathophysiologic discoveries. RLS/WED has a well-defined phenotype, one accessible and well-defined environmental vector (iron), and dramatic response to increasing activity of one neurotransmitter system (dopamine). Studies based on these 3 pillars of RLS/WED found a complex underlying biology almost the opposite of expectations. The well-defined phenotype enabled important genetic discoveries for RLS. In sleep medicine, only RLS/WED and narcolepsy have well-defined genetic factors, and both have well defined phenotypes missing for the other sleep disorders. Study of the environmental vector of iron deficiency found an underlying iron pathophysiology. The dopamine treatment response drove studies of dopamine pathophysiology.

This article includes sections focused on pathophysiologic findings from each of these 3 areas: genetics, cortical-spinal excitability, and iron and dopamine. There are other less well-developed features of RLS/WED pathophysiology that could be considered, particularly cortical excitability, neuroanatomical considerations, and other neurotransmitter/neuromodulators. The summary in the last section includes a brief note of these.

Disclosures: Dr R.P. Allen in the last 2 years has served as a consultant for UCB pharma, Xenoport. Luipold pharmceuticals and has had research support from NIH (NINDS R01 NS075184, NIA PO1-AG21190), Pharmacosmos and UCB Pharma.

Department of Neurology, Johns Hopkins University, Asthma & Allergy Building, 1B76b, 5501 Hopkins Bayview Boulevard, Baltimore, MD 21224, USA

E-mail address: rallen6@jhmi.edu

GENETICS AND RESTLESS LEG SYNDROME/WILLIS-EKBOM DISEASE PATHOPHYSIOLOGY

The well-defined RLS/WED phenotype enabled successful genomewide association studies (GWAS) that have now identified RLS/WED risk alleles on 5 specific genomic regions for MEIS1, BTBD9, PTPRD, MAP2k/SKOR1, and TOX3/BC034767 and on an intergenic region on chromosome 2 (rs6747972).[1–3] Most of these variants also seem to have some relation to the periodic leg movements (PLMS) motor sign of RLS/WED.[4] An RLS/WED risk allele on BTBD9 is also strongly associated with both increased PLMS independent of RLS/WED and with decreased peripheral iron stores (decreased serum ferritin).[5] Another BDBT9 allelic variant relates to RLS/WED diagnosis,[3] increased PLMS,[6] and greater decreases in peripheral iron stores with blood donations.[7] Functional relation of BTBD9 has been further indicated by findings of increased peripheral iron for a BDBT9-mutant mouse[8] and murine ventral midbrain iron content associated with a quantitative trait loci that includes BDBT9.[9] Besides these findings relating in general BDBT9 to iron deficiency in RLS/WED, there has been no significantly substantial discovery of potential genetics pathways to RLS/WED pathophysiology. This commonly occurs for results from GWAS for common diseases, suggesting the need for different approaches.

IRON PATHOPHYSIOLOGY

RLS/WED has one major, well-defined primary environmental factor of iron deficiency. This deficiency was noted in the seminal RLS/WED studies of Ekbom[10] and Nordlander.[11] RLS/WED severity increases with decreased peripheral iron,[12] and its prevalence is about 9 times greater in iron-deficient anemia than general populations.[13] All conditions that compromise iron status have been associated with increased risk of RLS/WED (eg, pregnancy and end-stage renal disease). Moreover, in these cases, aggressive treatment of the iron deficiency reduces RLS/WED severity. But most RLS/WED patients have normal serum ferritin and little indication for abnormal peripheral iron stores. The pathophysiology appears to be less peripheral and more about central nervous system iron status. Reduced cerebrospinal fluid (CSF) ferritin was reported in 2 separate studies for RLS/WED patients who had normal peripheral iron measures.[14,15]

The single best-documented biological abnormality for RLS/WED is brain iron deficiency. Initial reports showed decreased brain iron based on magnetic resonance imaging (MRI) of the substantia nigra and red nucleus as shown in **Fig. 1**.[16] Brain iron deficiency for RLS/WED has now been confirmed in 6 studies using different methods in different laboratories.[16–21] The brain areas most consistently showing the reduced iron include the substantia nigra and, to a lesser extent, the putamen and caudate. Recent studies with more sensitive measures have documented low iron in the thalamus.[20] The iron deficiency seems to be more regional than global, and the affected regions include not only iron rich areas such as the substantia nigra but also iron-poor areas, particularly the thalamus. Some iron-rich areas have not consistently shown decreased iron for RLS/WED (eg, cerebellar dentate nucleus). Thus, the pathophysiology seems to involve a regional brain iron deficiency present in most RLS/WED patients despite normal iron status.

Changes in iron regulatory proteins from RLS/WED autopsy studies present a surprisingly complicated interaction. H-ferritin but not L-ferritin is increased in the RLS/WED brains. The H-ferritin

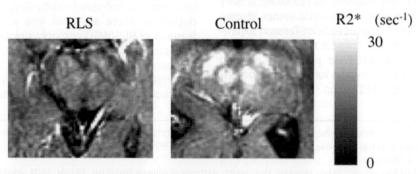

Fig. 1. R2* images in a 70-year-old RLS patient and a 71-year-old control subject. Much lower R2* relaxation rates are apparent in the RLS case in both red nucleus and substantia nigra. (*Adapted from* Allen RP, Barker PB, Wehrl F, et al. MRI measurement of brain iron in patients with restless legs syndrome. Neurology 2001;56(2):263–5; with permission.)

more than L-ferritin provides transport and storage of iron. In neuromelanin cells of the substantia nigra, transferrin receptor is decreased, contrary to expected response to reduced iron status. This finding may relate to a decreased activity of iron regulatory protein-1.[22] The transport of iron into the brain shows a more complete picture. Autopsy evaluation of motor cortex microvessels found decreased iron regulatory protein-1 activity with associated decreased iron intake/storage proteins of transferrin receptor, transferrin, and H-ferritin but no change in the iron export protein, ferroportin. Thus, we have a consistent pattern of impaired iron transport into the brain and, more specifically, into neuromelanin cells of the substantia nigra.[23] The failure of iron transport to the brain also occurs in the choroid plexus. The epithelial cells show decreased iron and H-ferritin consistent with iron deficiency, but they also show increased mitochondrial ferritin indicating increased mitochondrial iron uptake. The iron regulatory proteins in the choroid plexus are increased for the cellular iron intake (transferrin receptor, transferrin) but also iron export (ferroportin).[23] Thus, these cells show a pattern consistent with a higher turnover of iron feeding an increased mitochondrial iron status. The increased mitochondrial ferritin was also found in the cells of the substantia nigra but not the putamen.[24] In these cells there seemed to be more mitochondria and increased iron demand. Thus, the mitochondria seem to have acquired their iron surplus at the expense of cytosolic iron and overall cytosolic cellular iron deficiency.

Overall, the RLS/WED regional brain iron deficiency involves a failure to provide adequate iron transport across the blood-brain barrier compounded by a regional failure to import adequate iron into critical neuronal cells (eg, neuromelanin cells of the substantia nigra). A curious and possibly important finding of increased mitochondrial ferritin and iron turnover in the choroid plexus and possibly the substantia nigra may represent a fundamental feature of the iron pathophysiology deserving further consideration.

CONSEQUENCES OF IRON DEFICIENCY: HYPOXIC PATHWAY ACTIVATION AND MYELIN LOSS

The 2 major expected pathophysiologic consequences of brain iron deficiency have been documented: hypoxia and myelin loss. Oxygen transport depends on iron, and decreased iron should signal potential hypoxia. The hypoxic inducible factor 1-alpha has been found increased in the RLS/WED substantia nigra. The hypoxic inducible factor 2-alpha and the vascular endothelial growth factor were increased in the microvessels.[25] These differences occurred despite the lack of any significant indication of actual hypoxia. Activation of these hypoxic pathways would be expected to lead to increased dopaminergic activity as described in later discussion.

Two studies found hypoxia in the leg muscles of RLS/WED patients that is not explained by levels of activity. These could represent a sequelae of a general iron regulation problem.[26,27] Some recent studies have suggested an increased difference between morning and evening blood flow[28] and relative hypoxia in leg muscles of RLS/WED patients.[29] It may be that hypoxia or hypoxic pathway activation is one pathway to RLS/WED symptoms. This finding would explain the high prevalence of RLS/WED with chronic obstructive pulmonary disease.[30–32]

Myelin synthesis depends on iron, and brain iron deficiency in animals reduces myelin proteins, lipids, and cholesterol.[33,34] The brain iron deficiency of RLS/WED would be expected to produce a mild but significant myelin deficit. This was confirmed by imaging showing significant decreases in white matter in the corpus callosum, anterior cingulum, and precentral gyrus. Postmortem analyses also found a 25% decrease in myelin proteins.[35] This degree of myelin deficit could contribute to the RLS/WED symptoms, particularly in relation to sensorimotor integration that has time-dependent signaling.

DOPAMINE PATHOPHYSIOLOGY

The dramatic and immediate treatment benefits from levodopa led to a general view that RLS/WED has a significant brain dopamine deficiency. The search to document the dopamine abnormalities in RLS/WED turned out to be much more difficult than expected and produced surprising results. The initial CSF analyses showed no differences between RLS/WED and controls for the major proteins related to dopamine.[36,37] A repeat analysis of 3-orthymethyl dopamine (3-OMD) found significant increases in the CSF in 2 independent samples (**Fig. 2**).[38] Moreover, the increases correlated with the dopamine metabolite, homovanillic acid (HVA). Given the metabolic pathways from tyrosine hydroxylase to dopamine (see **Fig. 2**), the increase in both 3-OMD and HVA is best explained as an increase in tyrosine hydroxylase activity leading to increased dopamine production.

Brain imaging produced somewhat contradictory results. The early PET and single-photon emission computerized tomography studies found clear decreases in striatal D2 receptors,[39,40] but

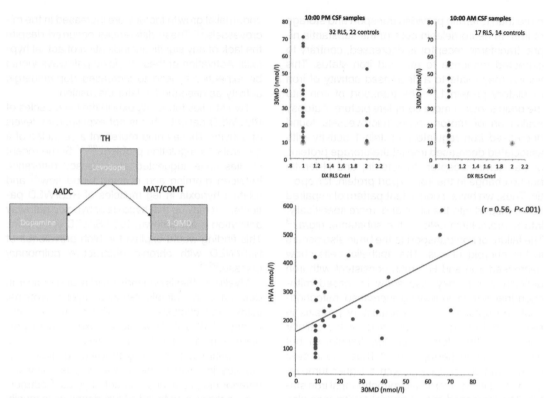

Fig. 2. RLS CSF samples show 3-OMD is increased and correlated with increased HVA. Top right panel shows increase in 2 separate sets of RLS patients for samples from evening and morning. Left panel shows metabolic pathways for levodopa to 3-OMD and HVA. Bottom right panel shows correlation of these 2 metabolites of levodopa from different metabolic pathways. The values correlate for both metabolites indicating likely increased levodopa rather than abnormalities in the 2 different metabolic pathways. These data are compatible with the autopsy data showing increased tyrosine hydroxylase in the substantia nigra. (*Adapted from* Allen RP, Connor JR, Hyland K, et al. Abnormally increased CSF 3-Ortho-methyldopa (3-OMD) in untreated restless legs syndrome (RLS) patients indicates more severe disease and possibly abnormally increased dopamine synthesis. Sleep Med 2009;10(1):124, 127; with permission.)

this would be most consistent with a response to increased synaptic dopamine. A later study reported increased D2 receptor binding, indicating the opposite of a decreased synaptic dopamine, but that study had mostly mildly affected patients.[41] The fluoro-L-dopa (fDOPA) studies, in contrast, have consistently shown decreased striatal fDOPA uptake. Given no cell loss in RLS/WED, the decreased fDOPA uptake would indicate a fast turnover of dopamine consistent with increased dopamine production. The final and probably most important imaging findings involve the dopamine transporter (DAT). Iron-deficient rodents show decreased D2 receptors similar to that seen in RLS/WED[42]; they also show a decreased DAT, mostly membrane-bound DAT.[43] Initial single-photon emission computerized tomography studies of total DAT generally found no significant differences between RLS/WED and controls,[39] but membrane-bound DAT was found

decreased in 2 separate studies reported together.[44] The decreased DAT was found with methylphenidate binding (**Fig. 3**). Thus, overall, the brain imaging studies also indicate increased striatal dopamine, not the expected decrease.[45]

DOPAMINE PATHOPHYSIOLOGY: BASIS FOR RESTLESS LEG SYNDROME/WILLIS-EKBOM DISEASE TREATMENT AUGMENTATION

The obvious problem arises: if the RLS/WED brain dopamine is already abnormally increased, how does increasing this further by levodopa reduce the symptoms? Resolving this apparent contradiction requires appreciating the strong circadian aspect of both dopaminergic activity and RLS/WED symptoms. Increased dopaminergic stimulation will produce a postsynaptic down-regulation likely at both receptor and internal cellular function. The general pattern of

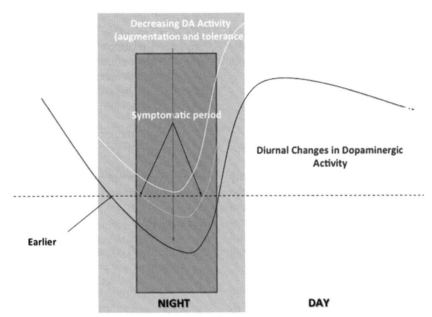

Fig. 3. Conceptualized basis for RLS augmentation. The dotted line indicates the critical postsynaptic dopamine signal level, decreasing below this produces RLS symptoms. The light white line is the RLS before treatment with symptoms at night. The dark white line represents initial treatment success with no symptoms. The red line represents the adjustment to the increased evening dopamine producing earlier and more intense RLS symptoms lasting longer during the night. Note that the morning and day stay protected from RLS symptoms. (*Adapted from* Earley CJ, Allen RP, Connor JR, et al. The dopaminergic neurons of the A11 system in RLS/WED autopsy brains appear normal. Sleep Med 2009;10:1155–7; with permission.)

decreased D2 receptors, especially for the more severe cases may represent part of this down-regulation of response. But dopamine has a clear circadian activity pattern decreasing in the evening and night and increasing in the morning. The RLS/WED postsynaptic adjustment to increased dopamine stimulation suffices for the daytime but seems to overcompensate when dopamine levels are lower during the evening and night. This produces a relative evening and nighttime dopamine deficit despite the overall dopamine increase. Thus, there is a circadian pattern of evening and night RLS/WED symptoms with, if anything, hyper-alertness and arousal in the morning preventing the expected sleepiness for the short and disrupted RLS/WED sleep.

A small dose of dopamine in the evening and night serves to correct for this relative evening decrease in dopamine, but this is to some extent adding coals to the fire. The treatment with increased dopamine stimulation leads to increasing the down-regulation beyond that already occurring with the disease, thus making the underlying RLS/WED disease worse and augmenting the symptoms. The eventual adjustment to the treatment leads to a need for adding even more stimulation and higher doses to be effective.

This initially looks like tolerance to the medication, but in this situation tolerance is essentially a worsening of the underlying pathology or augmentation. It is important to appreciate that tolerance and augmentation appear to be biologically the same for dopamine treatment of RLS. Tolerance is the first step.[46] Eventually, over time, the adjustment of the system to even more increased dopamine produces a gradual worsening of the RLS. The dopamine agents continue to help sleep a little, leaving the patient struggling with increased daytime symptoms and dependent on the medications to avoid significant withdrawal symptoms. **Fig. 3** demonstrates this problem. Thus, the pathophysiology of dopamine for RLS/WED indicates dopamine treatment needs to be done carefully at low doses. Because shorter-acting medications tend to require higher peek levels to support adequate duration, they tend to produce worse augmentation. Using longer-acting medications, particularly the continuous release transdermal rotigotine (Neupro, UCB pharma, Germany) reduces the risk and severity of RLS/WED augmentation. But even here the higher doses will produce significant augmentation (eg, rotigotine produces little augmentation over 5 years at the lower doses of 2 to 3 mg/24h but has significant augmentation at the 4-mg and higher doses).[47] Overall, the RLS/WED pathophysiology of dopamine indicates that dopamine medications often have a limited life-span for effective treatment, and other agents will be needed.

OTHER PATHOPHYSIOLOGIC FINDINGS IN RESTLESS LEG SYNDROME

Studies have found a range of other possible biological abnormalities in RLS/WED that have somewhat limited scientific support. Cortical excitability is one major exception. Transcranial magnetic stimulation (TMS) of the motor cortex for control of hand muscles has consistently shown decreased thresholds for response and reduced paired-pulse inhibition.[48–51] The increased cortical excitability is partially reduced by dopamine treatment.[52–54] The significance of these findings remains somewhat unclear. The increased cortical excitability has not been consistently related to any of the clinical features of RLS/WED.

Loss of cells has not generally been reported (eg, A11 dopamine cells[55]) except in one study that reported a decrease in thalamic cells staining for beta endorphin.[56] This, finding, however, needs to be confirmed. Evaluations of amounts of gray matter have produced conflicting results.[57–61] Overall, RLS/WED does not seem to be a neurodegenerative disorder, nor is there any convincing evidence of reduced number or death of cells. There are, however, consistent reports of regional white matter decrease in RLS/WED consistent with the expected effects of iron deficiency as noted before.[35,62,63]

An anatomic locus significant for RLS/WED symptoms has been suggested based on theoretic considerations and findings of dopamine, iron abnormalities, TMS, and MRI abnormalities. Much has been made of a "spinal theory" of RLS/WED involving abnormalities in the A11 descending dopamine system, but scant data have been provided supporting any abnormality in this system. The iron and brain imaging studies indicate changes in substantia nigra and striatum, particularly the putamen. The TMS findings indicate sensorimotor pathway abnormalities. Similarly, the MRI findings of white matter decreases seem to suggest abnormalities in cerebral sensorimotor pathways.[63]

SUMMARY

RLS/WED pathophysiology occurs in a wide range of locations and systems. It seems to have largely metabolic abnormalities mostly involving iron and the consequences of iron deficiency including increased dopamine. The iron-related abnormalities have even been found in the lymphocytes.[64] But iron is probably not the whole picture. RLS/WED like other common diseases may have multiple pathways to disease, some less common than others (eg, hypoxia without iron deficiency producing tyrosine hydroxylase and dopamine increases).

The major pathophysiologic findings for RLS/WED have provided guidance for treatment advances for reducing the risk of dopamine augmentation and emphasizing the importance of developing better methods for iron treatment.

REFERENCES

1. Schormair B, Kemlink D, Roeske D, et al. PTPRD (protein tyrosine phosphatase receptor type delta) is associated with restless legs syndrome. Nat Genet 2008;40(8):946–8.
2. Winkelmann J, Czamara D, Schormair B, et al. Genome-wide association study identifies novel restless legs syndrome susceptibility loci on 2p14 and 16q12.1. PLoS Genet 2011;7(7):e1002171.
3. Winkelmann J, Schormair B, Lichtner P, et al. Genome-wide association study of restless legs syndrome identifies common variants in three genomic regions. Nat Genet 2007;39(9):1000–6.
4. Moore H 4th, Winkelmann J, Lin L, et al. Periodic leg movements during sleep are associated with polymorphisms in BTBD9, TOX3/BC034767, MEIS1, MAP2K5/SKOR1, and PTPRD. Sleep 2014;37(9):1535–42.
5. Stefansson H, Rye DB, Hicks A, et al. A genetic risk factor for periodic limb movements in sleep. N Engl J Med 2007;357(7):639–47.
6. Vilarino-Guell C, Soto AI, Young JE, et al. Susceptibility genes for restless legs syndrome are not associated with Parkinson disease. Neurology 2008;71(3):222–3.
7. Sorensen E, Grau K, Berg T, et al. A genetic risk factor for low serum ferritin levels in Danish blood donors. Transfusion 2012;52(12):2585–9.
8. Deandrade MP, Johnson RL Jr, Unger EL, et al. Motor restlessness, sleep disturbances, thermal sensory alterations and elevated serum iron levels in Btbd9 mutant mice. Hum Mol Genet 2012;21(18):3984–92.
9. Jellen LC, Unger EL, Lu L, et al. Systems genetic analysis of the effects of iron deficiency in mouse brain. Neurogenetics 2012;13(2):147–57.
10. Ekbom KA. Restless legs. Stockholm (Sweden): Ivar Haeggströms; 1945. p. 123.
11. Nordlander NB. Therapy in restless legs. Acta Med Scand 1953;145:453–7.
12. Sun ER, Chen CA, Ho G, et al. Iron and the restless legs syndrome. Sleep 1998;21(4):371–7.

13. Allen RP, Auerbach S, Bahrain H, et al. The prevalence and impact of restless legs syndrome on patients with iron deficiency anemia. Am J Hematol 2013;88(4):261–4.

14. Earley CJ, Connor JR, Beard JL, et al. Abnormalities in CSF concentrations of ferritin and transferrin in restless legs syndrome. Neurology 2000;54(8): 1698–700.

15. Mizuno S, Mihara T, Miyaoka T, et al. CSF iron, ferritin and transferrin levels in restless legs syndrome. J Sleep Res 2005;14(1):43–7.

16. Allen RP, Barker PB, Wehrl F, et al. MRI measurement of brain iron in patients with restless legs syndrome. Neurology 2001;56(2):263–5.

17. Earley CJ, Barker BP, Horska A, et al. MRI-determined regional brain iron concentrations in early- and late-onset restless legs syndrome. Sleep Med 2006;7(5):458–61.

18. Godau J, Klose U, Di Santo A, et al. Multiregional brain iron deficiency in restless legs syndrome. Mov Disord 2008;23(8):1184–7.

19. Moon HJ, Chang Y, Lee YS, et al. T2 relaxometry using 3.0-tesla magnetic resonance imaging of the brain in early- and late-onset restless legs syndrome. J Clin Neurol 2014;10(3):197–202.

20. Rizzo G, Manners D, Testa C, et al. Low brain iron content in idiopathic restless legs syndrome patients detected by phase imaging. Mov Disord 2013; 28(13):1886–90.

21. Schmidauer C, Sojer M, Seppi K, et al. Transcranial ultrasound shows nigral hypoechogenicity in restless legs syndrome. Ann Neurol 2005;58(4): 630–4.

22. Connor JR, Wang XS, Patton SM, et al. Decreased transferrin receptor expression by neuromelanin cells in restless legs syndrome. Neurology 2004; 62(9):1563–7.

23. Connor JR, Ponnuru P, Wang XS, et al. Profile of altered brain iron acquisition in restless legs syndrome. Brain 2011;134(Pt 4):959–68.

24. Snyder AM, Wang X, Patton SM, et al. Mitochondrial ferritin in the substantia nigra in restless legs syndrome. J Neuropathol Exp Neurol 2009;68(11): 1193–9.

25. Patton SM, Ponnuru P, Snyder AM, et al. Hypoxia-inducible factor pathway activation in restless legs syndrome patients. Eur J Neurol 2011;18(11): 1329–35.

26. Larsson BW, Kadi F, Ulfberg J, et al. Skeletal muscle morphology in patients with restless legs syndrome. Eur Neurol 2007;58(3):133–7.

27. Wahlin-Larsson B, Ulfberg J, Aulin KP, et al. The expression of vascular endothelial growth factor in skeletal muscle of patients with sleep disorders. Muscle Nerve 2009;40(4):556–61.

28. Oskarsson E, Wahlin-Larsson B, Ulfberg J. Reduced daytime intramuscular blood flow in patients with restless legs syndrome/Willis-Ekbom disease. Psychiatry Clin Neurosci 2014;68(8):640–3.

29. Salminen AV, Rimpila V, Polo O. Peripheral hypoxia in restless legs syndrome (Willis-Ekbom disease). Neurology 2014;82(21):1856–61.

30. Benediktsdottir B, Janson C, Lindberg E, et al. Prevalence of restless legs syndrome among adults in Iceland and Sweden: lung function, comorbidity, ferritin, biomarkers and quality of life. Sleep Med 2010;11(10):1043–8.

31. Kaplan Y, Inonu H, Yilmaz A, et al. Restless legs syndrome in patients with chronic obstructive pulmonary disease. Can J Neurol Sci 2008;35(3):352–7.

32. Lo Coco D, Mattaliano A, Coco AL, et al. Increased frequency of restless legs syndrome in chronic obstructive pulmonary disease patients. Sleep Med 2009;10:572–6.

33. Yu GS, Steinkirchner TM, Rao GA, et al. Effect of prenatal iron deficiency on myelination in rat pups. Am J Pathol 1986;125(3):620–4.

34. Ortiz E, Pasquini JM, Thompson K, et al. Effect of manipulation of iron storage, transport, or availability on myelin composition and brain iron content in three different animal models. J Neurosci Res 2004;77(5):681–9.

35. Connor JR, Ponnuru P, Lee BY, et al. Postmortem and imaging based analyses reveal CNS decreased myelination in restless legs syndrome. Sleep Med 2011;12(6):614–9.

36. Stiasny-Kolster K, Mignot E, Ling L, et al. The role of CNS dopaminergic, serotonergic and hypocretin (orexin) systems in restless legs syndrome. Sleep 2003;26:A325–6.

37. Stiasny-Kolster K, Moller JC, Zschocke J, et al. Normal dopaminergic and serotonergic metabolites in cerebrospinal fluid and blood of restless legs syndrome patients. Mov Disord 2004;19(2):192–6.

38. Allen RP, Connor JR, Hyland K, et al. Abnormally increased CSF 3-Ortho-methyldopa (3-OMD) in untreated restless legs syndrome (RLS) patients indicates more severe disease and possibly abnormally increased dopamine synthesis. Sleep Med 2009;10(1):123–8.

39. Michaud M, Soucy JP, Chabli A, et al. SPECT imaging of striatal pre- and postsynaptic dopaminergic status in restless legs syndrome with periodic leg movements in sleep. J Neurol 2002;249(2):164–70.

40. Turjanski N, Lees AJ, Brooks DJ. Striatal dopaminergic function in restless legs syndrome: 18F-dopa and 11C-raclopride PET studies. Neurology 1999;52(5):932–7.

41. Cervenka S, Palhagen SE, Comley RA, et al. Support for dopaminergic hypoactivity in restless legs syndrome: a PET study on D2-receptor binding. Brain 2006;129(Pt 8):2017–28.

42. Erikson KM, Jones BC, Hess EJ, et al. Iron deficiency decreases dopamine D1 and D2

receptors in rat brain. Pharmacol Biochem Behav 2001;69(3–4):409–18.

43. Erikson KM, Jones BC, Beard JL. Iron deficiency alters dopamine transporter functioning in rat striatum. J Nutr 2000;130(11):2831–7.

44. Earley CJ, Kuwabara H, Wong DF, et al. The dopamine transporter is decreased in the striatum of subjects with restless legs syndrome. Sleep 2011;34(3):341–7.

45. Earley CJ, Kuwabara H, Wong DF, et al. Increased synaptic dopamine in the putamen in restless legs syndrome. Sleep 2013;36(1):51–7.

46. Winkelman JW, Johnston L. Augmentation and tolerance with long-term pramipexole treatment of restless legs syndrome (RLS). Sleep Med 2004;5(1):9–14.

47. Oertel W, Trenkwalder C, Benes H, et al. Long-term safety and efficacy of rotigotine transdermal patch for moderate-to-severe idiopathic restless legs syndrome: a 5-year open-label extension study. Lancet Neurol 2011;10(8):710–20.

48. Gunduz A, Adatepe NU, Kiziltan ME, et al. Circadian changes in cortical excitability in restless legs syndrome. J Neurol Sci 2012;316(1–2):122–5.

49. Lanza G, Cantone M, Lanuzza B, et al. Distinctive patterns of cortical excitability to transcranial magnetic stimulation in obstructive sleep apnea syndrome, restless legs syndrome, insomnia, and sleep deprivation. Sleep Med Rev 2015;19C:39–50.

50. Lanza G, Lanuzza B, Arico D, et al. Direct comparison of cortical excitability to transcranial magnetic stimulation in obstructive sleep apnea syndrome and restless legs syndrome. Sleep Med 2015;16(1):138–42.

51. Scalise A, Cadore IP, Gigli GL. Motor cortex excitability in restless legs syndrome. Sleep Med 2004;5(4):393–6.

52. Gorsler A, Liepert J. Influence of cabergoline on motor excitability in patients with restless legs syndrome. J Clin Neurophysiol 2007;24(6):456–60.

53. Scalise A, Pittaro-Cadore I, Janes F, et al. Changes of cortical excitability after dopaminergic treatment in restless legs syndrome. Sleep Med 2010;11(1):75–81.

54. Rizzo V, Arico I, Mastroeni C, et al. Dopamine agonists restore cortical plasticity in patients with idiopathic restless legs syndrome. Mov Disord 2009;24(5):710–5.

55. Earley CJ, Allen RP, Connor JR, et al. The dopaminergic neurons of the A11 system in RLS/WED autopsy brains appear normal. Sleep Med 2009;10:1155–7.

56. Walters AS, Ondo WG, Zhu W, et al. Does the endogenous opiate system play a role in the Restless Legs Syndrome?: a pilot post-mortem study. J Neurol Sci 2009;279(1–2):62–5.

57. Unrath A, Juengling FD, Schork M, et al. Cortical grey matter alterations in idiopathic restless legs syndrome: an optimized voxel-based morphometry study. Mov Disord 2007;22(12):1751–6.

58. Chang Y, Chang HW, Song H, et al. Gray matter alteration in patients with restless legs syndrome: a voxel-based morphometry study. Clin Imaging 2014;39(1):20–5.

59. Celle S, Roche F, Peyron R, et al. Lack of specific gray matter alterations in restless legs syndrome in elderly subjects. J Neurol 2010;257(3):344–8.

60. Comley RA, Cervenka S, Palhagen SE, et al. A comparison of gray matter density in restless legs syndrome patients and matched controls using voxel-based morphometry. J Neuroimaging 2012;22(1):28–32.

61. Hornyak M, Ahrendts JC, Spiegelhalder K, et al. Voxel-based morphometry in unmedicated patients with restless legs syndrome. Sleep Med 2007;9(1):22–6.

62. Chang Y, Paik JS, Lee HJ, et al. Altered white matter integrity in primary restless legs syndrome patients: diffusion tensor imaging study. Neurol Res 2014;36(8):769–74.

63. Unrath A, Muller HP, Ludolph AC, et al. Cerebral white matter alterations in idiopathic restless legs syndrome, as measured by diffusion tensor imaging. Mov Disord 2008;23(9):1250–5.

64. Earley CJ, Ponnuru P, Wang X, et al. Altered iron metabolism in lymphocytes from subjects with restless legs syndrome. Sleep 2008;31(6):847–52.

Neuroimaging in Restless Legs Syndrome

Federica Provini, MD, PhD[a,b],*, Giacomo Chiaro, MD[a]

KEYWORDS

- Restless legs syndrome • Willis-Ekbom disease • Neuroimaging • MRI • PET
- Single-photon emission computed tomography • Voxel-based morphometry
- Diffusion tensor imaging

KEY POINTS

- RLS pathophysiology excludes structural neurodegenerative processes, as shown by structural neuroimaging and autoptic studies.
- Both structural and functional neuroimaging studies showed that RLS is probably associated with changes in thalamus, sensorimotor cortical areas, and cerebellum.
- MRI and ultrasonography studies are consistent with a central iron deficiency in patients with RLS, mostly located in the SN.
- Functional studies point at a subcortical dopaminergic hypoactivity, which can be found in the striatum at both presynaptic and postsynaptic levels in patients with RLS.

INTRODUCTION

The pathophysiology of restless legs syndrome (RLS) still represents a puzzle of multiple interacting mechanisms involving cortical and subcortical brain structures, the spinal cord, the peripheral nervous system, and multiple biochemical pathways and neurotransmitters.

Over the last few years, various neuroimaging techniques have been used to study putative alterations in patients with RLS. Structural brain abnormalities in RLS have been studied by means of MRI in the form of voxel-based morphometry (VBM), diffusion tensor imaging (DTI), relaxometry, and transcranial ultrasonography (TCS) (**Table 1**). The neural mechanisms underlying RLS dysfunctions in central pathways have been investigated by means of functional MRI (fMRI), proton magnetic resonance spectroscopy (H-MRS), PET, and single-photon emission computed tomography (SPECT) imaging studies (**Table 2**).

Specifically, research attention focused on iron metabolism and the dopaminergic system. More recently, several radiographic studies have broadened the acknowledged pathophysiologic boundaries to other systems, including the serotoninergic, glutamatergic, and opiatergic circuitry. The few published works available have yielded different and sometimes inconsistent results, thus leaving open opportunities for further observations. This overview provides a critical literature review of all neuroimaging studies conducted on RLS, highlighting the most relevant findings.

BRAIN MRI

MRI studies showed no structural brain lesions in patients with RLS. Regarding iron concentration, although a universal agreement has not been reached yet, most studies are consistent with the view that a central iron deficiency plays a role in

Funding Sources: None.
Conflict of Interests: None.
[a] Department of Biomedical and Neuromotor Sciences, Bellaria Hospital, University of Bologna, Via Altura 3, Bologna 40139, Italy; [b] IRCCS Institute of Neurological Sciences of Bologna, Bologna, Italy
* Corresponding author. Department of Biomedical and NeuroMotor Sciences, Bellaria Hospital, University of Bologna, Via Altura 3, Bologna 40139, Italy.
E-mail address: federica.provini@unibo.it

1556-407X/15/$ – see front matter © 2015 Elsevier Inc. All rights reserved.

sleep.theclinics.com

Table 1
Structural neuroimaging of RLS

Results	Imaging Technique	No. Patients/Control Individuals	International RLS Study Group Rating Scale (Mean Score; Severity)	Medication	Author
GM and WM Volume Changes					
GM increase in dorsal thalamus	MRI/VBM	51/51	29; S	Y	Etgen et al,[13] 2005
GM increase in hippocampus and orbitofrontal gyrus	MRI/VBM	14/14	26; S	N	Hornyak et al,[14] 2007
GM decrease in primary sensorimotor cortex	MRI/VBM	63/40	27; S	Y	Unrath et al,[15] 2007
GM decrease in left hippocampus, parietal lobes, medial frontal areas, lateral temporal areas, and cerebellum	MRI/VBM	46/46	27; S	13/46	Chang et al[16]
GM anomalies in ACC	MRI/VBM	34/18	20; S	N	Pan et al,[21] 2014
WM changes near sensorimotor and thalamic areas	MRI/DTI	45/30	28; S	Y	Unrath et al,[22] 2008
WM decrease in corpus callosum, ACC, precentral gyrus Myelin decrease	MRI/VBM Autopsy Myelin WB	23/23	24; S	—	Connor et al,[11] 2011

Iron studies

Iron concentration decrease	MRI/R2	5/5	—	Y	Allen et al,[3] 2001
Iron concentration decrease in eRLS right striatum and GPi	MRI/R2	11/11	18; M	N	Margariti et al,[8] 2012
Iron concentration decrease in SN of eRLS	MRI/R2	41/39	—	N	Earley et al,[4] 2006
Iron concentration decrease in SN, thalamus, caudate	MRI/R2	6/19	—	N	Godau et al[6]
Iron concentration decrease in SN	TCS	20/20	—	Y	Schmidauer et al,[48] 2005
Iron concentration decrease in SN	TCS	49/49	—	Y	Godau et al,[49] 2007
Low iron index in SN	MRI/R2	37/40	25; S	12/37	Moon et al,[5] 2014
No difference	MRI/VBM; MRI/DTI	20/20	22; S	N	Rizzo et al,[19] 2012
No difference	MRI/VBM	11/11	18; M	N	Margariti et al,[8] 2012
No difference	MRI/VBM	17/54	16; M	N	Celle et al,[17] 2010
No difference	MRI/VBM	16/16	18; M	N	Comley et al,[18] 2012
No difference	MRI	12/12	—	8/12	Knake et al,[12] 2010

International RLS Study Group rating scale: very severe (VS), 31–40 points; severe (S), 21–30 points; moderate (M), 11–20 points; mild (Mi), 1–10 points; none (N), 0 points.

Abbreviations: ACC, anterior cingulate cortex; eRLS, early-onset RLS; GM, gray matter; GPi, globus pallidus internal; R2, relaxometry; SN, substantia nigra; WB, Western blot; WM, white matter.

Table 2
Functional neuroimaging in restless legs syndrome

Results	Imaging Technique	No. Patients/Control Individuals	International RLS Study Group Rating Scale (Mean Score; Severity)	Medication	Author
Cortical and Subcortical Activation Patterns					
Cerebellum and thalamus activation	fMRI	19/15	—	N	Bucher et al,[24] 1997
Sensorimotor cortex activation	fMRI	7	25; M	N	Spiegelhalder et al,[25] 2008
Abnormal thalamocortical connectivity	fMRI	25/25	13; Mi	N	Ku et al,[26] 2014
Diffuse cortical and subcortical activation	fMRI	36/23	—	N	Margariti et al,[8] 2012 Astrakas et al,[7] 2008
Neural Metabolite Abnormalities					
Reduced NAA/Cr ratio in medial thalamus	H-MRS	23/19	22; M	N	Rizzo et al,[20] 2012
Increased Glx/Cr ratio in thalamus	H-MRS	28/20	—	N	Allen et al,[28] 2013
Increased NAA in ACC	H-MRS	18	23; M	N	Winkelman et al,[29] 2014
Dopaminergic Function					
Increased D$_2$R BP in striatum and extrastriatal regions	PET	16/16	18; Mi	N	Cervenka et al,[36] 2006
Increased DAT density in striatum, caudate, putamen	SPECT	13/12	17; Mi	N	Kim et al,[44] 2012
Reduced [18F]dopa uptake and D$_2$R BP in putamen and caudate	PET	13/14	—	5/13	Turjanski et al,[33] 1999
Reduced [18F]dopa uptake in caudate and putamen and reduced D$_2$R BP in striatum	PET	9/23	—	N	Ruottinen et al,[34] 2000

Finding	Modality				Study
Reduced DAT BP in striatum	PET	31/36	—	21/31	Earley et al,[35] 2011
Reduced D2R BP in putamen and caudate but not in striatum; D2R density and affinity increase in striatum at night	PET	31/36	—	17/31	Earley et al,[39] 2013
Reduced D2R BP in striatum	SPECT	10/10	—	N	Michaud et al,[46] 2002
No difference in DAT and D2R BP	SPECT	25/20	—	11/25	Eisensehr et al,[41] 2001
No difference in DAT and D2R BP	SPECT	14/9	23; M	N	Tribl et al,[42] 2002
No difference in DAT and D2R BP	SPECT	14/10	23; M	Y	Tribl et al,[43] 2004
Normal dopaminergic function	SPECT	10/10	—	Y	Mrowka et al,[45] 2005
Opiatergic Function					
Negative correlations between opioid receptor BP and RLS severity	PET	15/12	25; M	8/15	Von Spiczak et al,[40] 2005
Serotoninergic Function					
Negative correlation between SERT availability and RLS symptoms	SPECT	16/16	17; Mi	No	Jhoo et al,[47] 2010

International RLS Study Group rating scale: very severe (VS), 31–40 points; severe (S), 21–30 points; moderate (M), 11–20 points; mild (Mi), 1–10 points; none (N), 0 points.

Abbreviations: ACC, anterior cingulate cortex; BP, binding potential; D2R, dopamine 2 receptor; DAT, dopamine transporter; Glx/Cr, glutamate/creatine ratio; NAA/Cr, N-acetylaspartate/creatine-phosphocreatine ratio; SERT, serotonin transporter.

patients with RLS, especially in the most severe forms.

The first use of standard T1-weighted and T2-weighted brain MRI showed that there are no structural lesions in RLS.[1] These data have been further confirmed by means of tyrosine hydroxylase (TH) staining, regional assessment of gliosis, or general histologic examination in autoptic specimens, which also excluded any neurodegenerative processes involving hypothalamic A11 cell bodies.[2]

A decrease in regional brain iron concentration in the substantia nigra (SN) and the putamen was first found in 5 patients with RLS compared with control individuals. Decrements were proportionate to RLS severity.[3] These findings have been later confirmed in a larger group of patients, documenting a more specific iron concentration decrease in early-onset compared with late-onset RLS.[4] Recently, Moon and colleagues detected a significantly lower SN mean iron index in the late-onset RLS compared with control individuals.[5] In addition, Godau and colleagues[6] showed a decreased iron concentration also in the thalamus and caudate nucleus. Reduction in brain iron content in the SN of patients with RLS was also confirmed by means of fMRI (**Fig. 1**).[7,8]

RLS brain autopsy is in agreement with both structural and functional results. Markedly reduced iron, H-ferritin staining, and transferrin receptor staining in the SN were found in 7 cerebral specimens from individuals with RLS. RLS tissue also showed significant increases in TH in the SN.[9,10] A decrease in D_2 dopamine receptor concentration in the putamen, a reduced expression of myelin proteins, and significant small decreases in white matter (WM) volume (corpus callosum, anterior cingulum, and precentral gyrus) were also found. The investigators stated that the evidence of less myelin and loss of myelin integrity in RLS brains, coupled with decreased ferritin and transferrin in the myelin fractions, should be regarded as a compelling argument for brain iron insufficiency in RLS.[11]

Only 1 study found no significant differences in T2 signal intensity values in 12 regions of interest (SN, pallidum, caudate head, thalamus, occipital WM, and frontal WM bilaterally) and in 2 reference regions (cerebrospinal fluid and bone).[12]

Voxel-Based Morphometry MRI

VBM MRI was used to evaluate volumetric differences in gray matter (GM) regions of patients with RLS. The few studies conducted with this technique yielded different results, ranging from an increase in GM density in thalamic regions to a decrease in GM density in various cortical regions to no difference in GM density between patients with RLS and control individuals.

Increases in GM density were found in the pulvinar bilaterally,[13] in both hippocampi, and in the orbitofrontal gyrus bilaterally.[14] The investigators suggested that the involvement of thalamic structures might either be part of the pathogenesis of RLS or reflect a consequence of chronic increase in afferent input of behaviorally relevant information. Hippocampal alterations might occur because of an increase in sensory input (as a result of the urge to move and the related unpleasant sensation). Involvement of the orbitofrontal gyrus should be considered for its role in modulating or inhibiting neural responses to aversive stimuli.

On the contrary, Unrath and colleagues[15] observed voxel clusters of significantly decreased GM density in the primary somatosensory cortex bihemispherically, also affecting primary motor areas (precentral gyrus). Similarly, 2 studies by Chang and colleagues[16] showed significant regional decreases of GM volume in the left hippocampal gyrus, both parietal lobes, medial frontal areas, lateral temporal areas, and left cerebellum. Analyses adjusted for age and gender detected significant negative correlations between symptom severity and the culmen of the cerebellum, as well as negative correlations between disease duration and some brain areas. The investigators argued that structural changes of the

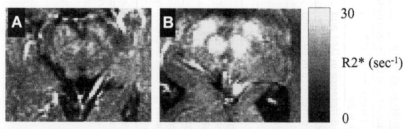

30

R2* (sec^{-1})

0

Fig. 1. R2* images in (*A*) a 70-year-old patient with RLS and (*B*) a 71-year-old control individual. Lower R2* relaxation rates are apparent in the RLS case in both red nucleus and SN. (*From* Allen RP, Barker PB, Wehrl F, et al. MRI measurement of brain iron in patients with restless legs syndrome. Neurology 2001;56:264; with permission.)

somatomotor cortices might be secondary to the involvement of A11 neurons and their long projection fibers.

No difference in GM density between RLS and control individuals was found in 5 of 9 studies conducted on smaller-sized groups.[8,17–20] Only a single study investigated both depressed and nondepressed drug-naive patients with RLS, showing no difference in GM density between patients with RLS and control individuals. Only depressed patients with RLS showed significantly decreased GM density in the bilateral anterior cingulate cortex (ACC).[21]

Diffusion Tensor Imaging MRI

Of 3 DTI MRI studies, 2 showed a reduction in fractional anisotropy (FA) in regions related functionally and anatomically to motor and somatosensory cortical areas. One study found no difference in DTI parameters.

No differences in FA, mean diffusivity, axial diffusivity, and radial diffusivity were found in any brain region. No correlations between tissue volume or DTI parameters and clinical parameters were found.[19]

Multiple clusters of regional FA decreases were observed in frontal and parietal WM of both hemispheres, most of them with functional and anatomic connections to motor/premotor and somatosensory cortical areas. In detail, 3 functional complexes could be delineated. The first complex consisted of subcortical areas adjacent to the bilateral precentral gyrus, the superior frontal gyrus, the thalamus, and the fiber projection network. The second complex was part of the somatosensory functional network and consisted of areas adjacent to the postcentral gyrus bilaterally. The third was observed as adjacent to the left hemispheric ACC as a part of the limbic functional system. Whether such alterations are primary is still unknown.[22] These findings have been further confirmed in the genu of the corpus callosum and frontal WM adjacent to the inferior frontal gyrus in patients with RLS compared with control individuals,[23] suggesting that loss of axonal density and myelin may account for WM changes seen in previous studies.

Functional MRI

fMRI studies suggest an involvement of thalamocortical sensorimotor pathways as well as of additional structures (including cerebellum) in the pathophysiology of RLS.

Patients with RLS were scanned during periods of sensory leg discomfort. During these symptomatic periods, fMRI showed a bilateral activation of the cerebellum and a contralateral activation of the thalamus. Associated involuntary periodic limb movements (PLMs) induced activation in subcortical areas (red nuclei and brainstem), whereas mimicked PLMs produced no subcortical activation but rather an involvement of the motor cortex and the globus pallidus, suggesting a subcortical origin for PLMs.[24]

Recently, a study used fMRI with simultaneous electromyography (EMG) to assess brain responses associated with tonic EMG. Tonic EMG was found inversely correlated with subjective sensory leg discomfort, thereby providing an objective reflection of RLS symptoms. Tonic EMG was also positively correlated with fMRI activation in sensorimotor cortical areas (ACC, precuneus, occipital cortex) and negatively correlated with the cerebellum.[25] A further involvement of thalamocortical sensorimotor pathways has also been confirmed in a study by Ku and colleagues.[26]

Considering the different circadian pattern of RLS, fMRI studies performed at night detected increased activation in the midbrain, pons, dorsolateral prefrontal cortex, ACC, left precentral gyrus, posterior central gyrus, pars opercularis, ventral anterior cingulum, right caudate body, inferior and superior parietal lobules, and putamen.[7,8] The investigators inferred that the increased activation of the prefrontal and ACC might be related to the hyperfunctioning of the system involved in the initiation and control of self-generated behaviors. They further interpreted these findings either as a primary disorder of the prefrontal and ACC resulting in amplified autoactivation behavior expressed as RLS symptoms or as a disorder secondary to low iron content or dysfunction of the dorsoposterior hypothalamic dopaminergic A11 cell group.[27]

Proton Magnetic Resonance Spectroscopy

H-MRS studies detected abnormalities of mainly 3 metabolites, namely aspartate, glutamate, and γ-aminobutyric acid (GABA), in the thalamus of patients with RLS.

A thalamic neuronal dysfunction in patients with RLS (presumably not caused by a degenerative process, because no structural changes were detected in thalamic areas) was confirmed by H-MRS studies. A significantly reduced N-acetylaspartate (NAA)/creatine-phosphocreatine (Cr) ratio and NAA concentration at the level of the medial thalamus was found in patients with RLS compared with control individuals. Lower NAA concentrations were also associated with a positive family history of RLS (**Fig. 2**).[20]

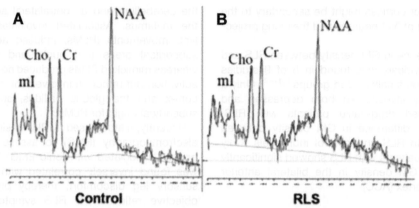

Fig. 2. Typical medial thalamic ^{1}H-MR spectra obtained from a control individual (*A*) and a patient with RLS (*B*). Note the lower NAA peak in the patient with RLS compared with the control individual. Cho, choline-containing compounds; Cr, creatine-phosphocreatine; ml, myoinositol. (*From* Rizzo G, Tonon C, Testa C, et al. Abnormal medial thalamic metabolism in patients with idiopathic restless legs syndrome. Brain 2012;135:3716; with permission.)

Glutamatergic hyperactivity has been proposed as a putative cause of disrupted and shortened sleep in RLS, because dopaminergic treatments fail to reduce arousals during sleep. A combined MRS and polysomnographic study showed that the thalamic glutamate (Glx)/Cr ratio (a combination of mostly glutamate and glutamine assessed as a ratio to the total Cr level) was higher for patients with RLS than control individuals. This ratio correlated significantly with the wake time during the sleep period and all other RLS-related polysomnographic sleep variables except for PLMs index. These data provide a consistent pattern indicating a significant increase in thalamic glutamatergic activity, which could produce hyperarousal in patients with RLS.[28]

Additional data suggested that known cerebellar–thalamic interactions may modulate the intensity of RLS sensory and motor symptoms.[29] It has been hypothesized that GABA levels would be lower in RLS in the thalamus and ACC because these areas participate in ascending central nervous system (CNS) pain modulatory systems, as well as in the cerebellum, a functionally active structure during RLS-related leg dysesthesias and movements.[8,30,31]

POSITRON EMISSION TOMOGRAPHY

PET studies have been used in association with various radioligands to assess neurotransmission abnormalities in the dopaminergic and opiate systems. The hypothesis of a central nigrostriatal presynaptic and postsynaptic dopaminergic hypofunction has been confirmed by means of [^{18}]

fluorodopa and [^{11}C]methylphenidate, whereas studies with [^{11}C]raclopride showed either a decreased or an increased D$_2$ receptor (D$_2$R) binding potential (BP). Regarding opiate systems, only 1 study conducted with [^{11}C]diprenorphine showed no opioid receptor binding difference between patients with RLS and control individuals.

Except for an early small study,[32] most findings supported the hypothesis of a central dopaminergic dysfunction in patients with RLS. Turjanski and colleagues[33] found a mildly reduced mean caudate and a significantly reduced putamen [^{18}F]dopa uptake as well as a significantly reduced mean D$_2$R binding in both the putamen and caudate, with no differences between L-dopa-naive and L-dopa-treated patients with RLS. A nigrostriatal presynaptic dopaminergic hypofunction has been confirmed in a group of patients suffering from both PLM disorder and RLS. The investigators found a marked (>80%) reduction of mean [^{18}F]dopa uptake in the caudate and putamen and a lower mean striatal D$_2$R BP compared with control individuals.[34] Similarly, presynaptic dopaminergic hypofunction has been assessed in the putamen and caudate of patients with RLS during both night and day scans by means of [^{11}C]methylphenidate binding to DAT.[35]

Hypoactivity in dopaminergic neurotransmission has also been determined by means of [^{11}C] raclopride. BP values in the striatum were significantly higher in patients with RLS than control individuals, and measurements in extrastriatal regions (thalamus subregions and the ACC) by means of [^{11}C]FLB 457 yielded similar results as a result of receptor upregulation, probably in response to hypoactivity in dopaminergic neurotransmission. The specific anatomic location of extrastriatal findings may reflect a disturbance of the central processing of sensory input in RLS.[36,37] These data, collected from drug-naive patients, are in contrast with previous findings in patients with RLS chronically exposed to dopaminergic treatments.[33] Chronic D_2R stimulation caused by dopaminergic treatment has been shown to induce receptor downregulation, resulting in lower radioligand binding.[38]

A more dynamic assessment of D_2R function by means of [^{11}C]raclopride was conducted considering all of the 3 interacting factors that constitute D_2R BP (the density of receptors on the membrane [β_{max}], the receptor affinity [K_d], and the amount of extracellular dopamine) in relation to the circadianity of RLS symptoms. On the one hand, patients with RLS showed equally lower D_2R BP in the putamen and caudate, but not in the ventral striatum, during both night and day measurements. On the other hand, receptor density and affinity increased only in the ventral striatum during nighttime (**Fig. 3**).[39]

Recent clinical evidence suggested a possible role of opioids in the pathophysiology of RLS with respect to sensory and motor symptoms. Opioid receptor binding by means of [^{11}C]diprenorphine detected no mean group differences between patients and control individuals. However, regional negative correlations between ligand binding and RLS severity in areas serving the medial pain system were found, suggesting that the more severe the RLS, the greater the release of endogenous opioids might be.[40]

SINGLE-PHOTON EMISSION COMPUTED TOMOGRAPHY

Generally, all SPECT studies investigating dopaminergic function detected no difference between patients with RLS and control individuals. Despite slight differences in the techniques used and the selected regions of interest, SPECT studies showed consistent results toward a normal striatal dopaminergic function. This finding is strikingly in contrast with PET studies, which have sometimes produced different, if not opposite, results. The opiatergic and serotoninergic function has also been assessed.

Presynaptic striatal DAT binding and density and postsynaptic D_2R binding examined with [^{123}I]-(N)-(3-iodopropen-2-yl)-2 β-carbomethoxy-3β-(4-chlorophenyl)-tropane SPECT, and striatal dopamine D_2R density with [^{123}I]-(S)-2-hydroxy-3-iodo-6-methoxy-[(1-ethyl-2-pyrrolidinyl)methyl] benzamide ([^{123}I]IBZM) were similar between drug-naive, levodopa-treated patients with RLS and control individuals.[41–43] In 1 recent study, DAT density was higher in the caudate, posterior putamen, and the entire striatum of RLS compared with control individuals, but D_2R receptor density was not. The investigators attempted to explain this increased DAT density as a compensatory upregulation secondary to an increase in dopamine release from presynaptic neurons or as a consequence of the

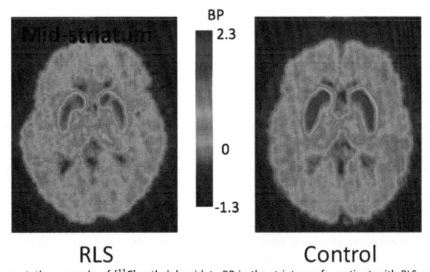

Fig. 3. Representative example of [^{11}C]methylphenidate BP in the striatum of a patient with RLS and a control individual. (*From* Earley CJ, Kuwabara H, Wong DF, et al. The dopamine transporter is decreased in the striatum of subjects with restless legs syndrome. Sleep 2011;34:344; with permission.)

accelerated clearance of dopamine from the synaptic cleft.[44]

Another study with [^{123}I]2-β-carbomethoxy-3-β-4-iodophenyl-tropane did not show significant reductions in caudate-to-cortex or putamen-to-cortex ratios between groups, but putamen ratios were significantly lower than caudate ratios only in patients with RLS. The investigators argued the usefulness of the method, which could not detect any definite signs of modified central dopaminergic function in patients with RLS.[45]

Slightly different results came from a study in which the median striatal [^{123}I]IBZM binding was significantly reduced in patients compared with control individuals. Nine of 10 patients showed a mean striatal D_2R binding lower than the control group mean. This last study was the only one to be carried out during nighttime and to show dopamine dysfunction through a decrease in [^{123}I]IBZM binding.[46]

Overall, a discrepancy between PET and SPECT findings is evident. Some investigators argue that SPECT results should be cautiously taken into account, because, as a result of long technical times, the ligand might have already been internalized by the time BP is determined. If this is the case, then, findings represent essentially a gross determination of the total D_2R pool and do not reflect the short-term state of membrane-bound D_2R. PET techniques, on the other hand, identify membrane-bound D_2R in real time.[35] Therefore, further imaging studies performed at other times of the day and perhaps focusing on other CNS regions, would be highly warranted.

According to the hypothesis of an increased serotoninergic transmission as exacerbating or causing RLS, only 1 study[47] investigated the role of serotonin in the pathogenesis of RLS. The severity of symptoms was negatively correlated with serotonin transporter availability.

TRANSCRANIAL ULTRASONOGRAPHY

All 4 TS studies of patients with RLS reported hypoechogenicity in the SN of patients compared with control individuals.

Patients with RLS showed a significant hypoechogenicity of the SN region compared with control individuals, and an even more markedly reduced echogenicity compared with patients with Parkinson disease.[48] Such hypoechogenicity is even more common in idiopathic rather than secondary RLS and it correlates significantly with severity of RLS symptoms.[49,50] Other brainstem abnormalities, such as red nucleus hyperechogenicity and brainstem raphe hypoechogenicity

were more prevalent in patients with RLS than in control individuals.[51]

SUMMARY

Despite the unassailable importance of neuroimaging studies in defining the pathophysiology of RLS, differences in results could be caused by multiple factors, either in study design (eg, small sample sizes, demographic differences between groups, insufficient washout periods in patients under treatment) or in focusing only on a few aspects of a real complex disease such as RLS (eg, overlooking the circadian nature of RLS or researching only the nigrostriatal dopaminergic system). Nevertheless, it can be generally inferred that neuroimaging findings suggest that RLS is a disease involving 3 main brain areas: the thalamus, the sensorimotor cortex, and the cerebellum. MRI confirmed a central iron deficiency as a cornerstone in RLS pathophysiology, and functional studies detected a main dopaminergic dysfunction in both striatal and extrastriatal regions. Further studies are needed to both confirm these findings and build new knowledge about unexplored aspects of RLS.

REFERENCES

1. Bucher SF, Trenkwalder C, Oertel WH. Reflex studies and MRI in the restless legs syndrome. Acta Neurol Scand 1996;94:145–50.
2. Earley CJ, Allen RP, Connor JR, et al. The dopaminergic neurons of the A11 system in RLS autopsy brains appear normal. Sleep Med 2009;10:1155–7.
3. Allen RP, Barker PB, Wehrl F, et al. MRI measurement of brain iron in patients with restless legs syndrome. Neurology 2001;56:263–5.
4. Earley CJ, B Barker P, Horska A, et al. MRI-determined regional brain iron concentrations in early- and late-onset restless legs syndrome. Sleep Med 2006;7:458–61.
5. Moon HJ, Chang Y, Lee YS, et al. T2 relaxometry using 3.0-tesla magnetic resonance imaging of the brain in early- and late-onset restless legs syndrome. J Clin Neurol 2014;10:197–202.
6. Godau J, Klose U, Di Santo A, et al. Multiregional brain iron deficiency in restless legs syndrome. Mov Disord 2008;23:1184–7.
7. Astrakas LG, Konitsiotis S, Margariti P, et al. T2 relaxometry and fMRI of the brain in late-onset restless legs syndrome. Neurology 2008;71:911–6.
8. Margariti PN, Astrakas LG, Tsouli SG, et al. Investigation of unmedicated early onset restless legs syndrome by voxel-based morphometry, T2 relaxometry, and functional MR imaging during the night-time hours. AJNR Am J Neuroradiol 2012;33:667–72.

9. Connor JR, Wang XS, Allen RP, et al. Altered dopaminergic profile in the putamen and substantia nigra in restless leg syndrome. Brain 2009;132:2403–12.

10. Connor JR, Boyer PJ, Menzies SL, et al. Neuropathological examination suggests impaired brain iron acquisition in restless legs syndrome. Neurology 2003;61:304–9.

11. Connor JR, Ponnuru P, Lee BY, et al. Postmortem and imaging based analyses reveal CNS decreased myelination in restless legs syndrome. Sleep Med 2011;12:614–9.

12. Knake S, Heverhagen JT, Menzler K, et al. Normal regional brain iron concentration in restless legs syndrome measured by MRI. Nat Sci Sleep 2010; 2:19–22.

13. Etgen T, Draganski B, Ilg C, et al. Bilateral thalamic gray matter changes in patients with restless legs syndrome. Neuroimage 2005;24:1242–7.

14. Hornyak M, Ahrendts JC, Spiegelhalder K, et al. Voxel-based morphometry in unmedicated patients with restless legs syndrome. Sleep Med 2007;9: 22–6.

15. Unrath A, Juengling FD, Schork M, et al. Cortical grey matter alterations in idiopathic restless legs syndrome: an optimized voxel-based morphometry study. Mov Disord 2007;22:1751–6.

16. Chang Y, Chang HW, Song H, et al. Gray matter alteration in patients with restless legs syndrome: a voxel-based morphometry study. Clin Imaging 2015;39:20–5.

17. Celle S, Roche F, Peyron R, et al. Lack of specific gray matter alterations in restless legs syndrome in elderly subjects. J Neurol 2010;257:344–8.

18. Comley RA, Cervenka S, Palhagen SE, et al. A comparison of gray matter density in restless legs syndrome patients and matched controls using voxel-based morphometry. J Neuroimaging 2012; 22:28–32.

19. Rizzo G, Manners D, Vetrugno R, et al. Combined brain voxel-based morphometry and diffusion tensor imaging study in idiopathic restless legs syndrome patients. Eur J Neurol 2012;19:1045–9.

20. Rizzo G, Tonon C, Testa C, et al. Abnormal medial thalamic metabolism in patients with idiopathic restless legs syndrome. Brain 2012;135(Pt 12):3712–20.

21. Pan PL, Dai ZY, Shang HF, et al. Gray matter anomalies in anterior cingulate cortex as a correlate of depressive symptoms in drug-naive idiopathic restless legs syndrome. Neuroscience 2014;277:1–5.

22. Unrath A, Muller HP, Ludolph AC, et al. Cerebral white matter alterations in idiopathic restless legs syndrome, as measured by diffusion tensor imaging. Mov Disord 2008;23:1250–5.

23. Chang Y, Paik JS, Lee HJ, et al. Altered white matter integrity in primary restless legs syndrome patients: diffusion tensor imaging study. Neurol Res 2014;36: 769–74.

24. Bucher SF, Seelos KC, Oertel WH, et al. Cerebral generators involved in the pathogenesis of the restless legs syndrome. Ann Neurol 1997;41:639–45.

25. Spiegelhalder K, Feige B, Paul D, et al. Cerebral correlates of muscle tone fluctuations in restless legs syndrome: a pilot study with combined functional magnetic resonance imaging and anterior tibial muscle electromyography. Sleep Med 2008;9:177–83.

26. Ku J, Cho YW, Lee YS, et al. Functional connectivity alternation of the thalamus in restless legs syndrome patients during the asymptomatic period: a resting-state connectivity study using functional magnetic resonance imaging. Sleep Med 2014;15:289–94.

27. Clemens S, Rye D, Hochman S. Restless legs syndrome: revisiting the dopamine hypothesis from the spinal cord perspective. Neurology 2006;67: 125–30.

28. Allen RP, Barker PB, Horska A, et al. Thalamic glutamate/glutamine in restless legs syndrome: increased and related to disturbed sleep. Neurology 2013;80:2028–34.

29. Winkelman JW, Schoerning L, Platt S, et al. Restless legs syndrome and central nervous system gamma-aminobutyric acid: preliminary associations with periodic limb movements in sleep and restless leg syndrome symptom severity. Sleep Med 2014;15: 1225–30.

30. Bucher SF, Seelos KC, Dodel RC, et al. Activation mapping in essential tremor with functional magnetic resonance imaging. Ann Neurol 1997;41: 32–40.

31. Shackman AJ, Salomons TV, Slagter HA, et al. The integration of negative affect, pain and cognitive control in the cingulate cortex. Nat Rev Neurosci 2011;12:154–67.

32. Trenkwalder C, Walters AS, Hening WA, et al. Positron emission tomographic studies in restless legs syndrome. Mov Disord 1999;14:141–5.

33. Turjanski N, Lees AJ, Brooks DJ. Striatal dopaminergic function in restless legs syndrome: 18F-dopa and 11C-raclopride PET studies. Neurology 1999;52:932–7.

34. Ruottinen HM, Partinen M, Hublin C, et al. An FDOPA PET study in patients with periodic limb movement disorder and restless legs syndrome. Neurology 2000;54:502–4.

35. Earley CJ, Kuwabara H, Wong DF, et al. The dopamine transporter is decreased in the striatum of subjects with restless legs syndrome. Sleep 2011;34: 341–7.

36. Cervenka S, Palhagen SE, Comley RA, et al. Support for dopaminergic hypoactivity in restless legs syndrome: a PET study on D2-receptor binding. Brain 2006;129:2017–28.

37. Price DD. Psychological and neural mechanisms of the affective dimension of pain. Science 2000;288: 1769–72.

38. Stanwood GD, Lucki I, McGonigle P. Differential regulation of dopamine D2 and D3 receptors by chronic drug treatments. J Pharmacol Exp Ther 2000;295:1232–40.

39. Earley CJ, Kuwabara H, Wong DF, et al. Increased synaptic dopamine in the putamen in restless legs syndrome. Sleep 2013;36:51–7.

40. von Spiczak S, Whone AL, Hammers A, et al. The role of opioids in restless legs syndrome: an [11C]diprenorphine PET study. Brain 2005;128:906–17.

41. Eisensehr I, Wetter TC, Linke R, et al. Normal IPT and IBZM SPECT in drug-naive and levodopa-treated idiopathic restless legs syndrome. Neurology 2001; 57:1307–9.

42. Tribl GG, Asenbaum S, Klosch G, et al. Normal IPT and IBZM SPECT in drug naive and levodopa-treated idiopathic restless legs syndrome. Neurology 2002;59:649–50.

43. Tribl GG, Asenbaum S, Happe S, et al. Normal striatal D2 receptor binding in idiopathic restless legs syndrome with periodic leg movements in sleep. Nucl Med Commun 2004;25:55–60.

44. Kim KW, Jhoo JH, Lee SB, et al. Increased striatal dopamine transporter density in moderately severe old restless legs syndrome patients. Eur J Neurol 2012;19:1213–8.

45. Mrowka M, Jobges M, Berding G, et al. Computerized movement analysis and beta-CIT-SPECT in patients with restless legs syndrome. J Neural Transm 2005;112:693–701.

46. Michaud M, Soucy JP, Chabli A, et al. SPECT imaging of striatal pre- and postsynaptic dopaminergic status in restless legs syndrome with periodic leg movements in sleep. J Neurol 2002;249:164–70.

47. Jhoo JH, Yoon IY, Kim YK, et al. Availability of brain serotonin transporters in patients with restless legs syndrome. Neurology 2010;74:513–8.

48. Schmidauer C, Sojer M, Seppi K, et al. Transcranial ultrasound shows nigral hypoechogenicity in restless legs syndrome. Ann Neurol 2005;58:630–4.

49. Godau J, Schweitzer KJ, Liepelt I, et al. Substantia nigra hypoechogenicity: definition and findings in restless legs syndrome. Mov Disord 2007;22: 187–92.

50. Pedroso JL, Bor-Seng-Shu E, Felicio AC, et al. Severity of restless legs syndrome is inversely correlated with echogenicity of the substantia nigra in different neurodegenerative movement disorders. a preliminary observation. J Neurol Sci 2012;319:59–62.

51. Godau J, Wevers AK, Gaenslen A, et al. Sonographic abnormalities of brainstem structures in restless legs syndrome. Sleep Med 2008;9:782–9.

The Molecular Genetics of Restless Legs Syndrome

David B. Rye, MD, PhD

KEYWORDS

- Restless legs • Periodic leg movements • Genetics • Molecular • Iron • Sleep

KEY POINTS

- Multiple genetic risk factors associating with restless legs syndrome (RLS) together account for a large proportion (≥80%) of the population risk for symptoms and signs of the disorder.
- In part because each disease allele's influence on increased risk for expressing RLS varies from roughly 20% to 70%, and the allele frequencies also vary greatly, a role for genetic testing has not been defined.
- *Drosophila*, murine, and zebra fish model systems implicate BTBD9 and MEIS1 as genes that cause RLS.
- BTBD9 and MEIS1 mediate iron and dopamine availability both directly and indirectly.
- Other gene candidates implicated in RLS require further study in animal and experimental model systems.
- Tissue-specific and brain region–specific gene expression profiling will hasten mechanistic understanding of RLS.

GENETIC EPIDEMIOLOGY, CANDIDATE GENE APPROACHES, AND LINKAGE STUDIES

Familial aggregation of restless legs syndrome (RLS) is well documented,[1–4] including Ekbom's[5] seminal description of the disorder in which he posited an autosomal dominant mode of inheritance.[5] Twin studies estimate the heritability of RLS (ie, the proportion of phenotypic variation that is attributable to genetic variation) at 54%[6] to 83%,[7] whereas in multiplex North American families it has been estimated at 60%.[8] Two independent segregation analyses propose dominant inheritance influenced by a highly penetrant (90%–100%) single gene in families with symptom onset at a young age, whereas a polygenic model best fits the onset of RLS in later life. RLS can also show anticipation (ie, earlier age of symptom onset in successive generations).[9,10] However, inheritance patterns and degrees of penetrance of RLS need to be interpreted with caution given the limitations in accurate assignment of affectation status. False-negatives, which are considerable confounders in genetic epidemiologic studies, can arise from symptom variability that can delay and even prevent presentation. Moreover, periodic leg movements of sleep (PLMs) in the absence of the defining compulsory sensory urges of RLS are a recognized endophenotype of RLS.[2] For example, PLMs occur as an asymptomatic condition in individuals who later develop classic RLS symptoms,[3] PLMs absent sensory complaints are more commonly encountered in families with RLS,[11] and alleles conferring risk for RLS revealed by genome-wide association studies (GWAS) also confer risk for PLMs[12,13] (discussed later). False-positive diagnoses are also problematic given the substantial number of conditions that can

Disclosure: In the past 3 years Dr D.B. Rye has consulted for or served on advisory committees for UCB Pharma Inc, Jazz Pharmaceuticals, and Xenoport, Inc.
Program in Sleep, Department of Neurology, Emory University School of Medicine, 12 Executive Park Drive Northeast, Atlanta, GA 30329, USA
E-mail address: drye@emory.edu

mimic RLS (eg, akathisia, paresthesias, and nocturnal leg cramps).

Pharmacologic agents acting at D_2 and D_3 dopamine receptors effectively treat both the sensory symptoms and PLMs, although there is no clear consensus as to whether a hypodopaminergic or hyperdopaminergic state is at the core of RLS/PLMs and which brain circuits are responsible.[3] This uncertainty has prompted testing for genetic variants in genes involved in dopamine's metabolism. Comparisons of single nucleotide polymorphisms (SNPs) within 8 genes (tyrosine hydroxylase [the rate-limiting enzyme for dopamine's synthesis], dopamine receptors 1–5, the dopamine transporter [the principal determinant of synaptic dopamine concentrations], and dopamine β-hydroxylase [the enzyme responsible for conversion of dopamine to noradrenaline]) in patients with RLS and controls reported no differences.[4] A polymorphism within the monoamine oxidase A gene promoter region that favors heightened enzymatic activity, and, in turn, more rapid elimination of synaptic dopamine, associates with RLS in women but not men.[14] The overall effect of this polymorphism is small, but it is one piece of evidence arguing that symptoms might reflect insufficient dopamine signaling.

A large number of genetic linkage studies have also been conducted in families with RLS to attempt to identify gene variants that segregate faithfully with the phenotype of interest (eg, variants that are not present in asymptomatic family members).[15,16] These approaches can be particularly insightful in monogenic versus polygenic disorders that respect mendelian patterns of inheritance. In RLS, linkage analyses are problematic. They rely on assuming a mode of inheritance that is not known and thereby is potentially incorrect; family members with PLMs but asymptomatic for RLS might be incorrectly classified as unaffected, and RLS as revealed by GWAS seems polygenic in origin (discussed later). However, 5 linkage regions for RLS have been reported and formally classified as loci RLS1 to RLS5,[15,16] with 2 additional novel loci identified since 2008.[17,18] For the most part, these studies are limited to only a few families, have not identified a causative gene, and have not been widely replicated. Moreover, given the assumptions that must be made about inheritance pattern, penetrance, allele frequency, and phenocopy rates for the purpose of these analyses, their significance is unclear. However, the RLS1 linkage locus on chromosome 12 remains of interest because it has been identified in a large number of families from multiple populations by independent investigators, at least 1 of which used nonparametric analysis.

GENOME-WIDE ASSOCIATION STUDIES

Knowledge of how variants in the sequence of the human genome confer risk of RLS/PLMs has advanced greatly with the advent and application of GWAS. Independent studies in diverse Northern European and North American populations point to involvement of 6 different genes that are widely expressed in the central nervous system and other organs: BTBD9, MEIS1, PTPRD (protein tyrosine phosphatase receptor type delta), MAP2K5, SKOR1, and TOX3.[12,19–23] Together, the allelic variants implicating these 6 genes account for nearly 80% of the population attributable risk for RLS. The at-risk SNPs are common and are located within noncoding, intronic, or intergenic regions. Association of the SNP rs3923809 in BTBD9 increases the risk of RLS and PLMs (even in the absence of RLS sensory symptoms) by 70% to 100%. Nearly one-half of those individuals of northern European ancestry are homozygous for this risk allele, so, by itself, it seems to play a role in at least 50% of RLS cases. A minor allele in MEIS1 nearly doubles a person's risk and is in a suspected cis-regulatory element potentially associated with reductions in MEIS1 messenger RNA (mRNA) and protein expression.[24,25] RLS susceptibility variants associated with PTPRD, MAP2K5, SKOR1, and TOX3 confer more modest risks. Almost nothing is known about how factors generally acknowledged to influence RLS expressivity (eg, female sex, advanced age, and iron decrements)[3] interact with these at-risk variants. Copy number and structural variants (eg, insertions or deletions) that might disrupt the function of the implicated genes have not been reported. Similarly, informative cis (local) or trans (distant) regulatory effects on gene and protein expression and splice variants associated with the at-risk alleles have not been reported.[12,19,20,24] The coding regions and exon-intron boundaries of BTBD9[4,26] and MEIS1[24,26,27] also lack any common functional polymorphisms. Several rare exonic variants in MEIS1 have been reported, but they do not segregate faithfully with the RLS phenotype.[26,27] Nonetheless, BTBD9 and MEIS1 are plausible contributors to disease pathophysiology because (1) each BTBD9 at-risk allele associates with a 13% lower serum ferritin level in a population enriched for RLS[12]; (2) an MEIS1 at-risk haplotype associates with aberrant iron homeostasis[28]; (3) the dosages of the BTBD9[12] and MEIS1 (Stefansson, unpublished observations, 2011) risk alleles are predictive of

PLMs number; (4) RLS can be modeled in animals by genetic disruptions of BTBD9[29,30]; (5) manipulations of BTBD9 in animals and cell culture disrupt iron and dopamine homeostasis (discussed later)[29,30]; and (6) in vitro and in vivo approaches in mice and zebra fish suggest that common and rare, loss-of-function intronic variants in MEIS1 may be sufficient to yield an RLS-like phenotype.[25,31] Furthermore, the frequencies of the at-risk alleles in different ethnic groups mirror the unique prevalences of RLS reported in different countries and continents.[23] For example, data from the International HapMap Project (http://www.hapmap.org) indicate that ~70% of individuals of northern European descent are carriers of the BTBD9 at-risk allele versus only ~35% of Japanese people (in whom the reported RLS prevalences are approximately half of those for northern European populations).

How the identified genetic susceptibility alleles ultimately lead to RLS remains elusive because (1) although the risk alleles account for substantial population attributable risk for RLS, they together have been estimated to account for only 7% of its heritability[22]; (2) RLS-related risk alleles are in noncoding regions that are generally thought to subserve regulatory functions such as influencing when and where genes are turned on and off; (3) there is evidence for pleiotropic and epigenetic effects; and (4) phenocopies of RLS/PLMs exist. Single genes can affect multiple traits, such as those comprising the RLS phenotypic spectrum (eg, pleiotropy). For example, decrements in mobilizable stores of iron considered an intermediate trait necessary for RLS to express itself, for example, may be modified by pleiotropic actions of the same genes that independently influence RLS. Decrements in mobilizable stores of iron might alternatively uniquely effect individuals who harbor RLS susceptibility gene variants. Although low serum ferritin levels associate with the BTBD9 at-risk allele in a population enriched for RLS,[12] for example, they do not seem to in the larger, general population.[32] The idea of allele-dependent epigenetic effects for iron finds further support in evidence that iron-deficient conditions reduce MEIS1 expression in cultured human cells.[28] Temporal dissociation of RLS sensory symptoms from its motor signs (eg, in PLMs that can reflect an asymptomatic forme fruste of RLS and that are affected by some of the same genetic factors) is also problematic. Therefore, further knowledge of the genetic architecture of RLS will demand comprehensive phenotyping that includes asymptomatic individuals with PLMs. An additional confounder is the potential for tissue-specific regulation of genes implicated

in RLS, as has been suggested for MEIS1.[28] Increased comorbidity of RLS-like symptoms with other medical conditions represents either an opportunity to identify biological factors that influence trait expressivity by way of the at-risk alleles or problematic phenocopies. For example, RLS/PLMs are exceedingly common in end-stage renal disease,[3] and are associated with BTBD9 and MEIS1 variants in northern Europeans,[33] and PTPRD variants in Taiwanese people[34]; however, these associations are not discernible in patients with multiple sclerosis experiencing RLS-like symptoms.[35]

EXPERIMENTAL STUDIES

Echoing a theme emerging from GWAS of many common diseases, the variants conferring susceptibility to RLS/PLMs do not provide a parsimonious explanation for how and why symptoms emerge. The at-risk SNPs in each instance implicate genes that are widely expressed in the central nervous system and other organs.

BTBD9

Although much is known of the versatile BTB domain–containing protein family, very little is known about the function of BTBD9 itself. The protein harbors 3 highly conserved peptide domains (in order from amino to carboxy terminus): a BTB domain, a BACK (BTB and C-terminal Kelch) domain, and several Kelch repeats. The BTB domain is a phylogenetically conserved protein-protein interaction motif named for the 3 Drosophila lines in which it was originally identified: broad complex, tramtrack, and bric-a-brack. It participates in a wide range of cellular functions, including transcriptional regulation, cytoskeleton dynamics, ion channel assembly and gating, and targeting proteins for ubiquitination.[36,37] The BACK domain is highly conserved across metazoan genomes, and may facilitate substrate orientation during ubiquitin ligation.[38,39] Kelch repeats interact with actin and play a role in cytoskeletal/microfilament orientation.[40]

Animal models have proved powerful in unraveling the molecular mechanisms of BTBD9's causative role in RLS.[29,30] The function of BTBD9 was unknown when it was revealed to harbor an at-risk allele for RLS/PLMs. Therefore, as a means of broad observation, traditional loss-of-function methodologies were the initial approaches undertaken despite a lack of evidence that protein expression was decreased in patients with RLS. Mutations of the Drosophila ortholog of BTBD9 (CG1826), either throughout the organism or limited to dopamine-containing neurons,[29] and murine knockouts of BTBD9[30] show RLS-like motor restlessness and sleep fragmentation[29,30] that disappear with dopamine receptor agonist administration.[29] Overexpression of BTBD9 in human embryonic kidney cells reduces iron regulatory protein-2 levels, which likely accounts for concomitant increases in ferritin, which is a storage form for mobilizable iron.[29] In BTBD9 knockout mice serum iron concentrations are increased.[30] Decrements in whole-head dopamine in the Drosophila mutants seem unmatched in the murine model, and not because of reductions in tyrosine hydroxylase levels (ie, the rate limiting, iron-dependent enzyme for dopamine synthesis). It would be worthwhile to examine dopaminergic neurotransmission at the synaptic level in these models considering that in vitro explorations using rat pheochromocytoma (PC12) cells suggest that BTBD9 may play a role in synaptic vesicle transport.[41] One proposed mechanism of RLS pathophysiology postulates that a deficiency in brain iron favors heightened synaptic dopaminergic signaling, thus accounting for the clinical efficacy of dopamine agonists via inhibitory autoreceptors.[3] Reconciling the influence of BTBD9 on iron and dopamine homeostasis with the prevailing heuristic model of RLS that posits iron and dopamine to be intermediate traits necessary for symptom expression[30] demands a more comprehensive accounting of BTBD9's interactors and molecular pathways.

Work primarily in Drosophila is beginning to provide the details of how BTBD9 might negatively affect dopamine signaling and, in so doing, fragment and curtail sleep such as is observed in RLS. BTBD9 seems to be a substrate adaptor for the Cullin-3 class of E3 ubiquitin ligases,[29] which itself regulates sleep and circadian rhythms.[42–44] Following genetic mutations in a BTB domain adaptor for Cullin-3 called insomniac (inc), flies showed fragmented sleep, markedly truncated sleep times, but normal circadian rhythms.[42] inc binds physically to Cullin-3 and pan-neuronal knockdown of Cullin-3 phenocopies the disrupted sleep of inc mutants.[42] Independent confirmation and extension come from demonstration that inc mutants lack rebound sleep following sleep deprivation, and that their reduced sleep times can be rescued by inhibiting dopamine's biosynthesis.[44] Candidate directed studies also implicate Cullin-3–dependent pathways in the modulation of circadian rhythms. These studies were founded on observations in Drosophila that Cullin-3 regulates the proteolytic processing of Cubitus interruptus,[45–47] a component of the hedgehog signaling pathway that is interconnected with the circadian oscillator.[48] Decreasing Cullin-3 expression in

Drosophila clock neurons, for example, reduces circadian oscillations in PERIOD and TIMELESS, attenuates the amplitude of the circadian rhythm, and modulates circadian period length.[43]

MEIS1

MEIS1 is a more studied homeobox gene whose Drosophila ortholog participates in distal limb formation and the patterning of motor neuron connectivity.[49,50] The Xenopus ortholog of MEIS1 specifies neural crest cell fate,[51] and is also essential to leukemogenesis and normal hematopoiesis[52] and vascular patterning/endothelial cell development in both mice[53] and zebra fish.[54] MEIS1 also seems to regulate substance P expression in the central amygdala, which is an important gateway by which descending forebrain influences can coordinate mood with autonomic nervous system activities[55]; two behavioral domains commonly affected by RLS.[3]

As in the case of BTBD9, the inter-relationships between MEIS1 and iron homeostasis seem complex, and are not readily incorporated into heuristic constructs that posit decrements in iron storage as a necessary intermediate trait through which risk for RLS is conferred. In the general population the at-risk haplotype in MEIS1 does not associate with low serum ferritin levels.[32] This haplotype associates with reductions in MEIS1 mRNA protein expression, and homozygosity increases light and heavy chain ferritin and the divalent metal iron transporter 1 gene and protein expression in the thalamus.[28] However, these findings were not observed in lymphoblasts or pontine brain regions, and occurred independent of changes in other major determinants of iron homeostasis in RLS brains.[28] In Caenorhabditis elegans, RNA interference–mediated knockdown of the MEIS1 ortholog unc-62 increases ferritin expression.[28] The potential for epigenetic effects also exists, because MEIS1 expression is attenuated in 2 cell lines cultured in media rendered iron deficient via chelators.[28]

PTPRD, MAP2K5, SKOR1, and TOX3

The molecular pathways through which PTPRD, MAP2K5, SKOR1, and TOX3 might influence RLS pathophysiology remain unexplored. PTPRD and MAP2K5 are intriguing candidates because of their known roles in movement-related neural circuitry. PTPRD functions in the guidance and termination of mammalian motor neuron axons,[56] and its expression is dampened in a dose-dependent fashion by estradiol.[57] MAP2K5, one of the mitogen-activated protein kinases, is implicated in muscle differentiation[58] and neuroprotection of dopaminergic neurons.[59] In contrast, *SKOR1* is primarily expressed in spinal dorsal horn interneurons during development[60] and cerebellar Purkinje cells,[61] and represses BMP signaling through binding to Smad1.[61] Thus, *SKOR1*'s potential role in RLS pathophysiology is likely to involve actions at spinal sensory and cerebellar motor circuits. *TOX3* belongs to the thymocyte selection–associated high mobility group (HMG)–box subfamily of chromatin binding proteins, regulates Ca^{2+}-dependent neuronal transcription, and seems essential to neural plasticity[62] and survival.[63] Although disruption of *TOX3* signaling is a proposed mechanism underlying cell proliferation in breast cancer,[64] the role by which *TOX3* may mediate RLS susceptibility is less clear.

SUMMARY

A substantial proportion of risk for RLS is explained by a few common SNPs. They reside in presumptive regulatory regions of genes that have not previously been suspected as candidates based on the prevailing biological and clinical knowledge of RLS. Tissue-specific, functional gene expression associations with the risk variants are unknown, but are a prerequisite to understanding a complex disease such as RLS. The challenge of translating the recent genetic discoveries has, therefore, fallen on more traditional experimental methodologies, especially reverse-genetics approaches of exploring *BTBD9* in *Drosophila*. The mechanistic details remain incomplete, but the rudimentary outlines of molecular pathways are emerging by which the implicated genes might influence RLS by way of functional interactions with iron and dopamine metabolism. Additional understanding is also likely to derive from investigations of how SNPs in noncoding regions regulate gene expression in a cell-specific and tissue-specific manner; for example, as recently shown through overlapping risk SNPs with transcription factor binding sites and chromatin modifications.[64,65]

REFERENCES

1. Allen RP, Picchietti D, Hening WA, et al. Restless legs syndrome: diagnostic criteria, special considerations, and epidemiology. A report from the Restless Legs Syndrome Diagnosis and Epidemiology Workshop at the National Institutes of Health. Sleep Med 2003;4(2):101–19.
2. Winkelman JW. Periodic limb movements in sleep–endophenotype for restless legs syndrome? [comment]. N Engl J Med 2007;357(7):703–5.
3. Rye D, Trotti L. Restless legs syndrome and periodic leg movements of sleep. In: Watts R, Obeso J, Standaert D, editors. Movement disorders. 3rd edition. New York: McGraw-Hill; 2012. p. 907–33.
4. Winkelmann J, Polo O, Provini F, et al. Genetics of restless legs syndrome (RLS): state-of-the-art and future directions. Mov Disord 2007;22(Suppl 18): S449–58.
5. Ekbom K. Restless legs. Acta Med Scand Suppl 1945;158:1–123.
6. Desai AV, Cherkas LF, Spector TD, et al. Genetic influences in self-reported symptoms of obstructive sleep apnoea and restless legs: a twin study. Twin Res 2004;7(6):589–95.
7. Ondo WG, Vuong KD, Wang Q. Restless legs syndrome in monozygotic twins: clinical correlates. Neurology 2000;55(9):1404–6.
8. Chen S, Ondo WG, Rao S, et al. Genomewide linkage scan identifies a novel susceptibility locus for restless legs syndrome on chromosome 9p. Am J Hum Genet 2004;74(5):876–85.
9. Trenkwalder C, Collado-Seidel V, Gasser T, et al. Clinical symptoms and possible anticipation in a large kindred of familial restless legs syndrome. Mov Disord 1996;11:389–94.
10. Lazzarini A, Walters AS, Hickey K, et al. Studies of penetrance and anticipation in five autosomal-dominant restless legs syndrome pedigrees [In Process Citation]. Mov Disord 1999;14(1):111–6.
11. Birinyi PV, Allen RP, Hening W, et al. Undiagnosed individuals with first-degree relatives with restless legs syndrome have increased periodic limb movements. Sleep Med 2006;7(6):480–5.
12. Stefansson H, Rye DB, Hicks A, et al. A genetic risk factor for periodic limb movements in sleep. N Engl J Med 2007;357(7):639–47.
13. Moore HT, Winkelmann J, Lin L, et al. Periodic leg movements during sleep are associated with polymorphisms in BTBD9, TOX3/BC034767, MEIS1, MAP2K5/SKOR1, and PTPRD. Sleep 2014;37(9): 1535–42.
14. Desautels A, Turecki G, Montplaisir J, et al. Evidence for a genetic association between monoamine oxidase A and restless legs syndrome. Neurology 2002;59:215–9.
15. Pichler I, Hicks AA, Pramstaller PP. Restless legs syndrome: an update on genetics and future perspectives. Clin Genet 2008;73(4):297–305.
16. Winkelmann J. Genetics of restless legs syndrome. Curr Neurol Neurosci Rep 2008;8(3):211–6.
17. Balaban H, Bayrakli F, Kartal U, et al. A novel locus for restless legs syndrome on chromosome 13q. Eur Neurol 2012;68(2):111–6.
18. Skehan EB, Abdulrahim MM, Parfrey NA, et al. A novel locus for restless legs syndrome maps to chromosome 19p in an Irish pedigree. Neurogenetics 2012;13(2):125–32.
19. Winkelmann J, Schormair B, Lichtner P, et al. Genome-wide association study of restless legs

syndrome identifies common variants in three genomic regions [see comment]. Nat Genet 2007; 39(8):1000–6.

20. Vilarino-Guell C, Farrer MJ, Lin SC. A genetic risk factor for periodic limb movements in sleep. N Engl J Med 2008;358(4):425–7.

21. Schormair B, Kemlink D, Roeske D, et al. PTPRD (protein tyrosine phosphatase receptor type delta) is associated with restless legs syndrome. Nat Genet 2008;40(8):946–8.

22. Winkelmann J, Czamara D, Schormair B, et al. Genome-wide association study identifies novel restless legs syndrome susceptibility loci on 2p14 and 16q12.1. PLoS Genet 2011;7(7):e1002171.

23. Mignot E. A step forward for restless legs syndrome [comment]. Nat Genet 2007;39(8):938–9.

24. Xiong L, Catoire H, Dion P, et al. MEIS1 intronic risk haplotype associated with restless legs syndrome affects its mRNA and protein expression levels. Hum Mol Genet 2009;18(6):1065–74.

25. Spieler D, Kaffe M, Knauf F, et al. Restless legs syndrome-associated intronic common variant in Meis1 alters enhancer function in the developing telencephalon. Genome Res 2014;24(4):592–603.

26. Vilarino-Guell C, Chai H, Keeling BH, et al. MEIS1 p.R272H in familial restless legs syndrome. Neurology 2009;73(3):243–5.

27. Schulte EC, Knauf F, Kemlink D, et al. Variant screening of the coding regions of MEIS1 in patients with restless legs syndrome. Neurology 2011; 76(12):1106–8.

28. Catoire H, Dion PA, Xiong L, et al. Restless legs syndrome-associated MEIS1 risk variant influences iron homeostasis. Ann Neurol 2011;70(1):170–5.

29. Freeman A, Pranski E, Miller RD, et al. Sleep fragmentation and motor restlessness in a Drosophila model of restless legs syndrome. Curr Biol 2012; 22(12):1142–8.

30. DeAndrade MP, Johnson RL Jr, Unger EL, et al. Motor restlessness, sleep disturbances, thermal sensory alterations and elevated serum iron levels in Btbd9 mutant mice. Hum Mol Genet 2012; 21(18):3984–92.

31. Schulte EC, Kousi M, Tan PL, et al. Targeted resequencing and systematic in vivo functional testing identifies rare variants in MEIS1 as significant contributors to restless legs syndrome. Am J Hum Genet 2014;95(1):85–95.

32. Oexle K, Schormair B, Ried JS, et al. Dilution of candidates: the case of iron-related genes in restless legs syndrome. Eur J Hum Genet 2013;21(4):410–4.

33. Schormair B, Plag J, Kaffe M, et al. MEIS1 and BTBD9: genetic association with restless leg syndrome in end stage renal disease. J Med Genet 2011;48(7):462–6.

34. Lin CH, Chen ML, Wu VC, et al. Association of candidate genetic variants with restless legs syndrome in end stage renal disease: a multicenter case-control study in Taiwan. Eur J Neurol 2014; 21(3):492–8.

35. Vavrova J, Kemlink D, Sonka K, et al. Restless legs syndrome in Czech patients with multiple sclerosis: an epidemiological and genetic study. Sleep Med 2012;13(7):848–51.

36. Perez-Torrado R, Yamada D, Defossez P. Born to bind: the BTB protein-protein interaction domain. Bioessays 2006;28:1194–202.

37. Bilic I, Ellmeier W. The role of BTB domain-containing zinc finger proteins in T cell development and function. Immunol Lett 2007;108(1):1–9.

38. Stogios P, Downs G, Jauhal J, et al. Sequence and structural analysis of BTB domain proteins. Genome Biol 2005;6:R82.

39. Stogios P, Privé G. The BACK domain in BTB-kelch proteins. Trends Biochem Sci 2004;29:634–7.

40. Adams J, Kelso R, Cooley L. The kelch repeat superfamily of proteins: propellers of cell function. Trends Cell Biol 2000;10:17–24.

41. Hashimoto Y, Muramatsu K, Kunii M, et al. Uncovering genes required for neuronal morphology by morphology-based gene trap screening with a revertible retrovirus vector. FASEB J 2012;26(11): 4662–74.

42. Stavropoulos N, Young MW. insomniac and Cullin-3 regulate sleep and wakefulness in Drosophila. Neuron 2011;72(6):964–76.

43. Grima B, Dognon A, Lamouroux A, et al. CULLIN-3 controls TIMELESS oscillations in the Drosophila circadian clock. PLoS Biol 2012;10(8):e1001367.

44. Pfeiffenberger C, Allada R. Cul3 and the BTB adaptor insomniac are key regulators of sleep homeostasis and a dopamine arousal pathway in Drosophila. PLoS Genet 2012;8(10):e1003003.

45. Ou CY, Lin YF, Chen YJ, et al. Distinct protein degradation mechanisms mediated by Cul1 and Cul3 controlling Ci stability in Drosophila eye development. Genes Dev 2002;16(18):2403–14.

46. Jiang J, Struhl G. Regulation of the Hedgehog and Wingless signalling pathways by the F-box/WD40-repeat protein Slimb. Nature 1998;391(6666):493–6.

47. Zhang Q, Zhang L, Wang B, et al. A hedgehog-induced BTB protein modulates hedgehog signaling by degrading Ci/Gli transcription factor. Dev Cell 2006;10(6):719–29.

48. Zhang EE, Liu AC, Hirota T, et al. A genome-wide RNAi screen for modifiers of the circadian clock in human cells. Cell 2009;139(1):199–210.

49. Casares F, Mann RS. Control of antennal versus leg development in Drosophila. Nature 1998;392(6677): 723–6.

50. Kurant E, Pai CY, Sharf R, et al. Dorsotonals/homothorax, the Drosophila homologue of meis1, interacts with extradenticle in patterning of the embryonic PNS. Development 1998;125(6):1037–48.

51. Maeda R, Mood K, Jones TL, et al. Xmeis1, a proto-oncogene involved in specifying neural crest cell fate in *Xenopus* embryos. Oncogene 2001;20(11):1329–42.

52. Argiropoulos B, Yung E, Humphries RK. Unraveling the crucial roles of Meis1 in leukemogenesis and normal hematopoiesis [comment]. Genes Dev 2007;21(22):2845–9.

53. Azcoitia V, Aracil M, Martinez AC, et al. The homeodomain protein Meis1 is essential for definitive hematopoiesis and vascular patterning in the mouse embryo. Dev Biol 2005;280(2):307–20.

54. Minehata K, Kawahara A, Suzuki T. meis1 regulates the development of endothelial cells in zebrafish. Biochem Biophys Res Commun 2008; 374(4):647–52.

55. Davidson S, Miller KA, Dowell A, et al. A remote and highly conserved enhancer supports amygdala specific expression of the gene encoding the anxiogenic neuropeptide substance-P. Mol Psychiatry 2006;11(4):323.

56. Uetani N, Chagnon MJ, Kennedy TE, et al. Mammalian motoneuron axon targeting requires receptor protein tyrosine phosphatases sigma and delta. J Neurosci 2006;26(22):5872–80.

57. Naciff JM, Overmann GJ, Torontali SM, et al. Gene expression profile induced by 17 alpha-ethynyl estradiol in the prepubertal female reproductive system of the rat. Toxicol Sci 2003;72(2):314–30.

58. Dinev D, Jordan BW, Neufeld B, et al. Extracellular signal regulated kinase 5 (ERK5) is required for the differentiation of muscle cells. EMBO Rep 2001;2(9):829–34.

59. Cavanaugh JE, Jaumotte JD, Lakoski JM, et al. Neuroprotective role of ERK1/2 and ERK5 in a dopaminergic cell line under basal conditions and in response to oxidative stress. J Neurosci Res 2006; 84(6):1367–75.

60. Mizuhara E, Nakatani T, Minaki Y, et al. Corl1, a novel neuronal lineage-specific transcriptional corepressor for the homeodomain transcription factor Lbx1. J Biol Chem 2005;280(5):3645–55.

61. Arndt S, Poser I, Moser M, et al. Fussel-15, a novel Ski/Sno homolog protein, antagonizes BMP signaling. Mol Cell Neurosci 2007;34(4):603–11.

62. Yuan SH, Qiu Z, Ghosh A. TOX3 regulates calcium-dependent transcription in neurons. Proc Natl Acad Sci U S A 2009;106(8):2909–14.

63. Dittmer S, Kovacs Z, Yuan SH, et al. TOX3 is a neuronal survival factor that induces transcription depending on the presence of CITED1 or phosphorylated CREB in the transcriptionally active complex. J Cell Sci 2011;124(Pt 2):252–60.

64. Cowper-Sal lari R, Zhang X, Wright JB, et al. Breast cancer risk-associated SNPs modulate the affinity of chromatin for FOXA1 and alter gene expression. Nat Genet 2012;44(11):1191–8.

65. Trynka G, Sandor C, Han B, et al. Chromatin marks identify critical cell types for fine mapping complex trait variants. Nat Genet 2013;45(2):124–30.

Diagnosis of Restless Legs Syndrome/Willis-Ekbom Disease

Diagnosis of Restless Legs
Syndrome/Willis-Ekbom
Disease

Diagnosis of Restless Leg Syndrome (Willis-Ekbom Disease)

Philip M. Becker, MD[a,b],*

KEYWORDS

- Restless leg syndrome (RLS) • Willis-Ekbom disease (WED) • Diagnostic criteria
- Mimics • Ferritin in RLS

KEY POINTS

- Diagnosis of restless leg syndrome, or Willis-Ekbom disease, (RLS/WED) is based on 5 diagnostic criteria: urge to move, rest worsens the urge, movement provides relief, evening or night worsening of the urge, and the best or sole explanation is RLS/WED.
- Serum ferritin should be tested in patients with moderate-to-severe RLS/WED, established patients with acute worsening of symptoms, or patients with illness producing blood loss.
- Polysomnography or nerve conduction–electromyographic study is not indicated unless a patient has additional clinical symptoms to warrant such testing (hypersomnia or poorly characterized neuropathy or radiculopathy).
- Diagnosis of young children or elderly with cognitive impairment may need evaluation of supportive or associated features and information from parents or caregivers to determine the presence of definite, possible, or probable RLS/WED.

INTRODUCTION

Restless leg syndrome, or Willis-Ekbom disease, (RLS/WED) is a neurosensorimotor disorder that is diagnosed through focused questioning rather than any specific test.[1] Although any limb may be affected, most patients have initial symptoms in the lower extremities and commonly report sleep onset and early maintenance insomnia. RLS/WED affects 2% to 4% of adults in North America and Europe at least twice weekly and is more common in women.[2,3] It is estimated to affect more than 10 million adults in the United States[3] and an estimated 1.5 million children and adolescents.[4] The clinical course of RLS/WED is commonly chronic and progressive in moderate-to-severe primary cases. Early onset of RLS/WED before age 30 is often intermittent and variably problematic until the patient reaches middle age. Presentation after age 50 is usually more rapid and clinically more troublesome.[5–7] On occasion, RLS/WED can be intermittent and enter remission.[8] Sleep onset and maintenance insomnia is often the primary reason for medical consultation.[5,9] Unless a patient has other symptoms of sleep disorder, particularly excessive daytime sleepiness, polysomnography is not needed for diagnosis of the sleep disturbance.[10] A patient with moderate-to-severe RLS/WED may average less than 5 hours of sleep per night. Interestingly, most RLS/WED patients with significant insomnia deny daytime sleepiness. For patients with mild

Author Disclosures: P.M. Becker discloses that in the prior 24 months he received grant-research support as a principal investigator from Apnicure and has received financial support for Speakers Bureau from Xenoport.
^a Sleep Medicine Associates of Texas, 5477 Glen Lakes Drive, Suite 100, Dallas, TX 75231, USA; ^b Department of Psychiatry, University of Texas Southwestern Medical Center, Dallas, TX, USA
* 5477 Glen Lakes Drive, Suite 100, Dallas, TX 75231.
E-mail address: pbecker@sleepmed.com

RLS/WED, sleep disturbance may be only a minor inconvenience.[11]

Challenges to diagnosis arise when the patient has other medical conditions, such as metabolic disease, neurologic dysfunction, musculoskeletal abnormalities, autoimmune disease, and/or psychiatric disorders. Patients may have difficulty characterizing the sensory discomfort but may use terms such as crawling, creeping, bugs, worms, electricity, energy, burning, pain, ache, or nervous. Symptoms present sitting in a chair, automobile, airplane, or lying down attempting to sleep. The practitioner must systematically question a patient about their sensory and motor experience in relationship to lifestyle, time of day, and concomitant medications to properly characterize the diagnosis in more complex patients. There may also be differences in the presentation of RLS/WED in children or the cognitively impaired.

DIAGNOSTIC CRITERIA

RLS/WED has been variously characterized as primary, familial, idiopathic, early onset, late onset, or secondary (eg, related to iron deficiency, anemia, pregnancy, or end-stage renal disease). Because the cause and genetics of RLS/WED remain under investigation, appropriate diagnosis focuses on symptom presentation. Consensus criteria for the diagnosis of restless leg syndrome were established through a National Institutes of Health conference and published in 2003.[1] Four criteria were defined to arrive at a diagnosis. In 2012, a fifth criterion was added by the International Restless Legs Syndrome Study Group (IRLSSG) to address the potential mimics that could complicate diagnosis.[12] In 2004, the acronym URGE came into

use to assist physicians in their diagnostic process. Subsequently, Lee and colleagues[13] added the fifth IRLSSG criteria that restless leg syndrome should be the sole or primary factor to account for the symptomatic complaint. The resulting acronym, URGES, stands for: (1) urge to move that is most commonly noted in the legs, (2) rest worsens the urge to move, (3) gyration or movement of the affected limb improves the urge, (4) evening and night intensification of the urge, and (5) the sole best explanation of the urge is RLS/WED. **Table 1** describes the 5 diagnostic criteria of URGES. The presenting symptom is the patient's urge to move because of a sensory disturbance that may prove difficult for the patient to describe. When the patient is at rest, the urge intensifies, while gyration or getting up to go (stretching or movement of the affected limbs) will at least temporarily provide relief of the urge to move. Unless the patient takes exacerbating medication or has the most severe presentation, the sensory component normally begins to intensify in the evening and first half of the night, lessening over the night and generally being of little problem in the morning hours. The diagnostic criteria have been incorporated in the *International Classification of Sleep Disorders*, 3rd edition, and in other diagnostic manuals.[14]

SPECIAL POPULATIONS: PEDIATRIC AND COGNITIVELY IMPAIRED

Pediatric diagnosis has been modified based on the ability of a child to describe the sensations.[15] The diagnosis is demarcated as definite, probable, or possible RLS/WED. The probable diagnosis of restless leg syndrome has been observed in

Table 1	
Diagnostic criteria using the acronym URGES	
Urge to move the limbs	Urge to move the legs (sometimes arms or other body parts) with or without dysesthesias
Rest-induced	Onset or exacerbation with both decreased motor activity and mental activation
	Motor and sensory symptoms most often develop during periods of rest or inactivity, such as sitting or lying
Gyration or movement improves urge	Relief with movement
	RLS symptoms are partially or totally relieved by movements such as walking or stretching
	High mental activation such as computer games may also reduce the urge
Evening or night worsening	Circadian pattern
	RLS symptoms usually occur or worsen in the evening or at bedtime
	Symptoms are generally minimal in the morning
Sole explanation for urge to move	Any other illness or disorder cannot explain the other 4 symptoms

infants based on observation by parents of poor sleep, especially when parents or siblings have RLS/WED. Between the ages 5 and 8, children begin to be able to report the 5 diagnostic features of the disorder, often using terms such as energy, hurting, spiders, or bugs in the legs to describe their attempt to fall asleep at night. **Box 1** presents the currently recommended diagnostic criteria for pediatric patients.

As can occur in the very young, the elderly patient with cognitive impairment may not be able to describe their symptoms. Dementia, aphasia, severe psychiatric disorder, or other cognitive impairment may prevent an accurate description by the patient. Past history from a caregiver is often the most helpful to increase diagnostic accuracy, although a therapeutic trial of levodopa may prove of diagnostic value. Levodopa 100 mg that reduces agitation and improves sleep provides a response that strongly suggests RLS/WED as the correct diagnosis.[16]

SUPPORTIVE AND ASSOCIATED CLINICAL FEATURES TO ASSIST DIAGNOSIS

When the core symptoms of RLS/WED cannot be established by history alone, the supportive and associated features, listed in **Box 2**, may be helpful. Positive family history of RLS/WED, periodic leg movements in sleep, a therapeutic response to dopaminergic therapy, sleep disturbance in the first half of the night, and a negative medical or neurologic workup increases the likelihood that the disorder is present. Based on findings in index patients, first-degree relatives have 3 to 7 times greater prevalence of RLS/WED than people without RLS/WED.[17,18] Nearly all patients with RLS/WED show at least an initial positive therapeutic response to either levodopa 100 mg or other dopaminergic agents.[16] Periodic limb movements in sleep (PLMS) are identified at a rate of greater than or equal to 5 leg movements per sleep hour in about 80% of people with RLS/WED and may assist in the diagnosis.[19] However, all that moves at night is not RLS/WED. PLMS are common in other disorders and among the elderly. Therefore, their presence in a polysomnogram should be considered to be only suggestive but

---

Box 1
Pediatric diagnostic criteria

Definite RLS

The child describes in his or her own words the adult criteria outlined in **Table 1**

Or, with the assistance of an adult observer, the child seemingly meets adult criteria

And 2 of the 3 following supportive criteria are met

1. There is a clinical sleep disturbance for age

2. A biological parent or sibling has definite RLS

3. A polysomnographic study has documented a periodic limb movement index of 5 or more per hour of sleep

Probable RLS

The child meets 3 adult criteria

1. The urge to move the legs

2. The urge to move begins or worsens with sitting or lying down

3. The urge to move is partially or totally relieved by movement

And the child has a biological parent or sibling with definite RLS

Or, the child shows signs of lower-extremity discomfort when sitting or lying down, with motor movement of the affected limbs; the discomfort has characteristics of worsening with rest and inactivity, relief with movement, and worsening during evening and nighttime hours

And the child has a biological parent or sibling with definite RLS

Possible RLS

The child has periodic limb movement disorder

And a biological parent or sibling has definite RLS but the child does not meet the criteria for definite or probable childhood RLS

Box 2
Supportive and associated clinical features

Supportive clinical features for RLS diagnosis

1. Positive family history

2. Positive response to dopaminergic therapy, such as brief levodopa trial

3. Presence of periodic limb movements on polysomnography.

Associated features

1. Clinical course is generally chronic and progressive

2. Sleep disturbance, particularly in the first half of the night

3. Normal neurologic examination in primary RLS, unless a comorbid condition exists

not diagnostic for RLS/WED.[20] Genetic studies indicate that PLMS and RLS/WED share a significant relationship in families.[21]

DISORDERS THAT MIMIC OR AFFECT THE DIAGNOSTIC PROCESS

There are disorders that have symptoms that mimic RLS/WED.[22] The most common are listed in **Box 3**. Confusion in the diagnostic process may arise with disorders that produce complaints of motor restlessness and those resulting in sensory symptoms of discomfort of the legs or feet. These disorders may meet some of the diagnostic criteria for RLS/WED.[22] There are also comorbid disorders, such as diabetic neuropathy or Parkinson disease, with RLS/WED.[23]

ALTERING AGENTS OR MEDICATIONS

Although not essential for diagnosis, it is important to recognize that various substances that are taken by patients with sleep disorders affect the presentation of RLS/WED, including caffeine, dopamine antagonists, antidepressants, antihistamines, decongestants, anticholinergics, and respiratory stimulants. A 2010 review assessed the evidence for exacerbation.[24] Anecdotal reports of caffeine exacerbation result in the recommendation that patients discontinue caffeine at noon.

Box 3
Mimics or comorbid disorders

- Neuroleptic-induced akathisia
- Fidgets
- Semiconscious leg jiggling
- Involuntary leg movements (PLM, propriospinal myoclonus at sleep onset, rhythmic movement disorder)
- Peripheral neuropathy
- Nocturnal leg cramps
- Vascular or neurogenic claudication
- Pruritus
- Arthritic leg discomfort
- Fibromyalgia
- Painful myopathies
- Varicose veins or venous insufficiency
- Deep vein thrombosis
- Fasciculations
- Positional discomfort
- Painful legs and moving toes

Neuroleptic agents are expected to increase RLS/WED symptoms, although other antagonists of dopamine, such as metoclopramide, also have proven problematic. Although there are variable reports on the impact of serotonin selective receptor inhibitors and serotonin-noradrenergic receptor inhibitors, it has been estimated that 30% to 40% of patients will experience exacerbation of symptoms on these agents. Decongestants, anticholinergics, and respiratory stimulants may also affect RLS/WED.

DIAGNOSTIC WORKUP

Again, history of the 5 diagnostic criteria directs diagnosis. Mimics also need to be assessed.[23]

Examination

The physical examination in primary RLS/WED is normal. The examination may detect secondary causes of RLS/WED or mimics. It is important to have the patient remove shoes and socks. To rule out peripheral neuropathy or radiculopathy, neurologic examination should include assessment of weakness, touch, pain, vibration, and position. Sensations of burning, tingling, and electric shocks are common in diabetes and renal disease in which RLS/WED and neuropathy may coexist. The comorbid presentation of both disorders may affect treatment decisions.[2] Arthritis, arterial insufficiency, venous disease, or varicosities may be a source of leg discomfort, so joints and pulses should be examined. Time of day also affects presentation. Examination in morning or early afternoon is unlikely to find the patient to be symptomatic. Later in the day, it may be possible to see the periodic flexion movements of the great toe or feet as the legs dangle from the examination table.

Laboratory Evaluation

There is no laboratory test for RLS/WED; however, assessment of iron deficiency, electromyogram, nerve conduction velocity, or polysomnographic studies may be considered in selected patients. Serum ferritin should be measured in patients with moderate or severe symptoms, recent exacerbation of RLS/WED, or risk factors for low iron stores.[25] Ferritin is an acute phase reactant. If a patient has had recent fever or suffers a chronic inflammatory disorder, it is also important to measure transferrin saturation and total iron-binding capacity. When serum ferritin levels are less than 50 μg/L, iron supplementation should be considered. When iron stores are abnormally low (ferritin <15 μg/L), iron repletion is indicated and an appropriate workup initiated. If symptoms warrant, assessment of peripheral neuropathy or renal failure should proceed.

Again, polysomnography is not recommended for primary RLS/WED.[26] Polysomnography may be appropriate if clinical symptoms of apnea are reported by the patient, there is excessive daytime sleepiness, or the patient has had sleep-related agitated behavior. Electromyography or nerve conduction testing of nerve function is only indicated for those patients in whom testing will affect treatment decisions.

A specialized study, the suggested immobilization test (SIT), has been used to research RLS/WED presentation and severity.[27] The patient receives monitoring of the anterior tibialis muscles for 60 minutes while resting in bed with head elevated. The SIT is usually administered in the late evening when RLS/WED symptoms intensify. The degree of discomfort is rated by the patient at 5-minute intervals while periodic leg movements of wakefulness (PLMW) are tallied. More than 40 PLMW per hour is considered diagnostic. The SIT has not seen broad clinical use because it is uncomfortable for the patient and offers only moderate sensitivity and specificity to diagnosis.

CONCLUSION

RLS/WED is a common neurosensorimotor disorder affecting millions of adults and children that is diagnosed using 5 clinical criteria (URGES). In patients with primary RLS/WED, diagnosis is usually straightforward based on the patient's symptomatic reports that meet the 5 criteria. When patients have comorbid conditions that include sensory or motor symptoms, diagnosis must include a thorough examination of sensory, motor, vascular, and joint signs to rule out other disorders that may mimic RLS/WED. A review of a patient's medication list is appropriate to assure that there are no agents that would be expected to exacerbate the disorder, such as dopamine antagonists, serotonergic or norepinephrine inhibitors, or stimulants such as decongestants or caffeine. The most helpful laboratory test is iron regulation, particularly serum ferritin at less than 50 ug/L, indicating potential value for iron supplementation. Routine polysomnographic, electromyogram, or nerve conduction velocity testing is not indicated unless the patient provides additional clinical complaints that would warrant the expense and alter the course of therapy. Appropriate diagnosis will be much appreciated by the RLS/WED patient who can receive an excellent therapeutic response from behavioral and pharmacologic interventions.

REFERENCES

1. Allen RP, Picchietti D, Hening WA, et al. Restless legs syndrome: diagnostic criteria, special considerations, and epidemiology. A report from the restless legs syndrome diagnosis and epidemiology workshop at the National Institutes of Health. Sleep Med 2003;4:101–19.
2. Allen RP, Stillman P, Myers AJ. Physician-diagnosed restless legs syndrome in a large sample of primary medical care patients in western Europe: Prevalence and characteristics. Sleep Med 2010;11:31–7.
3. Allen RP, Walters AS, Montplaisir J, et al. Restless legs syndrome prevalence and impact: REST population study. Arch Intern Med 2005;165(11):1286–92.
4. Picchietti D, Allen RP, Walters AS, et al. Restless legs syndrome: prevalence and impact in children and adolescents–the Peds REST study. Pediatrics 2007;120(2):253–66.
5. Allen RP, Earley CJ. Defining the phenotype of the restless legs syndrome (RLS) using age-of-symptom-onset. Sleep Med 2000;1(1):11–9.
6. Ondo W, Jankovic J. Restless legs syndrome: clinicoetiologic correlates. Neurology 1996;47(6):1435–41.
7. Allen RP. Controversies and challenges in defining the etiology and pathophysiology of restless legs syndrome. Am J Med 2007;120(1 Suppl 1):S13–21.
8. Walters AS, Hickey K, Maltzman J, et al. A questionnaire study of 138 patients with restless legs syndrome: the 'Night-Walkers' survey. Neurology 1996;46(1):92–5.
9. Silber MH, Becker PM, Earley C, et al. Willis-Ekbom Disease Foundation revised consensus statement on the management of restless legs syndrome. Mayo Clin Proc 2013;88(9):977–86.
10. Hornyak M, Feige B, Voderholzer U, et al. Polysomnography findings in patients with restless legs syndrome and in healthy controls: a comparative observational study. Sleep 2007;30(7):861–5.
11. Allen RP, Earley CJ. Restless legs syndrome: a review of clinical and pathophysiologic features. J Clin Neurophysiol 2001;18(2):128–47.
12. Allen RP, Picchietti DL, Garcia-Borreguero D, et al. Restless legs syndrome/Willis-Ekbom disease diagnostic criteria: updated International Restless Legs Syndrome Study Group (IRLSSG) consensus criteria–history, rationale, description, and significance. Sleep Med 2014;15(8):860–73.
13. Lee HB, Buchfuher M, Allen RP, et al, editors. Clinical management of restless legs syndrome. 2nd edition. New York: Professional Communications; 2013.
14. American Academy of Sleep Medicine. The international classification of sleep disorders: diagnostic – coding manual. 3rd edition. Westchester (IL): American Academy of Sleep Medicine; 2014.
15. Picchietti DL, Bruni O, de Weerd A, et al. Pediatric restless legs syndrome diagnostic criteria: an

update by the International Restless Legs Syndrome Study Group. Sleep Med 2013;14(12):1253–9.

16. Stiasny-Kolster K, Kohnen R, Möller JC, et al. Validation of the "L-DOPA test" for diagnosis of restless legs syndrome. Mov Disord 2006;21(9):1333–9.

17. Hening WA, Washburn M, Allen RP, et al. Blinded diagnoses confirm elevated frequency in relatives of restless legs syndrome (RLS) probands in a case-control family study of RLS (abstr). Mov Disord 2004;19(Suppl 9):S363.

18. Allen RP, La Buda MC, Becker P, et al. Family history study of the restless legs syndrome. Sleep Med 2002;3(Suppl):S3–7.

19. Michaud M, Paquet J, Lavigne G, et al. Sleep laboratory diagnosis of restless legs syndrome. Eur Neurol 2002;48(2):108–13.

20. Hening W. The clinical neurophysiology of the restless legs syndrome and periodic limb movements. Part I: diagnosis, assessment, and characterization. Clin Neurophysiol 2004;115(9):1965–74.

21. Stefansson H, Rye DB, Hicks A, et al. A genetic risk factor for periodic limb movements in sleep. N Engl J Med 2007;357(7):639–47.

22. Benes H, Walters AS, Allen RP, et al. Definition of restless legs syndrome, how to diagnose it, and how to differentiate it from RLS mimics [Review]. Mov Disord 2007;22(Suppl 18):S401–8.

23. Gemignani F, Brindani F, Vitetta F, et al. Restless legs syndrome in diabetic neuropathy: a frequent manifestation of small fiber neuropathy. J Peripher Nerv Syst 2007;12(1):50–3.

24. Hoque R, Chesson AL. Pharmacologically induced/exacerbated restless legs syndrome, periodic limb movements of sleep, and REM behavior disorder/REM sleep without atonia: literature review, qualitative scoring, and comparative analysis [Review]. J Clin Sleep Med 2010;6(1):79–83.

25. Sun ER, Chen CA, Ho G, et al. Iron and the restless legs syndrome. Sleep 1998;21(4):371–7.

26. Kushida CA, Littner MR, Morgenthaler T, et al. Practice parameters for the indications for polysomnography and related procedures: an update for 2005. Sleep 2005;28(4):499–521.

27. Michaud M. Is the suggested immobilization test the "gold standard" to assess restless legs syndrome? Sleep Med 2006;7(7):541–3.

The Role of Periodic Limb Movements During Sleep in Restless Legs Syndrome
A Selective Update

Stephany Fulda, PhD

KEYWORDS

- Periodic leg movements • Restless legs syndrome • Arousal • Treatment

KEY POINTS

- Periodic leg movements during sleep (PLMS) are a highly active research field.
- Recent studies have led to a re-evaluation of the role of PLMS with regard to arousals and sleep disturbances in restless legs syndrome (RLS).
- Dopaminergic and non-dopaminergic drug treatments differ in their effect on PLMS in RLS.
- PLMS may emerge as a new sleep-related cardiovascular risk factor and possible treatment target in RLS.

INTRODUCTION

Periodic leg movements during sleep (PLMS) are repetitive contractions of the tibialis anterior muscles occurring mainly during non–rapid eye movement sleep and are readily observed in polysomnographic recordings, which is a standard procedure in accredited sleep laboratories.[1] In patients with restless legs syndrome (RLS), many hundreds of such leg movements may be observed during a single night.[2]

Increased PLMS are also observed in a considerable proportion of patients with various sleep disorders[2] but they are also found in healthy subjects, with the prevalence sharply increasing with age.[3–6] However, the closest association with PLMS is found in patients with RLS; approximately 85% of these patients show frequent PLMS during nocturnal sleep.[7] Therefore, PLMS have been[8] and remain a supportive criterion for the diagnosis of RLS.[9] Nevertheless, recent accumulating evidence in this highly active research field is leading to changing views of several key aspects of the assumed role of PLMS in RLS, which are summarized in this article. In particular, this article focuses on the relationship of PLMS to cortical arousals and sleep disturbances in RLS, the effect of the newer non-dopaminergic drugs for RLS on PLMS, and recent evidence on the relationship between PLMS and transient nocturnal blood pressure increases.

PERIODIC LEG MOVEMENTS AND AROUSALS DURING SLEEP IN RESTLESS LEGS SYNDROME

During sleep, PLMS may co-occur with cortical arousals and this is usually quantified with the PLMS arousal index (ie, the number of PLMS that co-occur with an arousal divided by the number of hours with sleep).[10] However, the notion that PLMS cause these arousals and are therefore among the major causes of sleep disturbance in patients with RLS has been fundamentally re-evaluated based on recent studies. The 2014 updated diagnostic criteria for RLS still define PLMS as a

Disclosure: The author has nothing to disclose.
Sleep and Epilepsy Center, Neurocenter of Southern Switzerland, Civic Hospital (EOC) of Lugano, Via Tesserete 46, Lugano 6903, Switzerland
E-mail address: stephany.fulda@gmail.com

Sleep Med Clin 10 (2015) 241–248
http://dx.doi.org/10.1016/j.jsmc.2015.05.013
1556-407X/15/$ – see front matter

supportive feature for the diagnosis of RLS but state that, "contrary to initial expectations, PLMS are not directly related to the primary RLS/Willis-Ekbom disease (WED) morbidity of sleep disturbance, rather they may reflect some RLS/WED biology partially independent of that" [9(pp866)]. This statement is supported by several distinct lines of evidence.

For one, during sleep in patients with RLS, many instances of PLMS without cortical arousals or, vice versa, EEG arousals without PLMS might be observed.[11] **Table 1** lists those studies that quantified, in untreated patients with RLS, the number of PLMS, the number of PLMS associated with arousals, and the number of arousals per hour of sleep. A consistent finding across studies is that only about one-third of PLMS were associated with arousals[12–25] and also only one-third of arousals were associated with PLMS.[12–15,17,19] Therefore, most PLMS and arousals occur independently of each other.

In addition, even when PLMS and arousals occur together, the onset of the arousal precedes that of the onset of the PLM in only 40% to 50%,[26,27] which makes it difficult to claim a cause-effect relationship in most cases. Importantly, the lack of association in the studies mentioned earlier cannot be attributed to an overly restrictive definition for the association of PLMS and arousals.[27] The current standard criteria for the recording and scoring of PLMS state that PLMS are considered to be associated with an arousal when they are separated by less than 0.5 seconds between the end of one event and the onset of the other, regardless of which is first.[1,10,28] Even though these criteria were not evidence based, a recent study in patients with RLS has shown that, if PLMS and arousals occur anywhere near each other (within 10 seconds), then in almost all cases (ie, 98%) they overlap or are separated by less than 0.5 seconds.[27]

Another argument stems from a key study in this area that has been able to show that PLMS and arousals can be pharmacologically dissociated.[29] In this study, a group of patients with RLS were randomized to receive a single dose of the dopamine agonist pramipexole (0.25 mg), the benzodiazepine clonazepam (0.5 mg), or placebo. Both active drugs were effective on RLS sensory symptoms. Pramipexole strongly reduced PLMS without affecting the frequency of arousals, whereas clonazepam reduced arousals but had no effect on PLMS. This demonstration that a selective pharmacologic approach can dissociate PLMS from arousal events also further against a direct cause-effect relationship between the two

Table 1
PLMS and arousals in untreated patients with RLS

Study	Number	PLMS Index	PLMS Arousal Index	Arousal Index	PLMS Associated with Arousals (%)	Arousals Associated with PLMS (%)
Michaud et al,[12] 2002	100	28.2	5.2	15.8	18.43	32.91
Saletu et al,[13] 2002	12	39.70	12.80	31.80	32.24	40.25
Eisensehr et al,[14] 2003	27	26.4	9.5	21	35.98	45.23
Garcia-Borreguero et al,[15] 2004	30	25.02	13.09	37.96	52.31	34.48
Hornyak et al,[16] 2004	33[b]	36.65	13.50	—	36.83	—
Hornyak et al,[17] 2005	42[b]	36.90	12.60	29.30	34.14	43.00
Oertel et al,[18] 2006	40	58.67	20.20	—	34.42	—
Hornyak et al,[20] 2007	200[a]	33.29	12.84	—	38.57	—
Hornyak et al,[19] 2007	45	22.9	8.1	25.9	35.37	31.27
Boehm et al,[21] 2009	95	27.8	16.2	—	58.27	—
Jama et al,[22] 2009	107[a]	37.11	8.52	—	22.95	—
Inoue et al,[23] 2010	38[a]	32.55[c]	12.98[c]	—	39.87	—
Saletu et al,[24] 2010	80[a]	24.30	3.40	—	13.99	—
Winkelman et al,[25] 2011	131	46.70	13.20	—	28.26	—
Across studies weighted average					33.09	36.10

[a] In case more than 1 group of patients with RLS was described in the same study, values were averaged across groups.
[b] In case more than 1 night was recorded in patients with RLS, values were averaged across nights.
[c] Based on median.

phenomena. Based on these results it has been proposed that gamma-aminobutyric acid–ergic (GABAergic) agents and not dopamine agonists modulate cortical excitability during sleep and that PLMS are under dopaminergic but not GABAergic control, whereas RLS sensory symptoms are influenced by both GABAergic and dopaminergic drugs.[29]

In summary, both PLMS and arousals are common in patients with RLS. After recent studies it is now recognized that the two phenomena, rather than being connected by a simple reciprocal relationship, might be regulated by a more complex mechanism that includes them and possibly other sleep phasic events, such as transient heart rate and blood pressure increases. The finding that dopaminergic treatment, which strongly reduces PLMS, does not improve sleep instability, when present, in patients with RLS[29–32] has important implications for therapeutic management of sleep disorders in patients with RLS.[33]

DIFFERENTIAL DRUG TREATMENT EFFECTS ON PERIODIC LEG MOVEMENTS DURING SLEEP AND RESTLESS LEGS SYNDROME SYMPTOMS

Dopaminergic drugs have been the first-line treatments of RLS for a long time[34,35] and have been shown to be highly effective both for RLS symptoms and PLMS.[36] Indeed, a reduction of PLMS has often been chosen as a primary end point in polysomnographic clinical trials to assess the therapeutic response.[37–42] A first indirect clue that PLMS and RLS symptoms may respond differently to interventions is in the finding that the placebo response has been large for RLS symptoms but largely absent for PLMS.[43]

With the introduction of new pharmacologic treatments with a non-dopaminergic mode of action it has now become apparent that a decrease in PLMS is not a prerequisite for the successful treatment of RLS symptoms. The main non-dopaminergic drugs used, and by now also recommended,[33,44] for the treatment of RLS are the calcium channel alpha-2-delta ligands,[44] such as gabapentin, gabapentin enacarbil, and pregabalin. In **Table 2**, an overview of the effect of dopaminergic and non-dopaminergic drugs on PLMS is provided. It is readily apparent, as has long been known, that dopaminergic drugs have a consistent and strong effect on PLMS.[18,23,41,42,45] In contrast, the effect of non-dopaminergic drugs, even if not absent, is considerably smaller.[25,46–48] This difference is not only observable across studies but also, in those trials that have directly compared a dopaminergic with a non-dopaminergic agent,[24,49–51] the

decrease of PLMS was significantly smaller with non-dopaminergic substances.

It must be stressed that both drug classes have been shown to be effective in reducing RLS symptoms and that non-dopaminergic drugs, even when not affecting PLMS, often improved sleep quality to a greater extent that dopaminergic drugs.[24,49–51] Current international guidelines for the treatment of RLS now identify both dopaminergic and non-dopaminergic drugs as being first-line treatments of RLS.[33,44] At present, and as a consequence of these recent developments, the role of PLMS as a treatment target in RLS is undergoing a re-evaluation.

PERIODIC LEG MOVEMENTS DURING SLEEP AND TRANSIENT AUTONOMIC SYSTEM ACTIVATIONS

A consistent finding is the observation that PLMS are accompanied by transient increases in blood pressure[52–55] and heart rate.[56–63] The magnitude of these increases is modulated by sleep stage[57,58,61] and is increased when PLMS are bilateral[58,61] or accompanied by arousals.[53–56,61,63,64] Given that in patients with RLS many hundreds of PLMS may be observed in a single night, these frequent, repetitive nocturnal sympathetic system activations are the prime candidate mechanism for a possible pathophysiologic link between RLS and cardiovascular diseases. Indeed, PLMS, rather than RLS, are being discussed as a possible new sleep-related cardiovascular risk factor,[65] which might explain why the association of RLS with cardiovascular disease has been observed in many, but not all, studies.[66,67]

Concerning the specific role of PLMS in subjects with RLS, an important finding is that the magnitude of PLMS-associated increases in heart rate and blood pressure is significantly larger in patients with RLS compared with healthy controls with PLMS but without RLS.[54,62] In addition, a direct comparison between patients with RLS and healthy controls revealed no differences in various indicators of heart rate variability when periods of sleep without PLMS were compared between groups.[62] Together, this suggests a selective alteration of the phasic sympathetic activity rather than the sympathetic tone in RLS.

It is currently not well known whether in RLS this phasic sympathetic hyperactivation during sleep (ie, the larger activation compared with control subjects) is restricted to PLMS or also apparent for other phasic events of sleep, in particular arousals. The crucial question here is whether there is a generally increased number of autonomic nervous system activations during sleep in

Table 2
Change of PLMS with dopaminergic and non-dopaminergic treatment. Values are given as percentage of decrease from baseline unless otherwise specified

Study	Drug	Number	Duration Dosage	Decrease in PLMS (%)
Dopaminergic Drugs				
Allen et al,[42] 2004	Ropinirole	29	12 w 1.8 mg	76
Partinen et al,[41] 2006	Pramipexole	21	3 w 0.125 mg	94
		21	3 w 0.25 mg	91
		22	3 w 0.5 mg	91
		22	3 w 0.75 mg	57
Inuoe et al,[23] 2010	Pramipexole	20	6 w 0.75 mg	100
Oertel et al,[18] 2006	Cabergoline	20	5 w 2 mg	83
Oertel et al,[45] 2010	Rotigotine	41	7 w 3 mg	75
Dopaminergic and Non-dopaminergic Drugs				
Eisensehr et al,[49] 2004	SR levodopa	20	3 w 200 mg	53
	Valproic acid	20	3 w 600 mg	10
Garcia-Borreguero et al,[50] 2014	Pramipexole	76	4 w 0.5 mg	78
	Pregabalin	70	4 w 300 mg	39[a]
Happe et al,[51] 2003	Ropinirole	8	4 w 0.75 mg	73
	Gabapentin	8	4 w 750 mg	42
Saletu et al,[24] 2010	Ropinirole	40	1 d 0.5 mg	67[a]
	Gabapentin	40	1 d 300 mg	26[a]
Non-dopaminergic Drugs				
Garcia-Borreguero et al,[46] 2002	Gabapentin	22	6 w 1855 mg	47[a]
Garcia-Borreguero et al,[47] 2010	Pregabalin	30	12 w 337 mg	56
Kushida et al,[48] 2009	Gabapentin enacarbil	34	2 w 1800 mg	22
Winkelman et al,[25] 2011	Gabapentin enacarbil	131	4 w 1200 mg	27

Abbreviation: SR, slow release.
[a] Compared with placebo condition.

RLS that is restricted to PLMS or whether these may also be observed with the frequent non–PLMS-associated arousals or even occur as spontaneous activations unrelated to either PLMS or arousals. So far, all studies have chosen an event-related approach based on the PLMS and/or arousals and no study has quantified (1) how many of the PLMS or arousals are associated with a significant heart rate or blood pressure activation, or (2) how many of the activations are associated with PLMS or arousals in RLS. A major challenge in answering these questions is that so far there exists no published or accepted way to identify and classify the transient blood pressure and heart rate increases.

In this respect, the recently published methodology for the ENCORE study (Effects of Neupro on Cardiovascular Observations in Patients With Restless Legs Syndrome, NCT01455012), which was conducted to evaluate the effects of rotigotine on PLM-associated blood pressure excursion in RLS, represents a significant first step.[68] The double-blind, placebo-controlled, multicenter study included 89 patients with idiopathic RLS with a mean age of 57 years and an average PLMS index of 71. Continuous blood pressure monitoring was used and the investigators identified diastolic blood pressure (DBP) and systolic (SBP) blood pressure increases by an automated algorithm that identified all events with an average increase of greater than or equal to 2.5 mm Hg over 5 consecutive heartbeats. Results were given for time in bed and showed a high number of blood pressure increases, on average 788 SBP and 350 DBP increases during the course of the night. Because the study listed the average number of increases associated with PLMS and/or arousal, this allows to estimate how many BP increases were associated with PLMS and vice versa. For SBP, 33.5% of the 788 increases were associated with PLMS with (28.9%) or without arousal (4.6%), an additional 2.3% were associated to arousals without PLMS, but most (64.2%) were associated with neither PLMS nor arousals. A similar picture emerged for DBP increases, of which 40.8% were related to PLMS (34.0% without, 6.8% with arousal), 3.3% to arousals without PLMS, and 55.8% were unrelated to either. In contrast, 52% of all PLMS were associated with an SBP increase and 28% were associated with a DBP increase. Taken together, these numbers suggest that there is a close co-occurrence of PLMS with nocturnal blood pressure increases; however, even accounting for PLMS, there seems to be a large number of seemingly spontaneous blood pressure increases in patients with RLS. Results of the treatment part of the trial have so far only been reported in abstract form[69] but suggest that treatment with rotigotine led to a significant reduction of PLMS-associated BP increases.

If these promising results are confirmed, the next step will be to investigate whether such an effect on PLMS-associated nocturnal blood pressure activations also translates into a clinically meaningful impact on the cardiovascular risk profile in patients with RLS. If so, PLMS may be reborn as a significant treatment target in RLS.

SUMMARY AND OUTLOOK

Since the first polysomnographic recording of PLMS by Lugaresi and colleagues[70,71] in 1965 this enigmatic phenomenon has remained an active focus of research. As a result of this ongoing process, the role of PLMS in RLS is being re-characterized as more evidence accumulates. Major recent advances suggest that PLMS but not RLS symptoms are predominantly under dopaminergic control, whereas RLS symptoms respond to both dopaminergic and non-dopaminergic agents. This is supported by comparative treatment studies with dopaminergic and non-dopaminergic agents that show that the effect of non-dopaminergic compared with dopaminergic drugs on PLMS is considerably less or absent. At the same time, dopaminergic drugs have a smaller or absent effect on sleep disturbances and especially arousals in patients with RLS. Concurrently, PLMS are possibly emerging as a sleep-related cardiovascular risk factor owing to the association of these movements with the frequent, transient heart rate and blood pressure increases during the night. Should this new role of PLMS receive further support, PLMS may re-emerge as a clinically significant target of treatment in RLS.

REFERENCES

1. Iber C, Ancoli-Israel S, Chesson A, et al, American Academy of Sleep Medicine. The AASM manual for the scoring of sleep and associated events: rules, terminology and technical specifications. 1st edition. Westchester (IL): American Academy of Sleep Medicine; 2007.

2. Hornyak M, Feige B, Riemann D, et al. Periodic leg movements in sleep and periodic limb movement disorder: prevalence, clinical significance and treatment. Sleep Med Rev 2006;10:169–77.

3. Ancoli-Israel S, Kripke DF, Klauber MR, et al. Periodic limb movements in sleep in community-dwelling elderly. Sleep 1991;14:496–500.

4. Bixler EO, Kales A, Vela-Bueno A, et al. Nocturnal myoclonus and nocturnal myoclonic activity in the

normal population. Res Commun Chem Pathol Pharmacol 1982;36:129–40.

5. Morrish E, King MA, Pilsworth SN, et al. Periodic limb movement in a community population detected by a new actigraphy technique. Sleep Med 2002;3:489–95.

6. Scofield H, Roth T, Drake C. Periodic limb movements during sleep: population prevalence, clinical correlates, and racial differences. Sleep 2008;31:1221–7.

7. Trenkwalder C, Paulus W. Restless legs syndrome: pathophysiology, clinical presentation and management. Nat Rev Neurol 2010;6:337–46.

8. Allen RP, Picchietti D, Hening WA, et al. Restless legs syndrome: diagnostic criteria, special considerations, and epidemiology. A report from the restless Legs Syndrome Diagnosis and Epidemiology Workshop at the National Institutes of Health. Sleep Med 2003;4:101–19.

9. Allen RP, Picchietti DL, Garcia-Borreguero D, et al. Restless legs syndrome/Willis-Ekbom disease diagnostic criteria: updated International Restless Legs Syndrome Study Group (IRLSSG) consensus criteria – history, rationale, description, and significance. Sleep Med 2014;15:860–73.

10. Zucconi M, Ferri R, Allen R, et al. The official World Association of Sleep Medicine (WASM) standards for recording and scoring periodic leg movements in sleep (PLMS) and wakefulness (PLMW) developed in collaboration with a task force from the International Restless Legs Syndrome Study Group (IRLSSG). Sleep Med 2006;7:175–83.

11. El-Ad B, Chervin RD. The case of a missing PLM. Sleep 2000;23:450–1.

12. Michaud M, Paquet J, Lavigne G, et al. Sleep laboratory diagnosis of restless legs syndrome. Eur Neurol 2002;48:108–13.

13. Saletu B, Anderer P, Saletu M, et al. EEG mapping, psychometric, and polysomnographic studies in restless legs syndrome (RLS) and periodic limb movement disorder (PLMD) patients as compared with normal controls. Sleep Med 2002;3(Suppl):S35–42.

14. Eisensehr I, Ehrenberg BL, Noachtar S. Different sleep characteristics in restless legs syndrome and periodic limb movement disorder. Sleep Med 2003;4:147–52.

15. Garcia-Borreguero D, Larrosa O, de la Llave Y, et al. Correlation between rating scales and sleep laboratory measurements in restless legs syndrome. Sleep Med 2004;5:561–5.

16. Hornyak M, Riemann D, Voderholzer U. Do periodic leg movements influence patients' perception of sleep quality? Sleep Med 2004;5:597–600.

17. Hornyak M, Kopasz M, Feige B, et al. Variability of periodic leg movements in various sleep disorders: implications for clinical and pathophysiologic studies. Sleep 2005;28:331–5.

18. Oertel WH, Benes H, Bodenschatz R, et al. Efficacy of cabergoline in restless legs syndrome: a placebo-controlled study with polysomnography (CATOR). Neurology 2006;67:1040–6.

19. Hornyak M, Feige B, Voderholzer U, et al. Polysomnography findings in patients with restless legs syndrome and in healthy controls: a comparative observational study. Sleep 2007;30:861–5.

20. Hornyak M, Hundemer H-P, Quail D, et al. Relationship of periodic leg movements and severity of restless legs syndrome: a study in unmedicated and medicated patients. Clin Neurophysiol 2007;118:1532–7.

21. Boehm G, Wetter TC, Trenkwalder C. Periodic leg movements in RLS patients as compared to controls: are there differences beyond the PLM index? Sleep Med 2009;10:566–71.

22. Jama L, Hirvonen K, Partinen M, et al. A dose-ranging study of pramipexole for the symptomatic treatment of restless legs syndrome: polysomnographic evaluation of periodic leg movements and sleep disturbance. Sleep Med 2009;10:630–6.

23. Inoue Y, Hirata K, Kuroda K, et al. Efficacy and safety of pramipexole in Japanese patients with primary restless legs syndrome: a polysomnographic randomized, double-blind, placebo-controlled study. Sleep Med 2010;11:11–6.

24. Saletu M, Anderer P, Saletu-Zyhlarz GM, et al. Comparative placebo-controlled polysomnographic and psychometric studies on the acute effects of gabapentin versus ropinirole in restless legs syndrome. J Neural Transm 2010;117:463–73.

25. Winkelman JW, Bogan RK, Schmidt MH, et al. Randomized polysomnography study of gabapentin enacarbil in subjects with restless legs syndrome. Mov Disord 2011;26:2065–72.

26. Karadeniz D, Ondze B, Besset A, et al. EEG arousals and awakenings in relation with periodic leg movements during sleep. J Sleep Res 2000;9:273–7.

27. Ferri R, Rundo F, Zucconi M, et al. An evidence-based analysis of the association between periodic leg movements during sleep and arousals in restless legs syndrome. Sleep 2015;38:919–24.

28. Berry R, Brooks R, Gamaldo C, et al. The AASM manual for the scoring of sleep and associated events: rules, terminology and technical specifications, version 2.0.1. 2nd edition. Darien (IL): American Academy of Sleep Medicine; 2013.

29. Manconi M, Ferri R, Zucconi M, et al. Dissociation of periodic leg movements from arousals in restless legs syndrome. Ann Neurol 2012;71:834–44.

30. Ferri R, Manconi M, Aricò D, et al. Acute dopamine-agonist treatment in restless legs syndrome: effects on sleep architecture and NREM sleep instability. Sleep 2010;33:793–800.

31. Montplaisir J, Boucher S, Gosselin A, et al. Persistence of repetitive EEG arousals (K-alpha

complexes) in RLS patients treated with L-DOPA. Sleep 1996;19:196–9.

32. Tagaya H, Wetter TC, Winkelmann J, et al. Pergolide restores sleep maintenance but impairs sleep EEG synchronization in patients with restless legs syndrome. Sleep Med 2002;3:49–54.

33. Garcia-Borreguero D, Kohnen R, Silber MH, et al. The long-term treatment of restless legs syndrome/Willis-Ekbom disease: evidence-based guidelines and clinical consensus best practice guidance: a report from the International Restless Legs Syndrome Study Group. Sleep Med 2013;14:675–84.

34. Hening WA. Current guidelines and standards of practice for restless legs syndrome. Am J Med 2007;120:S22–7.

35. Trenkwalder C, Hening WA, Montagna P, et al. Treatment of restless legs syndrome: an evidence-based review and implications for clinical practice. Mov Disord 2008;23:2267–302.

36. Hornyak M, Trenkwalder C, Kohnen R, et al. Efficacy and safety of dopamine agonists in restless legs syndrome. Sleep Med 2012;13:228–36.

37. Brodeur C, Montplaisir J, Godbout R, et al. Treatment of restless legs syndrome and periodic movements during sleep with L-dopa: a double-blind, controlled study. Neurology 1988;38:1845–8.

38. Kaplan PW, Allen RP, Buchholz DW, et al. A double-blind, placebo-controlled study of the treatment of periodic limb movements in sleep using carbidopa/levodopa and propoxyphene. Sleep 1993;16:717–23.

39. Trenkwalder C, Hundemer HP, Lledo A, et al. Efficacy of pergolide in treatment of restless legs syndrome: the PEARLS Study. Neurology 2004;62:1391–7.

40. Ferini-Strambi L, Aarskog D, Partinen M, et al. Effect of pramipexole on RLS symptoms and sleep: a randomized, double-blind, placebo-controlled trial. Sleep Med 2008;9:874–81.

41. Partinen M, Hirvonen K, Jama L, et al. Efficacy and safety of pramipexole in idiopathic restless legs syndrome: a polysomnographic dose-finding study–the PRELUDE study. Sleep Med 2006;7:407–17.

42. Allen R, Becker PM, Bogan R, et al. Ropinirole decreases periodic leg movements and improves sleep parameters in patients with restless legs syndrome. Sleep 2004;27:907–14.

43. Fulda S, Wetter TC. Where dopamine meets opioids: a meta-analysis of the placebo effect in restless legs syndrome treatment studies. Brain 2008;131:902–17.

44. Garcia-Borreguero D, Ferini-Strambi L, Kohnen R, et al. European guidelines on management of restless legs syndrome: report of a joint task force by the European Federation of Neurological Societies, the European Neurological Society and the European Sleep Research Society. Eur J Neurol 2012;19:1385–96.

45. Oertel WH, Benes H, Garcia-Borreguero D, et al. Rotigotine transdermal patch in moderate to severe idiopathic restless legs syndrome: a randomized, placebo-controlled polysomnographic study. Sleep Med 2010;11:848–56.

46. Garcia-Borreguero D, Larrosa O, de la Llave Y, et al. Treatment of restless legs syndrome with gabapentin: a double-blind, cross-over study. Neurology 2002;59:1573–9.

47. Garcia-Borreguero D, Larrosa O, Williams A-M, et al. Treatment of restless legs syndrome with pregabalin: a double-blind, placebo-controlled study. Neurology 2010;74:1897–904.

48. Kushida CA, Walters AS, Becker P, et al. A randomized, double-blind, placebo-controlled, crossover study of XP13512/GSK1838262 in the treatment of patients with primary restless legs syndrome. Sleep 2009;32:159–68.

49. Eisensehr I, Ehrenberg BL, Rogge Solti S, et al. Treatment of idiopathic restless legs syndrome (RLS) with slow-release valproic acid compared with slow-release levodopa/benserazid. J Neurol 2004;251:579–83.

50. Garcia-Borreguero D, Patrick J, DuBrava S, et al. Pregabalin versus pramipexole: effects on sleep disturbance in restless legs syndrome. Sleep 2014;37:635–43.

51. Happe S, Sauter C, Klösch G, et al. Gabapentin versus ropinirole in the treatment of idiopathic restless legs syndrome. Neuropsychobiology 2003;48:82–6.

52. Ali NJ, Davies RJO, Fleetham JA, et al. Periodic movements of the legs during sleep associated with rises in systemic blood pressure. Sleep 1991;14:163–5.

53. Pennestri MH, Montplaisir J, Colombo R, et al. Nocturnal blood pressure changes in patients with restless legs syndrome. Neurology 2007;68:1213–8.

54. Pennestri M-H, Montplaisir J, Fradette L, et al. Blood pressure changes associated with periodic leg movements during sleep in healthy subjects. Sleep Med 2013;14:555–61.

55. Siddiqui F, Strus J, Ming X, et al. Rise of blood pressure with periodic limb movements in sleep and wakefulness. Clin Neurophysiol 2007;118:1923–30.

56. Winkelman JW. The evoked heart rate response to periodic leg movements of sleep. Sleep 1999;22:575–80.

57. Allena M, Campus C, Morrone E, et al. Periodic limb movements both in non-REM and REM sleep: relationships between cerebral and autonomic activities. Clin Neurophysiol 2009;120:1282–90.

58. Ferri R, Zucconi M, Rundo F, et al. Heart rate and spectral EEG changes accompanying periodic and non-periodic leg movements during sleep. Clin Neurophysiol 2007;118:438–48.

59. Ferrillo F, Beelke M, Canovaro P, et al. Changes in cerebral and autonomic activity heralding periodic limb movements in sleep. Sleep Med 2004;5:407–12.

60. Gosselin N, Lanfranchi P, Michaud M, et al. Age and gender effects on heart rate activation associated with periodic leg movements in patients with restless legs syndrome. Clin Neurophysiol 2003;114:2188–95.

61. Lavoie S, de Bilbao F, Haba-Rubio J, et al. Influence of sleep stage and wakefulness on spectral EEG activity and heart rate variations around periodic leg movements. Clin Neurophysiol 2004;115:2236–46.

62. Manconi M, Ferri R, Zucconi M, et al. Effects of acute dopamine-agonist treatment in restless legs syndrome on heart rate variability during sleep. Sleep Med 2011;12:47–55.

63. Sforza E, Nicolas A, Lavigne G, et al. EEG and cardiac activation during periodic leg movements in sleep: support for a hierarchy of arousal responses. Neurology 1999;52:786–91.

64. Sforza E, Juony C, Ibanez V. Time-dependent variation in cerebral and autonomic activity during periodic leg movements in sleep: implications for arousal mechanisms. Clin Neurophysiol 2002;113:883–91.

65. Alessandria M, Provini F. Periodic limb movements during sleep: a new sleep-related cardiovascular risk factor? Front Neurol 2013;4:116.

66. Ferini-Strambi L, Walters AS, Sica D. The relationship among restless legs syndrome (Willis-Ekbom Disease), hypertension, cardiovascular disease, and cerebrovascular disease. J Neurol 2014;261:1051–68.

67. Walters AS, Rye DB. Review of the relationship of restless legs syndrome and periodic limb movements in sleep to hypertension, heart disease, and stroke. Sleep 2009;32:589–97.

68. Cassel W, Kesper K, Bauer A, et al. Significant association between systolic and diastolic blood pressure elevations and periodic limb movements in patients with idiopathic restless legs syndrome. Sleep Med 2015. http://dx.doi.org/10.1016/j.sleep.2014.12.019.

69. Grieger F, Schollmayer E, Moran K, et al. The effect of rotigotine on nocturnal blood pressure changes and periodic limb movements of sleep in patients with idiopathic RLS: the encore study. Sleep Med 2013;14(Supplement 1):e304–5.

70. Lugaresi E, Coccagna G, Tassinari CA, et al. Polygraphic data on motor phenomena in the restless legs syndrome. Riv Neurol 1965;35:550–61 [in Italian].

71. Lugaresi E, Tassinari CA, Coccagna G, et al. Particulariés cliniques et polygraphiques du syndrome d'impatience des membres inférieurs. Rev Neurol 1965;13:545–55.

Differential Diagnoses of Restless Legs Syndrome/Willis-Ekbom Disease
Mimics and Comorbidities

Sudhansu Chokroverty, MD, FRCP[a,b,*]

KEYWORDS

- Restless legs syndrome • Differential diagnoses • Willis-Ekbom disease • Mimics • Comorbidities

KEY POINTS

- Restless legs syndrome (RLS) mimics cannot always be differentiated from RLS/Willis-Ekbom disease (WED) based on 4 essential criteria; hence, a fifth criterion has recently been established.
- RLS comorbidities (associated conditions) may provide us important clues for understanding the neurobiology of RLS/WED.
- Iron-dopamine connection, hypoxia pathway activation, and dopamine-opioid interaction are important pathophysiological mechanisms in RLS; this knowledge is derived from our understanding of RLS associations with a variety of medical, neurologic, and other conditions.
- Clinicians must formulate an RLS differential diagnosis based mainly on history and physical examination, but laboratory tests may sometimes be needed to arrive at a correct diagnosis.

Since establishing 4 essential diagnostic criteria for restless legs syndrome/Willis-Ekbom disease (RLS/WED)[1] in 1995 and then slightly modified in 2003,[2] it was realized based on scientific study that some conditions that mimic RLS/WED cannot be differentiated based on these 4 criteria. Hence, the International Restless Legs Syndrome Study Group added a fifth criterion[3] based on expert consensus Diagnostic Criteria of RLS (**Box 1**) to differentiate RLS/WED from these mimics. In addition, several conditions have been suggested to be associated with RLS/WED (symptomatic or secondary). Many of these conditions share an association with depleted iron stores (eg, iron-deficiency anemia, renal failure, pregnancy, rheumatoid arthritis), but others remain unexplored because of a single pathophysiologic diathesis. An intriguing question is whether these comorbid conditions are actually responsible for RLS/WED or the

recently reported RLS-specific genetic variants (eg, BTBD9, MEIS1) confer an increased risk of RLS/WED in these comorbid conditions. This article briefly summarizes the conditions mimicking RLS/WED in the first section, pointing out the distinction from true RLS/WED, as well as addressing these comorbid conditions in the second section so that corrective actions can be taken to alleviate or eliminate these associated conditions for optimal management of RLS/WED.

CONDITIONS MIMICKING RESTLESS LEGS SYNDROME/WILLIS-EKBOM DISEASE

Although these mimics do not cause RLS, it is important to be familiar with them to differentiate them from RLS/WED. These mimics can be classified into 4 major cases (**Box 2**):

1. Those that present with abnormal restlessness

[a] Department of Neurology, JFK Neuroscience Institute, Edison, NJ 08818, USA; [b] Department of Neuroscience, Seton Hall University, South Orange, NJ, USA

* Department of Neurology, JFK Neuroscience Institute, Edison, NJ 08818.

E-mail address: schok@att.net

Sleep Med Clin 10 (2015) 249–262
http://dx.doi.org/10.1016/j.jsmc.2015.05.021

Box 1
Five essential diagnostic criteria for RLS/WED

[a]Criterion 1. An urge to move the legs, usually but not always accompanied by uncomfortable sensations in the legs.

Criterion 2. The urge to move the legs with any accompanying unpleasant sensations begins or worsens during periods of inactivity or quiescence such as lying down or sitting.

Criterion 3. The urge to move the legs with any accompanying unpleasant sensations is partially or totally relieved by movement, such as walking or stretching, as long as the activity continues.

Criterion 4. The urge to move the legs with any accompanying unpleasant sensations during rest or inactivity only occurs or is worse in the evening or night than during the day.

Criterion 5. The above features are not accounted by another medical or behavioral condition (eg, myalgia, arthritis, venous stasis, leg cramps, positional discomfort or habitual foot tapping).

[a] The adult and the pediatric diagnostic criteria are merged together except that the description of these symptoms in criterion 1 should be in the child's own words.

Box 2
Conditions that can be confused with RLS/WED

Presenting with abnormal restlessness

- Akathisia
  - Neuroleptic induced
  - Related to central nervous system degenerative or infectious disease
- Disorders of abnormal muscular activity
  - Myokymia
  - Essential myoclonus
  - Orthostatic tremor
  - Orthostatic myoclonus
- Anxiety/depression
- Attention-deficit/hyperactivity disorder
- Orthostatic hypotensive restlessness while sitting
- Leg stereotypy disorder

Presenting with nocturnal leg discomfort or pain

- Growing pains
- Small fiber neuropathies
- Venous stasis–varicose veins
- Myalgias
- Arthritis
- Radiculopathies
- Delusional parasitosis

Presenting with combined unusual motor activity and leg discomfort or pain

- Painful muscle cramps, including nocturnal leg cramps
- Painful legs and moving toes syndrome
- Muscular pain–fasciculation syndrome
- Cramp-fasciculation syndrome
- Causalgia-dystonia syndrome
- Intermittent claudication

Presenting with nocturnal hypermotor activity

- Rhythmic movement disorder
- Periodic limb movement disorder
- Hypnagogic foot tremor
- Alternative leg muscle activation
- Hypnic jerks
- Propriospinal myoclonus at sleep onset

---

2. Those presenting with nocturnal leg discomfort or pain
3. Those presenting with combined unusual motor activity and leg discomfort or pain
4. Those presenting with nocturnal hypermotor activity

Akathisia

This condition can be mistaken for RLS/WED, but there are many differentiating features as shown in **Table 1**. The term *akathisia* is derived from the Greek word meaning "inability to sit." The term *akathisia* was first used in 1901 by Ludwig Haskov,[4] the Czech neuropsychiatrist ascribing this to hysteria. However, *akathisia* has emerged as an important side effect of neuroleptics in the second half of the twentieth century; neuroleptic-induced akathisia (NIA) remains the most familiar and acceptable term in contemporary writings.

Table 1
Differentiating features RLS/WED and Akathisia

Characteristics	RLS/WED	Akathisia
An urge to move	+	+
Motor restlessness	+ (Localized, usually to the legs, sometimes the arms except in augmentation when it could be generalized)	+ (Generalized or whole body)
Tasikinesia (forced walking)	−	+
Uncomfortable sensation	+ (Usually and localized to the legs)	−
Inner restlessness	−	+
Circadian pattern of symptoms	+	−
Relief by movement	+	−
Sleep disturbance (hyposomnia)	+ (Often severe)	− (Or mild)
Triggered by	Quiescence	Neuroleptics
PLMS	+ (>80% of cases)	+ (Occasionally)
Family history	+ in 50%–60%	−
Physical examination	Noncontributory except in secondary cases	Evidence of akathisia and sometimes drug-induced extrapyramidal manifestations
Best treatment	Dopamine agonist or alph-2-delta ligands	Anticholinergics or beta-adrenergic antagonists

−, Absent; +, Present.
Abbreviation: PLMS, periodic limb movements in sleep.

This condition can be acute, chronic, or tardive and related to withdrawal of neuroleptics. There are two essential clinical components: subjective feeling of inner restlessness and forced walking (tasikinesia) as objective evidence of motor restlessness. The US Food and Drug Administration Task Force,[5] in 1973, defined *akathisia* as "a subjective desire to be in constant motion" associated with "an inability to sit or stand still," and "a drive to pace up and down." The inner feeling of restlessness or fidgetiness results in motor manifestations consisting of difficulty sitting still, crossing and uncrossing legs, swaying and rocking of the whole body, marching in place, and constantly shifting body positions while sitting. These movements resemble chorea rather than the voluntary and myoclonic awake movements sometimes seen in patients with RLS/WED. These movements are uncontrollable and involuntary, although suppressible temporarily. These near-constant movements are present throughout the day and may become worse in the evening without relieving the intense desire to move and without any circadian pattern unlike those noted in RLS/WED. Although there are similarities, there are

distinct differences in the manifestations between NIA and RLS/WED as shown in **Table 1**.

Sometimes NIA manifests as focal *akathisia* or monoakathisia[6–8] characterized by rhythmic swaying of the leg while sitting and flexing the knee intermittently while standing up. Sometimes, patients with RLS/WED may also present with unilateral manifestation; therefore, using the term *focal akathisia* to describe RLS/WED features may create confusion. It is also important to remember that mild cases of NIA may show variability with intermittent manifestation similar to that noted in some patients with RLS/WED, particularly in the early stage of the illness. However, as seen in **Table 1**, other distinctive features[9] should clearly differentiate unilateral or early mild cases of RLS/WED from monoakathisia and mild NIA.

Essential Myoclonus

This condition may superficially resemble RLS/WED, causing some diagnostic confusion. Essential myoclonus usually appears in the first or second decade of life, and this can be familial or nonfamilial. The movements consist of sudden shocklike muscle jerks, which may be seen synchronously or asynchronously, symmetrically or asymmetrically, diffusely or focally, and rhythmically or arrhythmically.[10] Electromyography (EMG) burst duration, however, is much briefer than that noted in RLS or periodic limb movements in sleep (PLMS). In this condition, there are no urges to move the limbs and no preference for occurrence in the evening or during quiescence. Sometimes true myoclonic movements during rest and inactivity may be seen in patients with RLS, but the clinical and EMG characteristics differentiate essential myoclonus easily from RLS/WED.

Hypnic Jerks

Hypnic jerks or sleep starts are physiologic phenomena causing a sudden start or excitation of the motor center at the moment of sleep onset[11] experienced by up to 70% of the adult population sometime in their life. Intensified hypnic jerks denote accentuated hypnic jerks that may occur repeatedly causing sleep-onset insomnia.[12,13] These jerks may be triggered by stress, fatigue, or sleep deprivation; they are totally different from the essential diagnostic criteria of RLS.

Painful Legs and Moving Toes Syndrome

Painful legs and moving toes syndrome (PLMTS) is characterized by spontaneous, purposeless, and involuntary movements of the toes consisting of flexion, extension, abduction, and adduction accompanied by pain (deep aching or pulling) in the feet or the lower parts of the legs. Since the original description by Spillane and colleagues[14] in 1971, PLMTS has shown considerable variation. Patients may present with or without pain, unilaterally or bilaterally, and occasionally with similar manifestations in the arms; these presentations have been described in scattered case reports. The movements of the toes do not relieve the pain in contrast to that noted in RLS/WED. The movements are also not prominent during sleep and not particularly intense in the evening, thus differentiating it from RLS/WED by the absence of a circadian factor in this condition. Both central and peripheral mechanisms have been implicated as causation, but most cases result from a peripheral cause. Electrophysiological studies to characterize the EMG burst pattern have been limited; in one study,[15] 2 distinct EMG burst patterns have been described: synchronous activities in the agonist and antagonist muscles in the peripheral type and alternating EMG bursts in the agonist and antagonist muscles in the central type. In contrast, in our[16] physiologic observations, including polysomnographic study in several

patients, we noted a mixture of dystonic and myoclonic, synchronous, asynchronous, and rhythmic EMG bursts, which show a decrement during all stages of sleep but intermittent persistence during awake periods, non–rapid eye movement (NREM) sleep, particularly in the lighter stages, and occasionally in REM sleep. These findings are similar to other involuntary movements decreasing but not completely disappearing in sleep and reappearing during arousal and stage transitions. These electrophysiologic findings suggest a complex pathophysiology that may involve both peripheral afferent and supraspinal efferent control. The condition is present throughout the day without particular intensification during quiescence or evening in contrast to the findings in RLS/WED.

Muscular Pain/Fasciculation Syndrome

This rare condition is characterized by widespread fasciculation that has often been made worse by exercise, anxiety, or consumption of coffee accompanying occasional cramps at night and dull aching pain in the limbs.[17] Patients may complain of restlessness of the legs, but the symptoms do not necessarily improve on walking or with exercise; these findings clearly differentiate the condition from the essential diagnostic criteria of RLS/WED.

Cramp/Fasciculation Syndrome

This condition is another rare condition that resembles muscular pain/fasciculation syndrome; but this is characterized by hyperexcitability of the peripheral nerve, and patients present with calf fasciculation, muscle aching, cramps, stiffness, and exercise intolerance.[18] The characteristic EMG findings show afterdischarges after the main compound muscle action potentials, and these are abolished by regional curare but persist after nerve blocks suggesting an abnormal excitability in the distal motor axon. The condition resembles Isaac syndrome, and these patients improve following carbamazepine therapy. However, the clinical features of this condition are different from those in RLS/WED because these symptoms are present throughout the day and there is no circadian variation and no improvement on movements.

Causalgia-Dystonia Syndrome

This rare condition is characterized by dystonic muscle spasms usually in the legs in most of the cases, at least initially; but the arms may also be affected later.[19] Generally, causalgia and dystonia are noted simultaneously; the condition is often triggered by minor trauma. The patients complain of burning pain, allodynia, and hyperpathia accompanied by vasomotor and trophic skin changes. There is no circadian feature, and these clinical manifestations are easy to differentiate from RLS. The nature of the condition is unknown.

Myokymia

This condition is characterized by slow, vermicular, spontaneous contractions of broad strips of muscles that may or may not disappear during sleep depending on whether the condition resulted from a peripheral or a central nervous system disorder. Myokymia may be noted occasionally in normal individuals after fatigue, particularly the eyelid myokymia. Sometimes these movements in the calf muscles resemble restlessness of the legs. Masland[20] first noted an association between myokymia and RLS/WED. The characteristic features, however, of myokymia, the localized nature of the symptoms, and the lack of a clear relationship with quiescence or time of the day differentiate this from RLS.

Leg Stereotypy Disorder

This condition is not very well described in the literature and is often observed in people while they are sitting in meetings exhibiting stereotypic 1- to 2-Hz rhythmic flexion-extension movements of the hips with toes resting on the floor.[21] The movements may last from seconds to hours and go away when standing or walking. The individuals can stop the movements easily voluntarily. Many patients complain of an intense need to move the legs resulting from an inner restlessness feeling or an anxiety that is transiently relieved by the movement, thus superficially resembling RLS;

but this condition is present throughout the day and not particularly prominent in the evening, thus differentiating this from RLS. It is also not associated with any unpleasant sensations.

Painful Nocturnal Leg Cramps

Muscle cramps are very common, may occur from central or peripheral neurologic disorders, and symptoms may occur at rest or may be induced by exercise. A special variety of muscle cramp known as nocturnal leg cramp[22] is characterized by painful spasms of the legs usually in the calf but occasionally in the foot noted during sleep at night. The cramps may cause arousal from sleep and can be relieved by local massage or movement of the affected limb; thus, superficially, the condition resembles RLS/WED. Nocturnal leg cramps are not present during quiescence and are not necessarily present in the evening, and there is no urge to move the limbs. The cramps are often visible because of contractions of strips of muscles, and these painful leg cramps can be relieved by dorsiflexion of the foot. The electromyographic examination shows bursts of activities in the gastrocnemius muscles at random. The clinical features and the EMG should be able to differentiate the condition from RLS (**Table 2**). However, cramps can sometimes satisfy all four diagnostic essential criteria of RLS, which were initially established; therefore, the fifth criterion, established recently, specifically mentions that these symptoms should not be explained by another condition like cramps or positional discomfort. Muscle cramps can also occur in daytime; there are varieties of causes, including motor neuron disease, tetany, uremia, hypocalcemia, hyponatremia, hypomagnesemia, chronic polyneuropathy, and

Table 2
Differentiating features RLS/WED and nocturnal leg cramps

Characteristics	RLS/WED	Nocturnal Leg Cramps
An urge to move	+	−
Uncomfortable sensation	+ (Painful in up to 35%–40% of cases)	+ (Painful in 100% of cases)
Relief by	Any movement (usually of the legs)	Specific movement (eg, dorsiflexion of the foot in case of calf cramps)
Onset	Gradual	Sudden
Circadian pattern of symptoms	+	− (Always nocturnal)
Duration	Hours	Minutes
Distribution of symptoms	Usually in the legs but may be in the arms also	Localized to the calf with palpable contracting muscle
Response to dopaminergic drug	+	−

−, Absent; +, Present.

muscle diseases, such as myoglobinuria, myo-phosphorylase and phosphofructokinase defi-ciency, myotonia, stiff man syndrome, myokymia, tetanus, and neuromyotonia.

Orthostatic Hypotensive Restlessness

A distinct clinical syndrome has been described in patients with autonomic failure characterized by orthostatic hypotension and habitual, voluntary, transiently suppressible yet irresistible leg move-ments occurring only in the sitting position.[23] These symptoms are totally different from the essential diagnostic criteria of RLS. In addition, patients may complain of faint feelings in the up-right position along with restlessness of the legs. Recording of blood pressure in the supine and standing position will document significant ortho-static decrease of blood pressure. These symp-toms will improve when patients lie down in contrast to those seen in patients with RLS.

Orthostatic Tremor

Orthostatic tremor (OT) is a clinical syndrome characterized by tremulousness of the legs within seconds to minutes on standing up. The condition is sometimes called shaky legs syndrome, and this shakiness improves on walking. Because of restlessness or shakiness, the condition superfi-cially resembles RLS; improvement on walking also resembles RLS. However, this lacks all the essential diagnostic criteria of RLS, such as the urge to move and the circadian pattern of symp-toms. Also, when patients are lying down, there is no OT noted. Electromyographic study shows a characteristic tremor at a rate of 15 to 17 Hz prominent in the legs.[24] Since the term OT was coined by Heilman,[25] there has been a contro-versy about OT being a variant of essential tremor; but[26] the characteristic clinical features and the EMG findings differential OT from essen-tial tremor.

Intermittent Claudication

In this condition resulting from peripheral vascular disease, patients complain of pain and dysesthe-sia in the legs on walking but relieved by rest or on lying down, which are totally different from the symptoms of RLS present in quiescence and relieved by movement. In intermittent claudication, there is no urge to move and there is no circadian pattern. Patients usually do not complain of sleep disturbance, and the examination may reveal feeble pulsation in the peripheral arteries of the legs.

Attention-Deficit/Hyperactivity Disorder and Growing Pains

Many children with a diagnosis of growing pains may actually be having early symptoms of RLS, and several cases of childhood-onset of RLS have been described.[27] A subgroup of patients with growing pains has symptoms of attention-deficit/hyperactivity disorder (ADHD).[28] Some of these pa-tients with ADHD present with leg paresthesia; in fact, this could be a subgroup of childhood-onset RLS. These patients have nocturnal motor activity, and polysomnographic study may show an increased PLMS index in many of these patients. The painful symptoms in the condition of growing pains are relieved by massage rather than move-ment. However, some growing pains seemed to be a form of RLS or a precursor to adult RLS.[28]

Rheumatic Disorders

Because of pain and discomfort in the legs, arthritis may occasionally mimic RLS/WED. The symptoms, however, are localized to the joints and are aggravated by movement and walking without any circadian pattern, which are all in contrast to RLS/WED symptoms.

Periodic Limb Movements in Sleep

PLMS should not be equated with a diagnosis of RLS/WED because PLMS is a polysomnography (PSG) finding noted in sleep, whereas RLS is a dis-ease of quiescence during wakefulness. PLMS is characterized by periodically recurring stereo-typed limb movements, particularly dorsiflexion of the ankles and sometimes flexion of the knees and hips with a duration of EMG bursts of 0.5 to 10.0 seconds during predominantly NREM sleep occurring for at least 4 consecutive movements at an intermovement interval of 5 to 90 seconds (an average of 20–40 seconds).[22]

PLMS appears most commonly in RLS (at least in 80% of cases) but may also occur in several other medical, neurologic, and sleep disorders as well as with ingestion of medications (eg, selective serotonin reuptake inhibitors [SSRIs], tricyclic anti-depressants) and even in normal individuals, espe-cially in those aged 65 years or older. When PLMS (unassociated with RLS) is thought to cause repeated awakening and sleep fragmentation associated with impaired daytime functioning or excessive daytime sleepiness (not explainable by another medical, neurologic, psychiatric, or other sleep disorder), the condition is classified as peri-odic limb movement disorder in the current *Inter-national Classification of Sleep Disorders, Third*

Edition.[22] This entity is highly controversial, and many sleep specialists consider PLMS as simply a PSG physiologic phenomenon without a specific clinical significance.[29,30]

RESTLESS LEGS SYNDROME/WILLIS-EKBOM DISEASE COMORBIDITIES (SYMPTOMATIC OR SECONDARY CASES)

Several conditions have been suggested to be associated with RLS/WED, which are labeled as secondary or symptomatic cases, implying a causal relationship that remains to be determined and, hence, should be classified as comorbid conditions (**Box 3**).

Pregnancy and Restless Legs Syndrome/Willis-Ekbom Disease

A high prevalence of RLS symptoms was noted by Ekbom[31] in his original description. Subsequent case series and epidemiologic studies found that up to 20% to 27% of pregnant women have RLS/WED symptoms, most prominently in the third trimester.[32–39] In most women, symptoms appeared for the first time during pregnancy with subsequent resolution of symptoms within a week after delivery; but in some with previously diagnosed RLS, the symptoms worsened during pregnancy. There are several factors that are thought to be responsible for the occurrence or exacerbation of symptoms during pregnancy, such as iron and folate deficiencies, hormonal changes (eg, increased estrogen, progesterone, and prolactin levels), and mechanical factors causing vascular congestion in the legs.[35,37,40–42]

Polyneuropathies and Lumbosacral Polyradiculopathies

The prevalence of peripheral neuropathy in RLS/WED has been reported to be higher than that of the general population in some but not in all studies. For differentiating comorbid polyneuropathies and lumbosacral radiculopathies presenting with RLS-like symptoms from primary (idiopathic) RLS, particular attention should be paid to the nature of the sensory symptoms. The sensory symptoms of polyneuropathies or radiculopathies are present either intermittently or throughout the day and not necessarily worse in the evening and generally are not relieved by movements, thus differentiating these symptoms from evening worsening and relief of symptoms by movements in RLS/WED. Up to 35% to 40% of patients with RLS complain of actual pain that resembles central pain syndrome characterized by deep, disagreeable, unpleasant,

---

Box 3
RLS comorbidities (symptomatic or secondary disorders)

Medical disorders
- Iron deficiency and anemia
- Renal failure
- Rheumatologic disorders
- Diabetes mellitus
- Hypothyroidism
- Chronic obstructive pulmonary disease
- Congestive cardiac failure
- Hyperthyroidism
- Thrombophlebitis
- Magnesium deficiency
- Celiac disease
- Crohn disease
- Sjögren syndrome
- Obstructive sleep apnea

Neurologic disease
- Parkinson disease
- Multiple sclerosis
- Myelopathies
- Polyneuropathies
- Meralgia paresthetica
- Saphenous nerve entrapment
- Cortical and subcortical infarctions
- Lumbosacral radiculopathies
- Isaac syndrome
- Stiff man syndrome
- Spinocerebellar ataxia (SCA 3)
- Hyperekplexia

Surgical conditions
- Gastric reduction
- Lung transplantation

Medications
- Tricyclic antidepressants
- SSRIs
- Neuroleptics
- Dopamine antagonists
- Antihistamines (mostly H1 antagonists)
- Nonsteroidal antiinflammatory drugs

- Lithium
- Antinausea agents (eg metoclopramide)

Miscellaneous

- Pregnancy
- Blood donors
- ADHD/growing Pains
- Spinal anesthesia (transient RLS)

often nonlocalizable and nonradiating pain unaccompanied by objective sensory impairment in contrast to symptoms of tingling, numbness, burning, or stabbing (hyperalgesia) in a stocking-and-glove distribution or radiating along the root distribution accompanied by sensory impairment distally or along the root distribution in polyneuropathies or radiculopathies.

Gemignani and collaborators,[43,44] in several prospective and retrospective studies, postulated a frequent association of RLS with a subgroup of patients with painful polyneuropathies caused by nociceptive differentiation at the spinal level. RLS is also found to have a higher prevalence than controls in acquired, particularly dysimmune neuropathies (eg, chronic inflammatory demyelinating polyneuropathy) as well as in some inherited neuropathies (eg, Charcot-Marie-Tooth Type 1A).[45–49] There are, however, contradictory reports. In an earlier systematic study, Rutkove and collaborators,[50] in a consecutive series of patients with polyneuropathy, found a 5% frequency of RLS/WED, which is similar to that observed in the general population. Hattan and colleagues,[51] in a case-control series of 245 patients with polyneuropathies and 245 age- and sex-matched controls, observed that the overall prevalence of RLS after diagnostic confirmation did not differ between patients with neuropathy (12.2% vs controls 8.2%; $P = .14$). When classified by cause, however, these investigators noted a higher prevalence in patients with hereditary neuropathy than in acquired neuropathies and controls. RLS may also be particularly prevalent in certain types of neuropathies (eg, diabetic, cryoglobulinemic, or familial amyloid polyneuropathies[52]). Lim and colleagues,[53] based on their studies in 56 patients with idiopathic RLS and 36 age- and sex-matched controls, using quantitative sensory and sudomotor axon reflex tests concluded that abnormal sensory perception in patients with RLS/WED resulted from an impairment of central somatosensory processing rather than small fiber neuropathy. On the other hand, morphologic studies found evidence of subtle nerve damage.

Sural nerve biopsy findings[54] in 7 out of 8 patients with primary RLS were consistent with an axonal neuropathy, and skin punch biopsy[55] in the legs found evidence of subclinical small fiber neuropathy in 8 of 22 patients (36% with primary RLS). An explanation for these subtle morphologic changes may be age-related changes in these nerves and trauma caused by vigorous rubbing of the legs, resulting from an urge to move and rub to get relief from the uncomfortable sensation and urge. It is not clear why only a minority of patients with neuropathy, radiculopathies, or other lower motor neuron disorders develop RLS symptoms unless they are genetically predisposed.

Restless Legs Syndrome/Willis-Ekbom Disease, Iron Deficiency, and Anemia

There is strong evidence for iron deficiency, at least in one major subgroup of RLS/WED. Although Ekbom,[31] in his original description, mentioned iron deficiency, it was Nordlander[56] who in 1953 first demonstrated improvement of RLS symptoms in more than 90% of subjects after intravenous iron infusion. O'Keeffe and colleagues[57] revived the iron-deficiency theory in 1994 reporting low iron, measured by serum ferritin (the primary storage protein for iron) levels in patients with RLS. Subsequent elegant studies by the Johns Hopkins group of investigators[58–64] firmly established the role of iron in its pathogenesis and therapy. Iron is needed as a cofactor for tyrosine hydroxylase, the rate-limiting enzyme in the synthesis of dopamine; therefore, iron deficiency may interfere with the normal production of dopamine. Both iron and dopamine show a circadian rhythm, with the lowest levels occurring at night when RLS symptoms are worse. MRI of the brain[63] and limited pathologic findings[64] in patients with RLS clearly established brain iron acquisition and storage problems in the substantia nigra of these patients. The appearance of RLS symptoms after multiple blood donations[65,66] associated with iron-deficiency anemia, low serum hemoglobin and ferritin levels, and improvement after iron supplementation also point to the role of iron deficiency in the pathogenesis of RLS. Furthermore, iron deficiency may cause activation of hypoxic pathways (central and peripheral), another postulated pathogenetic mechanism for RLS symptoms.[67,68] However, not all iron-deficient states are associated with RLS and not all patients with RLS show iron deficiency. Therein lies the dilemma. Reports of failure[69,70] to find a significant difference in serum iron indices or hemoglobin between patients with RLS and control subjects with renal failure and pregnancy as well as a single report[71] failing to show a significant difference in RLS symptoms with iron supplementation after a randomized, double-blind, placebo-controlled, clinical trial pointed to the contradiction in the iron-deficiency theory. Thus, RLS seems to be a heterogeneous syndrome with several subtypes associated with separate neurobiological mechanisms.

Restless Legs Syndrome and Parkinson Disease

The prevalence studies of RLS in Parkinson disease (PD) are limited and somewhat contradictory. Pharmacologically, both PD and RLS benefit from dopaminergic treatment, although patients with RLS need much less medications than patients with PD. Neuroimaging studies of the brain show a mild striatal dysfunction in RLS[72,73] in contrast to severe nigrostriatal degeneration in PD. Decreased iron storage (hypoechogenicity) in the substantial nigra of patients with RLS contrasts with increased iron (hyperechogenicity) in PD. Absence of dopaminergic neuronal degeneration in limited neuropathological study of patients with RLS is in contrast to severe nigrostriatal degeneration in PD. The prevalence of RLS in PD has varied between 11.0% and 20.8% in limited studies.[74–77] In one prospective long-term study,[78] 15 out of 106 (14%) patients with de novo PD developed RLS. Ten out of 12 patients developed RLS within 24 months after starting dopaminergic medication suggesting that RLS may have developed through a mechanism of augmentation in these patients. The basic underlying mechanism, however, of increased incidence of RLS in PD remains unclear. There is one report of emergence of RLS after subthalamic deep brain stimulation (STN-DBS) in PD.[79] In this prospective observational study, 6 out of 31 patients with PD who were initially free from RLS developed RLS symptoms 6 months after bilateral chronic STN-DBS. The investigators suggested that overstimulation of the dopaminergic system as a result of the cumulative effects of dopamine agonists and STN-DBS led to an emergence of RLS in these patients.

Restless Legs Syndrome, Chronic Obstructive Pulmonary Disease, and Obstructive Sleep Apnea

In 1970, Spillane published a report for debate in the *British Medical Journal* documenting an association between RLS and chronic obstructive pulmonary disease (COPD) in 8 patients.[80] Subsequently, Chokroverty and Sachdeo[81] briefly reported an association among RLS, COPD, and sleep apnea; Schönbrunn and colleagues[82] questioned about RLS and sleep apnea as a random coincidence or a causal relation. These studies were reported before the essential diagnostic criteria for RLS/WED were established. The prevalence figure of 8.3% with RLS symptoms in 60 sequentially selected patients with PSG documented obstructive sleep apnea (OSA) reported by Lakshminarayanan and colleagues[83] is not dissimilar to the RLS prevalence figures in the general population. Improvement of sleep apnea and RLS symptoms in 17 patients with coexistent RLS and OSA following upper airway pressurization reported by Delgado Rodrigues and coworkers[84] raises question about RLS mimics in their patients. Kaplan and colleagues[85] compared 2 groups of patients with COPD: group 1 consisting of 133 patients with COPD with 39 (29.1%) fulfilling the diagnostic criteria of RLS and the second group of 65 age-matched patients with COPD without RLS. Group 1 with RLS had a longer duration of COPD and more marked hypoxemia/hypercapnia than the other group without RLS symptoms. It is plausible that longstanding nocturnal hypoxemia in OSA and both diurnal and nocturnal hypoxemia in patients with COPD played a role in the pathogenesis of RLS in view of the recent hypothesis of activation of hypoxic pathways in the pathogenesis of RLS/WED.

Renal Failure, Dialysis, and Restless Legs Syndrome

There is an increased prevalence of RLS (20%–50% and even higher) with end-stage renal disease (ESRD) on dialysis.[69,86–93] Iron deficiency and chronic kidney disease are the strongest predictors of RLS in older hospitalized patients, and serum ferritin less than 70 µg/L is the best cutoff for identifying possible iron deficiency.[94] Patients with ESRD with RLS showed an increased likelihood of cardiovascular and cerebrovascular events and mortality.[95] There are no specific biochemical risk factors identified with RLS except for low iron status as a predictor of poor outcome. Report of the disappearance of RLS after kidney transplantation suggests that some unknown biochemical or other factors are causing RLS symptoms in ESRD.[96] There is a report of a genetic influence on RLS in patients with ESRD, with BTBD 9 being significantly associated.[97]

Rheumatoid Arthritis and Restless Legs Syndrome

There is an increased prevalence of RLS/WED (25%–30%) in the rheumatoid arthritis population.[98–101] Factors responsible for increased association of sleep disorders, including RLS, in rheumatoid arthritis include iron deficiency, proinflammatory cytokines, and other immunomodulatory changes.

Medications and Restless Legs Syndrome

There are scattered case and anecdotal reports of exacerbation or causation of RLS symptoms after ingestion of antidepressants (tricyclic and SSRIs, neuroleptics, dopamine antagonists, antihistamines [mostly H1 antagonists], and lithium).[102,103] The role of antidepressants in RLS symptoms remains controversial. Berger[104] observed that 75% of patients with RLS on tricyclic antidepressants and SSRIs for depression in a single practice also had a history of regular intake of nonopioid analgesics, which, he suggested, enhanced the risk for RLS. This hypothesis is strengthened by a previous report from Leutgeb and Martus[105] who postulated that neither antidepressants nor neuroleptics but nonsteroidal antiinflammatory drugs used as analgesics seemed to be the major risk factor for RLS/WED. Following a retrospective chart review of 200 consecutive patients referred to their sleep disorder center, Brown and coinvestigators[106] also concluded that there was no statistically significant association between RLS symptoms and antidepressant medications.

Miscellaneous Other Conditions Associated with Restless Legs Syndrome/Willis-Ekbom Disease

There are a few scattered case reports of RLS/WED associated with varicose veins and thrombophlebitis, hypothyroidism,[107] hyperthyroidism,[108] hyperparathyroidism,[109] meralgia paraesthetica,[110] saphenous nerve entrapment,[111] multiple sclerosis, myelopathies, Isaac syndrome, stiff person syndrome, hyperekplexia,[102] spinal anesthesia[112] (causing transient RLS symptoms), cerebral and brainstem infarctions (cortical and subcortical strokes),[113–115] as well as in conditions associated with increased small intestinal bacterial overgrowth (eg, Celiac disease, Crohn disease).[116]

Approach to Restless Legs Syndrome/Willis-Ekbom Disease Mimics and Comorbidities

For the diagnosis of RLS/WED mimics and those conditions associated with (comorbidities) RLS/WED, salient clinical features, as summarized earlier, should help in arriving at the correct diagnosis. In addition to history and physical examination, laboratory tests (**Box 4**), which should be subservient to clinical information, may be needed to confirm the diagnosis of these other conditions

---

Box 4
Laboratory investigations for differential diagnosis

Overnight polysomnography
- To document presence of associated sleep apnea
- To show PLMS and PLMW qualitatively and quantitatively

Actigraphy
- To document PLM quantitatively and sleep efficacy as well as motor hyperactivity

EMG and nerve conduction study
- For possible polyneuropathies, including small fiber neuropathy (sympathetic skin response)

Clinical laboratory tests
- Serum ferritin, iron, hematocrit
- Serum folate and vitamin B12 levels
- Fasting blood glucose for diabetes mellitus and diabetes neuropathy
- Blood urea nitrogen and creatinine for possible renal failure

Neuroimaging tests
- MRI of the brain and spinal cord for suspected central nervous system disease

Miscellaneous tests
- Urinary drug screening for drug-induced RLS/WED
- Nerve biopsy for obscure neuropathy

---

superficially resembling or associated with RLS/WED. These tests may include an overnight PSG, multiple sleep latency tests, actigraphy, EMG and nerve conduction velocity (NCV) studies, hematological and biochemical tests in blood samples, urinalysis, drug screening, and neuroimaging investigations (see **Box 4**). Overnight PSG will document the presence of sleep-disordered breathing and PLMS. In atypical and unusual cases of RLS, recording PLMS may be important as a supporting feature. An overnight PSG is important to show associated sleep apnea in RLS/WED, which is important for optimal treatment decision.

Actigraphy

An actigraph or an actometer (an activity monitor) worn at the ankle may be useful to record PLMS after adjusting the settings. An advantage of this method is the ability to record for days in patients' homes or work places eliminating labor-intensive in-laboratory PSG recording. This device is also useful for monitoring treatment. The disadvantages include lack of standardization and specificity and failure to differentiate from other movements, including respiratory-related PLMS.

Electromyography and nerve conduction velocity

These studies are important to exclude polyneuropathies, lumbosacral radiculopathies, and other lower motor neuron disorders that may be associated with RLS/WED. Standard NCV will not be able to diagnose small fiber neuropathy (which may be an important comorbid condition in RLS), but sympathetic skin response can be performed using the standard EMG equipment to document autonomic and indirectly small fiber dysfunction suggesting small fiber neuropathy.

To diagnose iron deficiency (important in RLS/WED), iron status can be determined by obtaining serum iron level, hemoglobin, total iron-binding capacity, ferritin, percent iron saturation, and transferrin levels. The ideal ferritin level for patients with RLS/WED should be 50 to 70 μg/L or greater, but iron overload should be avoided as hemochromatosis (an iron storage disorder) and RLS may coexist on a genetic basis. Other important tests include serum folate and vitamin B12 levels, fasting blood glucose to exclude diabetes mellitus as a cause for neuropathy, blood urea nitrogen, and creatinine to exclude renal failure. Neuroimaging tests of the brain and spinal cord may be needed in those suspected to have an associated central neurologic disorder. Urinary drug screening may be needed in suspected cases. The role of nerve biopsy remains controversial. In most cases, nerve biopsy is not needed but may be obtained for research purposes and also when there is a strong suspicion of small fiber neuropathy.

REFERENCES

1. Walters AS. Toward a better definition of the restless legs syndrome. The International Restless Legs Syndrome Study Group. Mov Disord 1995; 10:634–42.
2. Allen RP, Picchietti D, Hening WA, et al. Restless legs syndrome: diagnostic criteria, special considerations, and epidemiology. A report from the restless legs syndrome diagnosis and epidemiology workshop at the National Institutes of Health. Sleep Med 2003;4:101–19.
3. Allen RP, Picchietti DL, Garcia-Borreguero D, et al. Restless legs syndrome/Willis-Ekbom disease diagnostic criteria: updated International Restless Legs Syndrome Study Group (IRLSSG) consensus criteria–history, rationale, description, and significance. Sleep Med 2014;15(8):860–73.
4. Haskovec L. L'akathisie. Rev Neurol 1901;9:1107–9.
5. American College of Neuropsychopharmacology—Food and Drug Administration Task Force. Neurological syndromes associated with antipsychotic drug use. N Engl J Med 1973;289:20–3.
6. Yamashita H, Horiguchi J, Mizuno S, et al. A case of neuroleptic-induced unilateral akathisia with periodic limb movements in the opposite side during sleep. Psychiatry Clin Neurosci 1999;53:291–3.
7. Hermesh H, Munitz H. Unilateral neuroleptic-induced akathisia. Clin Neuropharmacol 1990;13: 253–8.
8. Carrazana E, Rossitch E Jr, Martinez J. Unilateral "akathisia" in a patient with AIDS and a toxoplasmosis subthalamic abscess. Neurology 1989;39: 449–50.
9. Walters AS, Hening W, Rubinstein M, et al. A clinical and polysomnographic comparison of neuroleptic-induced akathisia and the idiopathic restless legs syndrome. Sleep 1991;14:339–45.
10. Chokroverty S, Manocha MK, Duvoisin RC. A physiologic and pharmacologic study in anticholinergic-responsive essential myoclonus. Neurology 1987;37:608–15.
11. Oswald I. Sudden bodily jerks on falling asleep. Brain 1959;82:92–103.
12. Broughton R. Pathological fragmentary myoclonus, intensified sleep starts and hypnagogic foot tremor: three unusual sleep related disorders. In: Koella WP, editor. Sleep 1986. New York: Fischer-Verlag; 1988. p. 240–3.
13. Chokroverty S, Bhat S, Gupta D. Intensified hypnic jerks: a polysomnographic and polymyographic analysis. J Clin Neurophysiol 2013;30(4):403–10.
14. Spillane JD, Nathan PW, Kelly RE, et al. Painful legs and moving toes. Brain 1971;94:541–56.
15. Schoenen J, Gonce M, Delwaide PJ. Painful legs and moving toes: a syndrome with different physiopathologic mechanisms. Neurology 1984;34:1108–12.
16. Reddy R, Siddiqui F, Dinar AH, et al. A polymyographic and polysomnographic analysis of painful and painless legs moving toes syndrome [abstract]. Mov Disord 2005;20(supp. 10):S64.
17. Hudson AJ, Brown WF, Gilbert JJ. The muscular pain-fasciculation syndrome. Neurology 1978;28: 1105–9.
18. Tahmoush AJ, Alonso RJ, Tahmoush GP, et al. Cramp-fasciculation syndrome: a treatable hyperexcitable peripheral nerve disorder. Neurology 1991;41(7):1021–4.
19. Bhatia KP, Bhatt MH, Marsden CD. The causalgia-dystonia syndrome. Brain 1993;116:843–51.
20. Masland RL. Myokymia: a cause of restless legs. JAMA 1947;134:1298.

21. Patel N, Jankovic J, Hallett M. Sensory aspects of movement disorders. Lancet Neurol 2014;13(1):100–12.
22. American Academy of Sleep Medicine. The international classification of sleep disorders. 3rd edition diagnostic and coding manual. Darien (IL): American Academy of Sleep Medicine; 2014.
23. Cheshire WP Jr. Hypotensive akathisia: autonomic failure associated with leg fidgeting while sitting. Neurology 2000;55:1923–6.
24. Sander HW, Masdeu JC, Tavoulaeas G, et al. Orthostatic tremor: an electrophysiological analysis. Mov Disord 1998;13:735–8.
25. Heilman KM. Orthostatic tremor. Arch Neurol 1984;41:880–1.
26. Papa S, Gershanik OS. Orthostatic tremor: an essential tremor variant. Mov Disord 1988;3:97–108.
27. Picchietti DL, Underwood DJ, Farris WA, et al. Further studies on periodic limb movement disorder and restless legs syndrome in children with attention-deficit hyperactivity disorder. Mov Disord 1999;14:1000–7.
28. Rajaram SS, Walters AS, England SJ, et al. Some children with growing pains may actually have restless legs syndrome. Sleep 2004;27:767–73.
29. Mahowald MW. Periodic limb movements are NOT associated with disturbed sleep. Con. J Clin Sleep Med 2007;3(1):15–7.
30. Mendelson WB. Are periodic leg movements associated with clinical sleep disturbance? Sleep 1996;19(3):219–23.
31. Ekbom KA. Restless legs: a clinical study. Acta Med Scand Suppl 1945;158:1–123.
32. Goodman JD, Brodie C, Ayida GA. Restless leg syndrome in pregnancy. BMJ 1988;297:1101–2.
33. Suzuki K, Ohida T, Sone T, et al. The prevalence of restless legs syndrome among pregnant women in Japan and the relationship between restless legs syndrome and sleep problems. Sleep 2003;26:673–7.
34. Manconi M, Govoni V, De Vito A, et al. Pregnancy as a risk factor for restless legs syndrome. Sleep Med 2004;5:305–8.
35. Manconi M, Ulfberg J, Berger K. When gender matters: restless legs syndrome. Report of the "RLS and woman" workshop endorsed by the European RLS Study Group. Sleep Med Rev 2012;16(4):297–307.
36. Alves DA, Carvalho LB, Morais JF, et al. Restless legs syndrome during pregnancy in Brazilian women. Sleep Med 2010;11(10):1049–54.
37. Chen PH, Liou KC, Chen CP, et al. Risk factors and prevalence rate of restless legs syndrome among pregnant women in Taiwan. Sleep Med 2012;13(9):1153–7.
38. Balendran J, Champion D, Jaaniste T, et al. A common sleep disorder in pregnancy: restless legs syndrome and its predictors. Aust N Z J Obstet Gynaecol 2011;51(3):262–4.
39. Shang X, Yang J, Guo Y, et al. Restless legs syndrome among pregnant women in China: prevalence and risk factors. Sleep Breath 2014. [Epub ahead of print].
40. Picchietti DL, Hensley JG, Bainbridge JL, et al. Consensus clinical practice guidelines for the diagnosis and treatment of restless legs syndrome/Willis-Ekbom disease during pregnancy and lactation. Sleep Med Rev 2015;22 [pii:S1087-0792(14)00119-1].
41. Hübner A, Krafft A, Gadient S, et al. Characteristics and determinants of restless legs syndrome in pregnancy: a prospective study. Neurology 2013;80(8):738–42.
42. Minár M, Košutzká Z, Habánová H, et al. Restless legs syndrome in pregnancy is connected with iron deficiency. Sleep Med 2015;16(5):589–92.
43. Gemignani F, Brindani F, Vitetta F, et al. Restless legs syndrome and painful neuropathy-retrospective study. A role for nociceptive deafferentation? Pain Med 2009;10(8):1481–6.
44. Gemignani F, Vitetta F, Brindani F, et al. Painful polyneuropathy associated with restless legs syndrome. Clinical features and sensory profile. Sleep Med 2013;14(1):79–84.
45. Gemignani F, Brindani F, Negrotti A, et al. Restless legs syndrome and polyneuropathy. Mov Disord 2006;21(8):1254–7.
46. Rajabally YA, Shah RS. Restless legs syndrome in chronic inflammatory demyelinating polyneuropathy. Muscle Nerve 2010;42(2):252–6.
47. Luigetti M, Del Grande A, Testani E. Restless leg syndrome in different types of demyelinating neuropathies: a single-center pilot study. J Clin Sleep Med 2013;9(9):945–9.
48. Boentert M, Knop K, Schuhmacher C, et al. Sleep disorders in Charcot-Marie-Tooth disease type 1. J Neurol Neurosurg Psychiatry 2014;85(3):319–25.
49. Gemignani F, Marbini A, Di Giovanni G, et al. Charcot-Marie-Tooth disease type 2 with restless legs syndrome. Neurology 1999;52:1064–6.
50. Rutkove SB, Matheson JK, Logigian EL. Restless legs syndrome in patients with polyneuropathy. Muscle Nerve 1996;19:670–2.
51. Hattan E, Chalk C, Postuma RB. Is there a higher risk of restless legs syndrome in peripheral neuropathy? Neurology 2009;72(11):955–60.
52. Cho YW, Na GY, Lim JG, et al. Prevalence and clinical characteristics of restless legs syndrome in diabetic peripheral neuropathy: comparison with chronic osteoarthritis. Sleep Med 2013;14(12):1387–92.
53. Lim YM, Chang SE, Chung S, et al. Small fiber function in drug naïve patients with idiopathic restless legs syndrome. J Clin Neurosci 2012;19(5):702–5.

54. Iannaccone S, Zucconi M, Marchettini P, et al. Evidence of peripheral axonal neuropathy in primary restless legs syndrome. Mov Disord 1995;10:2–9.

55. Polydefkis M, Allen RP, Hauer P, et al. Subclinical sensory neuropathy in late-onset restless legs syndrome. Neurology 2000;55:1115–21.

56. Nordlander NB. Therapy in restless legs. Acta Med Scand 1953;145:453–7.

57. O'Keeffe ST, Gavin K, Lavan JN. Iron status and restless legs syndrome in the elderly. Age Ageing 1994;23:200–3.

58. Sun ER, Chen CA, Ho G, et al. Iron and the restless legs syndrome. Sleep 1998;21:371–7.

59. Allen RP, Earley CJ. Restless legs syndrome: a review of clinical and pathophysiologic features. J Clin Neurophysiol 2001;18:128–47.

60. Allen R. Dopamine and iron in the pathophysiology of restless legs syndrome (RLS). Sleep Med 2004; 5:385–91.

61. Earley CJ, Heckler D, Allen RP. The treatment of restless legs syndrome with intravenous iron dextran. Sleep Med 2004;5:231–5.

62. Earley CJ, Connor JR, Beard JL, et al. Ferritin levels in the cerebrospinal fluid and restless legs syndrome: effects of different clinical phenotypes. Sleep 2005;28:1069–75.

63. Allen RP, Barker PB, Wehrl F, et al. MRI measurement of brain iron in patients with restless legs syndrome. Neurology 2001;56:263–5.

64. Connor JR, Boyer PJ, Menzies SL, et al. Neuropathological examination suggests impaired brain iron acquisition in restless legs syndrome. Neurology 2003;61:304–9.

65. Silber MH, Richardson JW. Multiple blood donations associated with iron deficiency in patients with restless legs syndrome. Mayo Clin Proc 2003;78:52–4.

66. Ulfberg J, Nystrom B. Restless legs syndrome in blood donors. Sleep Med 2004;5:115–8.

67. Patton SM, Ponnuru P, Snyder AM, et al. Hypoxia-inducible factor pathway activation in restless legs syndrome patients. Eur J Neurol 2011; 18(11):1329–35.

68. Salminen AV, Rimpilä V, Polo O. Peripheral hypoxia in restless legs syndrome (Willis-Ekbom disease). Neurology 2014;82(21):1856–61.

69. Collado-Seidel V, Kohnen R, Samtleben W, et al. Clinical and biochemical findings in uremic patients with and without restless legs syndrome. Am J Kidney Dis 1998;31:324–8.

70. Lee KA, Zaffke ME, Baratte-Beebe K. Restless legs syndrome and sleep disturbance during pregnancy: the role of folate and iron. J Womens Health Gend Based Med 2001;10:335–41.

71. Davis BJ, Rajput A, Rajput ML, et al. A randomized double-blind placebo-controlled trial of iron in restless legs syndrome. Eur Neurol 2000;43:70–5.

72. Ruottinen HM, Partinen M, Hublin C, et al. An FDOPA PET study in patients with periodic limb movement disorder and restless legs syndrome. Neurology 2000;54:502–4.

73. Michaud M, Soucy JP, Chabli A, et al. SPECT imaging of striatal pre- and postsynaptic dopaminergic status in restless legs syndrome with periodic leg movements in sleep. J Neurol 2002;249:164–70.

74. Ylikoski A, Martikainen K, Partinen M. Parkinson's disease and restless legs syndrome. Eur Neurol 2015;73(3–4):212–9.

75. Fereshtehnejad SM, Shafieesabet M, Shahidi GA, et al. Restless legs syndrome in patients with Parkinson's disease: a comparative study on prevalence, clinical characteristics, quality of life and nutritional status. Acta Neurol Scand 2015;131(4): 211–8.

76. Bhalsing K, Suresh K, Muthane UB, et al. Prevalence and profile of restless legs syndrome in Parkinson's disease and other neurodegenerative disorders: a case-control study. Parkinsonism Relat Disord 2013;19(4):426–30.

77. Verbaan D, van Rooden SM, van Hilten JJ, et al. Prevalence and clinical profile of restless legs syndrome in Parkinson's disease. Mov Disord 2010; 25(13):2142–7.

78. Calzetti S, Angelini M, Negrotti A, et al. A long-term prospective follow-up study of incident RLS in the course of chronic DAergic therapy in newly diagnosed untreated patients with Parkinson's disease. J Neural Transm 2014;121(5):499–506.

79. Marques A, Fantini ML, Morand D. Emergence of restless legs syndrome after subthalamic stimulation in Parkinson's disease: a dopaminergic overstimulation? Sleep Med 2015;16(5):583–8.

80. Spillane JD. Restless legs syndrome in chronic pulmonary disease. Br Med J 1970;4:796–8.

81. Chokroverty S, Sachdeo R. Restless limb-myoclonus sleep apnea syndrome [abstract]. Ann Neurol 1984;16:124A.

82. Schönbrunn E, Riemann D, Hohagen F, et al. Restless legs and sleep apnea syndrome—random coincidence or causal relation? Nervenarzt 1990; 61:306–11.

83. Lakshminarayanan S, Paramasivan KD, Walters AS, et al. Clinically significant but unsuspected restless legs syndrome in patients with sleep apnea. Mov Disord 2005;20:501–3.

84. Delgado Rodrigues RN, Alvim de Abreu E, Silva Rodrigues AA, et al. Outcome of restless legs severity after continuous positive air pressure (CPAP) treatment in patients affected by the association of RLS and obstructive sleep apneas. Sleep Med 2006;7:235–9.

85. Kaplan Y, Inonu H, Yilmaz A, et al. Restless legs syndrome in patients with chronic obstructive pulmonary disease. Can J Neurol Sci 2008;35(3):352–7.

86. Kutner N, Bliwise D. Restless legs complaint in African American and Caucasian hemodialysis patients. Sleep Med 2002;3:497–500.

87. Stefanidis I, Vainas A, Dardiotis E. Restless legs syndrome in hemodialysis patients: an epidemiologic survey in Greece. Sleep Med 2013;14(12):1381–6.

88. Lin CH, Wu VC, Li WY. Restless legs syndrome in end-stage renal disease: a multicenter study in Taiwan. Eur J Neurol 2013;20(7):1025–31.

89. Araujo SM, de Bruin VM, Nepomuceno LA. Restless legs syndrome in end-stage renal disease: clinical characteristics and associated comorbidities. Sleep Med 2010;11(8):785–90.

90. Aritake-Okada S, Nakao T, Komada Y, et al. Prevalence and clinical characteristics of restless legs syndrome in chronic kidney disease patients. Sleep Med 2011;12(10):1031–3.

91. Sakkas GK, Giannaki CD, Karatzaferi C, et al. Current trends in the management of uremic restless legs syndrome: a systematic review on aspects related to quality of life, cardiovascular mortality and survival. Sleep Med Rev 2015;21:39–49.

92. Giannaki CD, Hadjigeorgiou GM, Karatzaferi C, et al. Epidemiology, impact, and treatment options of restless legs syndrome in end-stage renal disease patients: an evidence-based review. Kidney Int 2014;85(6):1275–82.

93. Merlino G, Lorenzut S, Gigli GL, et al. A case-control study on restless legs syndrome in nondialyzed patients with chronic renal failure. Mov Disord 2010;25(8):1019–25.

94. Quinn C, Uzbeck M, Saleem I, et al. Iron status and chronic kidney disease predict restless legs syndrome in an older hospital population. Sleep Med 2011;12(3):295–301.

95. Lin CH, Sy HN, Chang HW, et al. Restless legs syndrome is associated with cardio/cerebrovascular events and mortality in end-stage renal disease. Eur J Neurol 2015;22(1):142–9.

96. Winkelmann J, Stautner A, Samtleben W, et al. Long-term course of restless legs syndrome in dialysis patients after kidney transplantation. Mov Disord 2002;17:1072–6.

97. Schormair B, Plag J, Kaffe M, et al. MEIS1 and BTBD9: genetic association with restless leg syndrome in end stage renal disease. J Med Genet 2011;48(7):462–6.

98. Salih AM, Gray RE, Mills KR, et al. A clinical, serological and neurophysiological study of restless legs syndrome in rheumatoid arthritis. Br J Rheumatol 1994;33:60–3.

99. Reynolds G, Blake DR, Pall HS, et al. Restless legs syndrome and rheumatoid arthritis. Br Med J (Clin Res Ed) 1986;292:659–60.

100. Taylor-Gjevre RM, Gjevre JA, Skomro R, et al. Restless legs syndrome in a rheumatoid arthritis patient cohort. J Clin Rheumatol 2009;15(1):12–5.

101. Taylor-Gjevre RM, Gjevre JA, Nair BV. Increased nocturnal periodic limb movements in rheumatoid arthritis patients meeting questionnaire diagnostic criteria for restless legs syndrome. BMC Musculoskelet Disord 2014;15:378.

102. Hening W, Allen R, Walters A, et al. Motor functions and dysfunctions of sleep. In: Chokroverty S, editor. Sleep disorders medicine: basic science, technical considerations and clinical aspects. Boston: Butterworth; 1999. p. 441–507.

103. Lesage S, Hening WA. The restless legs syndrome and periodic limb movement disorder: a review of management. Semin Neurol 2004;24:249–59.

104. Berger K. Non-opioid analgesics and the risk of restless legs syndrome—a spurious association? Sleep Med 2003;4:351–2.

105. Leutgeb U, Martus P. Regular intake of non-opioid analgesics is associated with an increased risk of restless legs syndrome in patients maintained on antidepressants. Eur J Med Res 2002;7:368–78.

106. Brown LK, Dedrick DL, Doggett JW, et al. Antidepressant medication use and restless legs syndrome in patients presenting with insomnia. Sleep Med 2005;6:443–50.

107. Bon E, Rolland Y, Laroche M, et al. Hypothyroidism on Colchimax revealed by restless legs syndrome. Rev Rhum Engl Ed 1996;63:304.

108. Tan EK, Ho SC, Eng P, et al. Restless legs symptoms in thyroid disorders. Parkinsonism Relat Disord 2004;10:149–51.

109. Lim LL, Dinner D, Tham KW, et al. Restless legs syndrome associated with primary hyperparathyroidism. Sleep Med 2005;6:283–5.

110. Ekbom KA. Restless legs. JAMA 1946;131:481.

111. Lewis F. The role of the saphenous nerve in insomnia: a proposed etiology of restless legs syndrome. Med Hypotheses 1991;34:331–3.

112. Högl B, Frauscher B, Seppi K, et al. Transient restless legs syndrome after spinal anesthesia: a prospective study. Neurology 2002;59(11):1705–7.

113. Lee SJ, Kim JS, Song IU, et al. Poststroke restless legs syndrome and lesion location: anatomical considerations. Mov Disord 2009;24(1):77–84.

114. Ruppert E, Kilic-Huck U, Wolff V, et al. Brainstem stroke-related restless legs syndrome: frequency and anatomical considerations. Eur Neurol 2015;73(1–2):113–8.

115. Gupta A, Shukla G, Mohammed A, et al. Restless legs syndrome, a predictor of subcortical stroke - a prospective study on 346 stroke patients. Sleep Med 2015, in Press.

116. Weinstock LB, Walters AS, Paueksakon P. Restless legs syndrome–theoretical roles of inflammatory and immune mechanisms. Sleep Med Rev 2012;16(4):341–54.

Management of Restless Legs Syndrome/Willis-Ekbom Disease

Preface

Management of Restless Legs Syndrome/Willis Ekbom Disease

Restless legs syndrome (RLS), or Willis Ekbom disease (WED), is a chronic, insidious disease with occasional remissions and frequent exacerbations. With a complete, lasting cure not yet in sight and the specter of augmentation overshadowing existing medications, managing the symptoms becomes the therapeutic goal.

The next few articles will summarize and review available data on managing RLS. The nonpharmacologic management of RLS includes lifestyle changes, old wives' tales/recommendations, behavioral and cognitive manipulations, supplements, and procedures. The merits of yoga have been mentioned in the literature and are considered here as well. The pharmacologic management of RLS using dopaminergics as well as its challenges, including augmentation, are extensively reviewed.

Other pharmacotherapies have been successfully used to control RLS symptoms. These include the α-2-δ ligands and the opioids. Among the α-2-ligands, pregabalin,[1,2] gabapentin,[3–6] and the extended-release gabapentin enacabril[7–10] have been extensively reviewed. The opioids may not have gotten their day in the news, possibly due to stigma and limited industry interest. Nevertheless, these are among the most successful medications used to control WED symptoms. These include oxycodone,[11] methadone,[12] and oxycodone + naloxone,[13] among others. Several articles focus on managing RLS in special populations and in specific settings.

Denise Sharon, MD, PhD, FAASM
Tulane University School of Medicine
1430 Tulane Avenue
New Orleans, LA 70112, USA

Advanced Sleep Center
2905 Kingman Street
Metairie, LA 70006, USA

E-mail address:
denisesharon@cox.net

REFERENCES

1. Garcia-Borreguero D, Patrick J, DuBrava S, et al. Pregabalin versus pramipexole: effects on sleep disturbance in restless legs syndrome. Sleep 2014;37(4):635–43. http://dx.doi.org/10.5665/sleep.3558.
2. Allen RP, Chen C, Garcia-Borreguero D, et al. Comparison of pregabalin with pramipexole for restless legs syndrome. N Engl J Med 2014;370(7):621–31.
3. Razazian N, Azimi H, Heidarnejadian J, et al. Gabapentin versus levodopa-c for the treatment of restless legs syndrome in hemodialysis patients: a randomized clinical trial. Saudi J Kidney Dis Transpl 2015;26(2):271–8.
4. Micozkadioglu H, Ozdemir FN, Kut A, et al. Gabapentin versus levodopa for the treatment of Restless Legs Syndrome in hemodialysis patients: an open-label study. Ren Fail 2004;26(4):393–7.
5. Happe S, Sauter C, Klösch G, et al. Gabapentin versus ropinirole in the treatment of idiopathic restless legs syndrome. Neuropsychobiology 2003;48(2):82–6.
6. Garcia-Borreguero D, Larrosa O, de la Llave Y, et al. Treatment of restless legs syndrome with gabapentin: a double-blind, cross-over study. Neurology 2002;59(10):1573–9.
7. Bogan RK, Lee DO, Buchfuhrer MJ, et al. Treatment response to sleep, pain, and mood disturbance and their correlation with sleep disturbance in adult patients with moderate-to-severe primary restless legs syndrome: pooled analyses from 3 trials of gabapentin enacarbil. Ann Med 2015;47:269–77.
8. Sun Y, van Valkenhoef G, Morel T. A mixed treatment comparison of gabapentin enacarbil, pramipexole, ropinirole and rotigotine in moderate-to-severe restless legs syndrome. Curr Med Res Opin 2014;30(11):2267–78. http://dx.doi.org/10.1185/03007995.2014.946124.
9. Kushida CA, Walters AS, Becker P, et al, XP021 Study Group. A randomized, double-blind, placebo-controlled, crossover study of XP13512/GSK1838262 in the treatment of patients with primary restless legs syndrome. Sleep 2009;32(2):159–68.

Sleep Med Clin 10 (2015) xix–xx
http://dx.doi.org/10.1016/j.jsmc.2015.07.003
1556-407X/15/$ – see front matter © 2015 Published by Elsevier Inc.

10. Ellenbogen AL, Thein SG, Winslow DH, et al. A 52-week study of gabapentin enacarbil in restless legs syndrome. Clin Neuropharmacol 2011;34(1):8–16. http://dx.doi.org/10.1097/WNF.0b013e3182087d48.

11. Walters AS, Winkelmann J, Trenkwalder C, et al. Long-term follow-up on restless legs syndrome patients treated with opioids. Mov Disord 2001;16(6):1105–9.

12. Ondo WG. Methadone for refractory restless legs syndrome. Mov Dis 2005;20(3):345–8.

13. Trenkwalder C, Beneš H, Grote L, et al, RELOXYN Study Group. Prolonged release oxycodone-naloxone for treatment of severe restless legs syndrome after failure of previous treatment: a double-blind, randomised, placebo-controlled trial with an open-label extension. Lancet Neurol 2013; 12(12):1141–50. http://dx.doi.org/10.1016/S1474-4422(13)70239-4 [Erratum appears in Lancet Neurol 2013;12(12):1133].

Nonpharmacologic Management of Restless Legs Syndrome (Willis-Ekbom Disease): Myths or Science

Denise Sharon, MD, PhD[a,b,*]

KEYWORDS

- Restless legs syndrome (RLS) • Periodic limb movements (PLMs)
- Periodic limb movements of sleep (PLMS) • Periodic limb movement disorder (PLMD)
- Nonpharmacologic management • Behavioral modifications • Supplements • Yoga

KEY POINTS

- Nonpharmacologic management of restless legs syndrome (RLS) is part of the overall treatment.
- There is limited peer-reviewed literature on nonpharmacologic options.
- Nonpharmacological treatment options for RLS include:
  - Behavioral modifications.
  - Lifestyle changes.
  - Substances, diets, and supplements.
  - Applications and procedures.
  - Cognitive behavioral treatment.

INTRODUCTION

Contrary to the (relative) bounty of randomized, double-blind, controlled studies of medications for restless legs syndrome (RLS) and evidence in favor of iron supplementation, there are very few studies on the nonpharmacologic management of this disease. Listening to patients' individual cures and old wives' tales, one can learn about the various ethnic and cultural practices. Limited scientific accounts left a void filled by superstitions, myths, and folk beliefs. Alas, it is the quest to verify and understand these phenomena that promotes science. When the world embraced the Internet, the field opened to many Web sites, blogs, and discussion boards giving an equal voice to everyone and promoting a plethora of (treatment) options. These Web sites may seem authoritative based on journalistic prowess, by reporting study results, or by quoting doctors and professors. Some of these promoted therapies for RLS are innocuous, but some can have significant side effects or become outright dangerous over time. It is, therefore, important that the clinician be familiar with the options in order to recommend and guide patients toward the most effective, nondetrimental treatment selection.

This review lists the different nonpharmacologic options for RLS based on a search of peer-reviewed literature listed on databases, reference lists of retrieved articles, examination of patients' charts, and Internet-based information. The nonpharmacologic management of RLS is important as treatment in itself in cases when patients are

Disclosure: The author has nothing to disclose.
[a] Tulane University School of Medicine, 1430 Tulane Avenue, New Orleans, LA 70112, USA; [b] Advanced Sleep Center, 2905 Kingman Street, Metairie, LA 70006, USA
* Advanced Sleep Center, 2905 Kingman Street, Metairie, LA 70006.
E-mail address: denisesharon@cox.net

Sleep Med Clin 10 (2015) 263–278
http://dx.doi.org/10.1016/j.jsmc.2015.05.018

not interested in medications, such as mild, inter-mittent cases; when medications are not indi-cated, such as in pregnancy; or as an adjuvant to pharmacologic treatment. It includes behavior modification and lifestyle changes, substances, diets and supplements, applications and proce-dures, as well as cognitive-behavioral treatment. Within each group, the supporting literature is pre-sented as well as anecdotal evidence, patients' re-ports, and Web-based testimonials in the hope to prompt the reader to separate the myths from the facts and improve on the science.

As with the pharmacologic treatment of RLS, there are individual differences in the effectiveness of the different options. These differences under-line the importance of tailoring a plan for the spe-cific individual. More often than not, different options and combinations might be effective at different times during the course of the disease requiring the clinician to be tuned to status changes.

BEHAVIOR MODIFICATIONS AND LIFESTYLE CHANGES
Sleep Hygiene

The term *sleep hygiene* was first introduced by Na-thaniel Kleitman and refers to healthy lifestyle prac-tices that improve sleep. It evolved into many variations of sleep rules and was included as a sleep disorder in earlier classifications.[1] Almost every sleep center developed its own version of sleep hygiene tips given routinely to every patient with a sleep disorder. These tips usually include several recommendations regarding sleep sche-dule and sleep environment, light exposure, bedroom activities, substance use, and exercise (**Box 1**). Adherence to the rules of good sleep hy-giene is part of the insomnia treatment, and many patients with RLS present with an insomnia complaint. Additional tips for patients with RLS are included in **Box 2**.[2] The effect of maintaining good sleep hygiene on RLS symptoms has yet to be established.

Physical Activity

Exercise is one of the practices addressed by sleep hygiene. Lack of exercise was associated with increased RLS prevalence,[3] even though symptoms of RLS were more frequent with phys-ical activity close to bedtime.[4] Aerobic and lower-body resistance training performed 3 times per week improved RLS symptoms as measured by the International Restless Legs Scale (IRLS) in a randomized 12-week trial.[5] The effect of exercise might be related to the increase in cardiac output (ie, blood flow).[6] Reduced daytime intramuscular

blood flow was noted in 8 female patients with RLS using laser Doppler flowmetry.[7] Peripheral hypoxia was associated with the appearance of RLS symptoms and showed a strong correlation

---

Box 1
Sleep hygiene instructions

1. Maintain a regular sleep routine.
2. Allow enough hours for sleep during the main sleeping period.
3. A 10- to 20-minute power nap can be sched-uled if needed.
4. Use the bed only for sleep and sex.
5. The bedroom should be conducive to sleep: cool, dark, and uncluttered.
6. Use a comfortable mattress and bedding.
7. Avoid heavy meals before sleep; a small snack is acceptable.
8. Avoid caffeine, alcohol, and nicotine close to sleep.
9. Avoid exercise or heavy physical activity close to sleep.
10. Avoid screen activity (TV, computer, hand-held device, phone, and so forth) close to sleep.
11. Avoid work or mentation close to sleep: thinking, planning, and reminiscing.
12. Establish a bedtime routine: calming and relaxing.
13. Enjoy good daylight exposure in the morning.

Box 2
Lifestyle tips to control RLS symptoms

No	Yes
Sleep deprivation	Consider delaying bedtime and wake time
Bed rest	Exercise moderately during the day, stretching in the evening
Relaxed sitting in the evening	Active relaxation: reading, card games, crossword puzzles, meaningful discussion, sexual activity
Extreme temperatures	Preferred ambient temperature
Tannins (coffee, tea, alcohol), sugars	Balanced diet
Frequent blood donation	Maintain adequate iron stores

with RLS severity, being reversed by dopaminergic treatment.[8]

The effect of exercise on reducing periodic limb movements of sleep (PLMS) can be a result of releasing endorphins, which are endogenous opioid compounds that produce analgesia.[9] Exercise was also noted to increase the release of dopamine while diminishing corticostriatal hyperexcitability.[10]

On a health-related forum, a self-identified patient with RLS reported that exercising the legs in bed by raising each leg from the knee 50 times, then relaxing, helps with sleep, in addition to limiting the use of medications. On another forum, a patient with RLS described how tightening for 15 seconds and releasing all body muscles for about 10 to 15 minutes enables sleep. Others reported that exercise or stretching and relaxing the lower extremities' muscles did not work for them. A menopause site touts the benefits of walking as a cure for RLS symptoms. It recommends walking 20 minutes a day. Stretching should precede walking according to the site to prevent injuries during exercise and to relieve RLS symptoms.

Obesity and Weight Loss

Obesity and high serum cholesterol have been associated with an increased risk of RLS[11]; this is also true for obesity and abdominal adiposity based on data from more than 80,000 overweight subjects.[12] However, there is no data on the effect of weight loss on RLS symptoms.

Hypertension and Hypertension Control

High blood pressure was more prevalent in middle-aged women with RLS from the Nurses' Health Study cohort.[13] This finding supports studies suggesting that PLMS during sleep are associated with increases in blood pressure.[14,15] The evidence that controlling hypertension improves the symptoms of RLS is lacking.

Medications That Can Trigger or Worsen Restless Legs Syndrome

Antihistamines,[16] antidepressants,[17–21] antiemetics,[22] and antipsychotics[23,24] are among the medications noted to trigger or worsen RLS symptoms. However, discontinuing these medications was not always associated with symptom relief.

Blood Donation

The effect of blood donation on RLS is arguable. Several studies showed that frequent and repeated blood donations are associated with increased RLS prevalence and worsening of the symptoms.[25–29] However, these results were not replicated in the United States[30]; reducing the frequency of blood donations did not seem to affect the prevalence of RLS.[31,32] Self-reported severity of RLS symptoms decreased with ceasing blood donations,[27] indicating that patients with RLS might benefit from counseling regarding donating blood, the frequency of the practice, and its potential impact on iron stores.

Seating Arrangements

High stools that allow feet to dangle and sitting on the floor were anecdotally reported to either help or trigger RLS symptoms. Other options include sitting on the floor with or without elevating the feet. On a travel Web site forum there is a recommendation for patients with RLS to choose aisle seats on planes. There are no evidence-based data on seating options or on choosing the aisle seats on planes and in theaters, but at least it can help the next seat neighbors.

Occupational Counseling

The role of occupational counseling in the treatment of RLS has yet to be established. Absenteeism was reported in association with RLS.[33] The effects of delaying work start hours, flexible schedules, and increasing activity in the evening hours have yet to be studied. Prolonged standing as well as prolonged sitting frequently triggers RLS symptoms. It is important to rule out venous insufficiency in cases when symptoms seem to be associated with prolonged standing. Occupational counseling and guidance toward occupations that may allow flexible schedules and involve less travel, less sitting, and more activity in the evening hours may play an important role in the management of adolescents and young adults with RLS.

SUBSTANCES
Tannins

Tannins are water-soluble polyphenols commonly found in most dark-colored fruits, nuts, legumes, chocolate, coffee, tea, and wine.[34] Tannins interfere with absorption of nonheme iron from plants,[35] which may partially explain the worsening of RLS symptoms.[36]

Alcohol

Alcohol may initially relieve restlessness and promote sedation; but once it is metabolized, a rebound sympathetic drive may worsen restlessness and interfere with sleep. Aldrich and

Shipley[37] reported worsening of RLS symptoms and a significant increase in periodic limb movements (PLMs) in patients who drank 2 or more alcoholic beverages per day. The prevalence of RLS, though, does not seem to be affected by alcohol, caffeine, or nicotine,[38–42] even though Rangarajan and colleagues[43] reported the contrary in a South Indian population. Interesting to note is that Cirillo and Wallace[44] observed that current alcohol consumption was associated with decreased RLS prevalence in the elderly.

Caffeine

The effects of caffeine are also inconsistent. Ohayon and Roth[4] reported that daily coffee intake was associated with periodic limb movement disorder (PLMD) in a large cross-sectional study in 5 European countries. Even before, in 1978, Lutz[45] described coffee as the major causative factor of RLS symptoms in 62 patients with RLS and associated anxiety. Coffee intake was a significant predictor of RLS in patients undergoing dialysis.[46]

Nicotine

Conversely, Chen and colleagues[47] found that smoking, but not coffee or tea, was associated with RLS in Taiwanese patients on long-term hemodialysis. This study supports previous findings that RLS is associated with smoking and with low alcohol consumption.[3] Patients with RLS were noted to have an increased nocturnal smoking habit,[48] and several case reports noted that RLS symptoms were relieved by smoking cessation.[49]

Lavigne and colleagues[50] reached a different conclusion. The group observed no difference in the prevalence of motor RLS and PLMS by smoking. Moreover, in several case reports nicotine was observed to improve restlessness. One case reported was of a 77-year-old woman with a 40-year history of RLS who experienced symptom relief for 20 to 30 minutes after smoking a cigarette.[51] Similar results with smoking were noted in 6 patients with Parkinson disease (PD) by Ishikawa and Miyatake.[52] Chewing tobacco seemed to also relieve RLS symptoms.[53] These observations suggest a possible protective effect of nicotine against nigrostriatal damage[54] and need more study.

DIETS
Sugars

Reports on impaired glucose tolerance tests in patients with RLS,[55,56] possibly caused by repeated arousals, triggered suggestions to avoid sugars after 3 PM. A randomized double-blind placebo-controlled trial in one patient assessed the effect of artificial sweeteners on RLS symptoms and noted an increase in symptom frequency while using saccharine or the combination of saccharine and cyclamate but not with cyclamate only.[57]

Monosodium Glutamate

Different forums suggest avoiding products with monosodium glutamate as it is considered an excitotoxin additive. Higher glutamate and glutamine to creatinine ratio was observed in the right thalamus of patients with RLS.[58] However, no relationship has been established between RLS and monosodium glutamate.

Gluten Free

A gluten-free diet was reported to decrease RLS symptoms on a celiac disease forum. Few studies investigated the high association of RLS with celiac disease[59] and the response of RLS symptoms to a gluten-free diet,[60] suggesting celiac disease as a possible cause for low serum ferritin in patients with RLS. On the other hand, the prevalence of antibodies in gluten-sensitive enteropathy was not increased in patients with RLS.[61]

Dairy Free

Casein is mentioned on many Web sites as a culprit for RLS. Testimonials report improvement in RLS symptoms with a dairy-free diet. There are no studies in support of a dairy-free diet for the management of RLS.

Aluminum

A few Web sites suggest avoiding aluminum hydroxide–containing antacids, such as Alumag, Mylanta, and Amphojel, and deodorants with aluminum. This suggestion might be the result of a report to the Food and Drug Administration (FDA) about an individual who developed RLS taking aluminum magnesium hydroxide. There is no data to support this recommendation.

SUPPLEMENTS
Iron

Iron plays an important role in the pathophysiology of RLS.[62–65] Iron supplementation when iron stores are reduced is a benchmark in RLS management[66] and has been extensively studied,[67–74] warranting a separate article.

Other Supplements (Separate or in Various Combinations)

Several classes of supplements were mentioned in association with RLS. These classes include vitamins, elements and electrolytes, herbs, and hormones. The available data are scarce or just nil. Reports from peer-reviewed literature are summarized in **Table 1**. **Box 3** lists supplements described or discussed on the Internet or in the lay press that our patients read. Some of them follow the recommendations. There are currently no scientific data to support their use.

Vitamins

Several types were studied or mentioned in relation with RLS. However, there are limited data on the effect of vitamin supplementation in general and even less in relation to RLS.[75] Vitamins are mostly acquired through nutrition and play a major role in the metabolism. Limited supply, malabsorption, and possibly circadian factors can affect their availability. One of the few studies was conducted by Earley and his colleagues[76] and showed large diurnal changes in tetrahydrobiopterin that is synthesized by vitamin B9 (folate) in patients with RLS. Sagheb and his group[78] assessed the effects of vitamin C, vitamin E, and combined vitamin C + E and compared them with placebo in a group of patients with end-stage renal disease (ESRD) comorbid with RLS. The severity of RLS symptoms was assessed using the IRLS. Compared with placebo, the severity of the RLS symptoms decreased by a mean of 10 points in each of the 3 treatment groups with no difference between them.

Elements

Calcium may play a role in RLS symptoms. An increased prevalence of RLS was noted in patients with ESRD on calcium antagonists,[84] despite finding no difference in serum calcium levels following their treatment (with calcium-channel blockers).[100] Also calcium levels were higher in patients undergoing hemodialysis diagnosed with RLS.[85]

Magnesium involvement in RLS treatment is debatable. Magnesium supplements are frequently mentioned on different Web sites as a cure for RLS with specific dose recommendations for men, women, pregnancy, and breastfeeding or for feet soaking. These sites quote a report by Popoviciu and colleagues[101] suggesting that some of the polysomnographic changes in sleep patterns of 10 patients with RLS are similar to other parasomnias caused by magnesium deficiency. Furthermore, Hornyak and colleagues[87] reported improved RLS symptoms and sleep and reduced PLMS with magnesium in another 10 patients group. Also intravenous magnesium sulfate given for preterm labor to a 26-week pregnant woman with a 13-year history of RLS resolved all of her symptoms.[88] However, Walters and his group,[89] using results of serum and cerebrospinal fluid studies, concluded that magnesium is not likely to play a role in RLS.

Melatonin

Circadian aspects of RLS symptoms and of PLMS raised questions about the possible circadian changes in cortical excitability.[102] It is not clear yet if the peak of the melatonin secretion precedes or follows the sensory and motor symptoms of RLS.[92,93] Reduced PLMS with melatonin was observed in patients with PLMD.[90] To the contrary, Whittom and colleagues[91] noted that PLMS worsen on the Suggested Immobilization Test (SIT) after patients received melatonin. RLS-related insomnia also seems Herbs to not be correlated to decreased melatonin.[94]

Herbs and Seeds

Valerian, drinks and concoctions, homeopathic remedies

Valerian is an herb with sedative properties. Cuellar and Ratcliffe[95] studied 37 participants in a randomized placebo-control triple blind study comparing valerian to placebo for 8 weeks. The authors did not find significant differences, but concluded that there is a trend toward improved IRLS score and sleep in the valerian group.

Patients' discussion boards often present suggestions for drinks and concoctions to relieve RLS symptoms. These drinks include poppy seed tea that has traces of opiate. Opiates can relieve RLS symptoms.[103–106] Another proposed drink is tonic water that has very small amounts of quinine. Quinine was used for the treatment of muscle cramps, but its use was discontinued because of severe side effects. Quinine did not relieve RLS symptoms.[107] Baking soda has been used as an antacid and to treat hypokalemia and tricyclic antidepressants overdose.[108] There are no studies documenting its efficacy for treating RLS symptoms. Apple cider vinegar is alkaline and is another suggested therapy for RLS with no clinical backing. Black strap molasses is rich in iron, which is an important factor in RLS and its management.

Homeopathic remedies that are frequently mentioned on the Internet as potential RLS symptom relievers include aconite, arsenicum, causticum, ignatia, rhus tox, sulfur, and zincum metallicum. There is no evidence supporting their use, and these can cause more harm than good because some are poisonous if accumulated in the body.

Table 1
Supplements and their potential association with RLS

Supplement	Role	Effect on RLS Prevalence	Effect on RLS Symptoms	Comments
Vitamin B3 (niacin)	Increases HDL cholesterol, reduces triglycerides, improves joint flexibility	—	Relieved in 1 case report[74]	—
Vitamin B9 (folate)	Synthesis of BH4 (tyrosine hydroxylase, dopamine) and many other functions	—	Improved in 6 women with RLS and depression[75] Improved symptoms on different forums	Large diurnal changes in BH4 in RLS[76]
Vitamin B12 (cobalamin)	Regulation and synthesis of DNA, synthesis of fatty acids and other functions	—	Improved in 1 case report[77] Improved symptoms on different forums	—
Vitamin C (ascorbic acid)	Improves iron and many other functions	—	Relieved in patients with ESRD by 10 points average (IRLS)[78]	—
Vitamin D	Calcium absorption, modulation of cell growth, neuromuscular and immune function, reduction of inflammation	1. Increased in vitamin D deficiency[79] 2. Serum vitamin D lower in RLS[80]	Improved with supplement[81]	Dopaminergic dysfunction caused by vitamin D deficiency consistent with protein profile of RLS[82]
Vitamin E	Antioxidant, supports the immune system	—	1. Relieved in placebo-controlled study in ESRD by 10 points average (IRLS)[78] 2. Relieved in 2 patients[83]	Relief of leg cramps in 22 pts[83]
Calcium	Propagation of neuromuscular activity, regulation of endocrine functions, blood coagulation, bone and teeth metabolism, and many other functions	1. Increased prevalence in pts with ESRD on calcium blockers[84] 2. Calcium levels higher in ESRD and RLS[85]	Improved symptoms on different forums	—

	Function		Beneficial evidence	Conflicting evidence
Iron	Dopamine synthesis and many other functions	Decreased iron stores associated with RLS	Improved or relieved on multiple studies (see text)	—
Magnesium	Phosphorylation of ATP, binding macromolecules to organelles,[86] among other functions	—	1. Improved: reduced PLMS in 10 pts[87] 2. Resolved in 1 case report of 26 wk pregnant woman with 13 y RLS[88]	No role in RLS by serum and cerebrospinal magnesium studies[89]
Melatonin	Circadian rhythms and many other functions	—	1. Reduced PLMS in pts with PLMD[90] 2. Worsening of PLMs on SIT after melatonin[91]	1. Peak of melatonin secretion vs sensory and motor symptoms[92,93] 2. RLS-related insomnia not correlated with decreased melatonin[94]
Valerian	Sedative herb	—	Improved: IRLS, sleepiness[95] Improved symptoms on different forums	—

Abbreviations: BH4, tetrahydrobiopterin; ESRD, end-stage renal disease; HDL, high-density lipoprotein; pts, patients.

Box 3
Supplements with questionable role in controlling but frequently mentioned on RLS websites

Vitamin B6 (pyridoxine) is involved in the production of serotonin, norepinephrine, and formation of myelin.

Iodine is required to synthesize thyroid hormones in order to maintain a euthyroid state. Iodine is added to table salt to prevent goiter but not to gourmet salts. The distance from the ocean affects the soil content of iodine.

Potassium regulates muscle and nerve excitability. Symptoms of potassium deficiency include muscle cramps, muscle fatigue, irritability, and insomnia.

Zinc is a cofactor in many enzymes. Zinc is involved in the regulation of dopamine by acting as a dopamine reuptake inhibitor.

L-Theanine is a glutamate analogue that increases the levels of dopamine. There are anecdotal reports that L-theanine worsens RLS symptoms. One report on a group of boys with attention-deficit/ hyperactivity disorder showed that it improves relaxation and sleep[96]

Omega-3 fatty acids have complex effects on most neurotransmitters and can affect dopamine levels.

Ribose is used to improve athletic performance and prevent muscle fatigue, cramping, pain, and stiffness.

Tyrosine is a precursor of dopamine.

Aesculus hippocastanum (horse chestnut) is used to improve venous drainage by enhancing prostaglandin; it improves symptoms of chronic venous insufficiency, but the evidence for controlling cramps is insufficient.[97]

Astragalus (milk vetch) may stimulate the immune system, but there are no clinical data to support it.

Bach Rescue is a homeopathic blend of 5 flowers with relaxing and sedative properties. Improved RLS symptoms were reported on different forums

Curcumin is a phenol in the ginger family. It was found to alter iron metabolism potentially causing iron deficiency

Ginger is an herb used to treat gastrointestinal problems. It is also used for pain relief from arthritis and muscle soreness. Different forums have reported on its ability to reduce RLS symptoms.

Ginkgo biloba improves endothelium-dependent vasodilatation and, consequently, blood flow to the brain. It acts as an antioxidant.

Kava is an herb with sedative and anesthetic properties. It also has significant side effects (cases of liver failure reported). It is touted as a cure for RLS on different Web sites and forums, but its potential for side effects overshadows its unproven clinical effect.

Passion flower is an herb with sedative and anesthetic properties. It is said to improve RLS symptoms

Poppy seed has opiate traces, and improvement in RLS symptoms was reported on different forums.

Ruscus aculeatus (butcher's broom) is a shrub with antiinflammatory, antithrombotic, and diuretic properties. A study on 148 patients with chronic venous insufficiency compared with placebo showed better results and good tolerability.[98]

St. John's wort is an herb that promotes dopamine and possibly ameliorates symptoms of RLS.[99]

Homeopathic remedies (aconite, arsenicum, causticum, ignatia, rhus tox, sulfur, and zincum metallicum) can be poisonous if accumulated in the body.

APPLICATIONS AND PROCEDURES
Soap Bar, Massage, Sensory Stimulation, Botulinum Toxin, Enhanced External Counter Pulsation, Endovenous Laser Ablation, Sclerotherapy

Old wives' tales suggest baths, massages, and the use of soap. Interestingly enough, even though water therapy is always discussed with or mentioned by the patients, there are only anecdotal reports to support it. Hot baths, cold baths, jet baths, foot baths, alternating hot and cold packs, adding hydrogen peroxide, Epsom salt, baking soda, sea salts, and essential oils are reported by patients with RLS symptoms as having different degrees of success. Keeping the legs warm or keeping them cold, avoiding heavy blankets, and the use of pillows positioned under or between the legs are frequent tips on different Internet forums and occasionally may find their way in the clinic, despite of only anecdotal evidence to support them.

The most far-fetched therapy is the soap bar in bed, under the sheets, between or near the legs, or even holding it during sleep. It is popular on many Web sites, even with health professionals, and was reported to successfully control RLS symptoms and nocturnal leg cramps by several readers but not for others. It was mentioned in one of Ann Landers columns in a daily newspaper. One proposed explanation besides a simplistic pure placebo effect is that bar soaps contain esters and oils that evaporate from the surface of the bar may induce vasodilatation.[109]

Massage might have been the first treatment for symptoms of RLS. It is based on our intuitive instinct to rub areas that hurt. The first known accounts date to about 2700 BC. Massage was noted to increase dopamine secretion as measured in urine.[110] Deep massage, but no light or superficial massage, was reported to relieve RLS symptoms in all 173 (72% female) Indian patients.[111] The massage was performed between the ankle and the knee by either a deep rub with the palm or by pressing the muscles leading to their sequential compression. In most cases, family members, usually the younger ones, performed the massage. The investigators mention that it is common practice in Indian families that younger members of the family give the elders a deep legs massage at bedtime. Several subjects in the study found that tying a rope or cloth on their legs tight enough to prevent blood flow provided more relief than massage. The continuous pressure on the legs might have reduced the excitability of spinal neurons, resulting in symptom relief. Tying the rope/cloth was more common among women (82%), possibly related to the patriarchal social culture.

A case report presented a twice-a-week massage protocol over 3 weeks that focused on the lower extremities, the piriformis, and hamstring muscles and used different techniques. It resulted in improvement in reported RLS symptoms, including tingling sensations, urge to move, and sleeplessness. The symptoms returned 2 weeks after treatment discontinuation.[112]

Bodywork tips for RLS on one Web site include piriformis release, myofascial release, trigger point therapy, deep tissue massage, and sports massage. Another Web site suggests tissue density restoration massage of the lower legs with warm cream. The use of alcohol and muscle ointments is also recommended on different forums, as is Reiki massage. Reflexology was reported on the Reflexology Success Web site to improve sleep in one case of RLS.

The hypothesis that sensory stimulation may improve RLS symptoms was tested by Rozeman and colleagues.[113] In the study, 36 patients with RLS were randomized to undergo 3 consecutive SITs under each of 3 conditions: no electrical stimulation, application of an external electrical stimulus to the posterior tibial nerve, and application of a similar stimulus a little aside from the nerve to limit the stimulus effect to the tactile sensory effect only. The results of the study showed only a small trend toward lower visual analog scale scores in patients with RLS receiving an electrical stimulus.[113]

Botulinum toxin (Botox) is a neurotoxic protein used to relax and paralyze a muscle for a period of 3 to 4 months. Its hypothesized effect on RLS might be attributed to reducing peripheral and central sensitization to pain when injected subcutaneously to the lower limbs.[114] A small series that included 3 patients received botulinum toxin type A intramuscular injections in both legs, and one patient that received an additional injection in the lumbar paraspinal muscles reported improvement in RLS symptoms. The patients reduced or discontinued oral therapy for RLS, and the effects lasted for 10 to 12 weeks.[115] The study, however, lacked measures of RLS severity. Another single-arm open-label pilot trial corroborated these results by showing a statistically significant improvement in IRLS during the first 4 weeks of treatment with botulinum toxin A.[116]

These promising results were contradicted by a double-blind placebo-controlled crossover pilot trial in 6 patients who showed no significant improvement in IRLS and mean Clinical Global Improvement scales with botulinum toxin.[117] Furthermore, an open-label noncomparative study showed no efficacy in alleviating RLS symptoms with botulinum toxin type A.[118]

Enhanced external counter pulsation (EECP) is used to treat refractory angina pectoris in patients who are not amenable to coronary revascularization. Coincidentally, it was found to significantly improve RLS symptoms as measured by the IRLS in 6 patients with angina or congestive heart failure and RLS.[119]

Hayes and colleagues[120] performed endovenous laser ablation on 35 patients with RLS with concurrent duplex-proven superficial venous insufficiency (SVI). An IRLS improvement by 15 or more points was reported in 89% of the patients, and 53% showed an IRLS score of 5 or less. Moreover, 31% had a score of zero, supporting the conclusion that SVI should be ruled out in all patients with an RLS diagnosis.

Sclerotherapy was associated with initial relief in 98% of patients with varicose vein disease and RLS. The investigator suggests that this subpopulation of patients with RLS be considered for lower-extremities phlebological evaluation.[121]

DEVICES

Relaxis (Sensory NeuroStimulation, Inc, San Clemente, CA) is the only RLS nonpharmacologic treatment to be approved by the FDA.[122] It is a pad designed to provide timed vibratory counter-stimulation and is available by prescription. The developers reported an improvement in medical outcomes study (MOS) and in inventory scores similar to the improvement achieved by dopaminergic medications.[123,124]

Compression stockings applied to the thigh and leg regions improved RLS symptoms as measured by the IRLS. A pilot study showed that patients who wore a pneumatic sequential compression device for 1 hour each evening before the onset of RLS symptoms showed either complete symptom resolution or a significant improvement.[125] A randomized double-blind sham-controlled trial in 35 patients corroborated the initial findings, with one-third showing complete relief and the rest a significant improvement.[126] The basis for this method is similar to EECP.

Near-infrared light (NIR) can generate nitric oxide in the endothelium similar to exercise. Following a successful case report[127] in which NIR was used to reduce symptoms of RLS, the Mitchell group randomized 34 patients to either the control or the treatment group. The treatment consisted of 12 sessions of 30-minute treatments with NIR to the lower legs. After 4 weeks the treatment group had a significantly greater reduction on the IRLS.[128] In yet another study, 25 patients with RLS were randomized to 2 different wavelengths and frequencies on the infrared devices. The patients received 30-minute treatments to the lower legs, 3 times per week for 4 weeks. Both groups showed a significant improvement in IRLS scores after 4 weeks regardless of the device used.[129]

Deep brain stimulation can improve sleep quality in PD.[130] Okun and colleagues[131] reported the case of a woman with generalized dystonia and RLS whose restless legs resolved after bilateral deep brain stimulation of the globus pallidus internus. Ondo and colleagues[132] implanted bilateral deep brain stimulation of the globus pallidus internus to test if the procedure can improve idiopathic RLS. The results showed that the patient had a good but incomplete response.

Stupar[133] reported a case of RLS symptoms being improved to 65% after 2 weeks of *chiropractic therapy*. The improvement persisted beyond 1 month.

Standard acupuncture reduced leg activity on actigraphy.[134] However, a review by Cui and colleagues[135] concluded that there is insufficient evidence to determine whether acupuncture is an efficacious and safe treatment of RLS. Acupuncture and Teding Diancibo Pu (TDP) radiation (from a special electromagnetic spectrum mineral lamp developed in China) had a better therapeutic effect on RLS when compared with L-dopa.[136]

Wang and Fan[137] presented a series of 50 cases of pediatric RLS successfully treated with the integrated method of Chinese herbal drugs and *auricular-plaster therapy*.

BEHAVIORAL AND COGNITIVE

Mental activities are usually recommended to control the symptoms of RLS. These activities can include crossword puzzles, reading, card games, and computer work.[138] Additional activities may include knitting and having a meaningful discussion.

Sexual activity or masturbation can be used to control symptoms of RLS.[139] However, men with PLMD had fewer maximum tumescent episodes and less frequent sexual thoughts.[140]

The role of *cognitive-behavioral therapy (CBT)* in RLS is suggested by the increase in dysfunctional attitudes and beliefs about sleep in these patients. Short-term effects of CBT on PLMD were compared with treatment with clonazepam.[141] Patients treated with CBT showed decreased daytime napping, and patients treated with clonazepam showed decreased periodic-leg-movements arousals. The effect of CBT on RLS symptoms has yet to be investigated.

The *placebo effect* of treatments over RLS symptoms has to be taken into consideration. A considerable placebo response that was associated with changes in the IRLS was noted in patients who underwent pharmacologic treatment.[142]

SUMMARY

In conclusion, although there are more holes than cheese in Swiss cheese, the nonpharmacologic treatments for RLS are worth considering given the limitations and partial success of the currently approved methods. Additional research to establish the efficacy of nonpharmacologic treatments for RLS and to separate the myths from the science is very much needed.

Yoga and RLS

Manvir Bhatia, MD (Medicine), DM (Neurology)
Director Sleep Medicine and Senior Consultant Neurology
Saket City Hospital and Neurology and Sleep Center
New Delhi, India

Yoga and meditation is recognized as a form of mind-body medicine that integrates an individual's physical, mental and spiritual components to improve aspects of health, particularly stress related illnesses.

The word *yoga* comes from a Sanskrit root *yuj*, which means union or yoke, to join, and to direct and concentrate one's attention. It is typically considered that yoga is composed of physical postures (asanas), breathing techniques (pranayama), and meditation (dhyana).

Therapeutic yoga is defined as the application of yoga postures and practice to the treatment of health conditions and involves instruction in yogic practices and teachings to prevent, reduce, or alleviate structural, physiologic, emotional and spiritual pain, suffering, or limitations.

Yoga nidra or "yogi sleep" is a sleeplike state that causes deep states of relaxation while still maintaining full consciousness.

RLS is known to be caused by a deficiency of dopamine, with triggers for worsening of RLS being anxiety and stress. In addition, there is coexisting depression in many patients.

Yogic techniques are known to balance the parasympathetic/sympathetic system and result in improvement of mood, anxiety, and so forth. Thus, logically, yoga should prove to be an effective, safe mode of treatment of RLS.

A study by Kjaer and colleagues[143] demonstrated a 65% increase in endogenous dopamine release in the ventral striatum during yoga nidra meditation. Increased dopamine tone was noted during meditation-induced change of consciousness.

Iyengar yoga is based on the 4 principles of Ashtanga yoga, with an emphasis on improving stamina, flexibility, concentration, and balance.[144]

Yama, the first principle, emphasizes abstinence from violence, which helps the body resist cravings and materialistic desires.

The second principle, Niyama, emphasizes cleansing the body and the mind of stress caused by unfulfilled desires.

The third principle is based on the asanas, which help the body improve strength and flexibility and combat physical malaise.

The fourth principle, pranayama, emphasizes deep, slow breathing. Pratyahara and Dhyana, the other principles incorporated into Iyengar yoga, emphasize quieting the mind and achieving unity with the divine.

With this practice, Iyengar targeted multiple ailments and disorders such as high blood pressure, depression, chronic neck and back pain, immunodeficiency, increase in concentration and focus, thereby helping to relieve the mind and body of stress.[145]

Innes and colleagues[146] enrolled 13 women with moderate to severe RLS in an 8-week Iyengar yoga program. The patients were drug naïve and had symptoms at least 2 days per week. The investigators reported a 49% decline in RLS symptoms overall and a 62% decrease in symptoms severity, along with significant sleep improvement.

In conclusion, yoga may be a safe alternative or complementary treatment of RLS. The underlying mechanism may be a decrease in sympathoadrenal and hypothalamic pituitary adrenal axis activation while restoring parasympathetic/sympathetic balance. Yoga may also promote a change in dopamine levels. Studies on yoga have also shown changes in the neurochemical system, which may promote beneficial changes in mood, sleep, autonomic nervous system function, and pain processing contributing to reduction of RLS symptoms.

REFERENCES

1. American Academy of Sleep Medicine. International classification of sleep disorders, revised: diagnostic and coding manual. Chicago: American Academy of Sleep Medicine; 2001.

2. Byrne R, Sinha S, Chaudhuri KR. Restless legs syndrome: diagnosis and review of management

options. Neuropsychiatr Dis Treat 2006;2(2): 155–64.

3. Phillips B, Young T, Finn L, et al. Epidemiology of restless legs symptoms in adults. Arch Intern Med 2000;160(14):2137–41.

4. Ohayon MM, Roth T. Prevalence of restless legs syndrome and periodic limb movement disorder in the general population. J Psychosom Res 2002;53(1):547–54.

5. Aukerman MM, Aukerman D, Bayard M, et al. Exercise and restless legs syndrome: a randomized controlled trial. J Am Board Fam Med 2006;19(5): 487–93.

6. Clifford PS, Hellsten Y. Vasodilatory mechanisms in contracting skeletal muscle [review]. J Appl Physiol (1985) 2004;97(1):393–403.

7. Oskarsson E, Wåhlin-Larsson B, Ulfberg J. Reduced daytime intramuscular blood flow in patients with restless legs syndrome/Willis Ekbom disease. Psychiatry Clin Neurosci 2014;68(8):640–3.

8. Salminen AV, Rimpilä V, Polo O. Peripheral hypoxia in restless legs syndrome. Neurology 2014;82(21): 1856–61.

9. de Mello MT, Lauro FA, Silva AC, et al. Incidence of periodic limb movements and of the restless legs syndrome during sleep following acute physical activity in spinal cord injury subjects. Spinal Cord 1996;34(5):294–6.

10. Petzinger GM, Fisher BE, Van Leeuwen JE, et al. Enhancing neuroplasticity in the basal ganglia: the role of exercise in Parkinson's disease. Mov Disord 2010;25(Suppl 1):S141–5.

11. De Vito K, Li Y, Batool-Anwar S, et al. Prospective study of obesity, hypertension, high cholesterol, and risk of restless legs syndrome. Mov Disord 2014;29(8):1044–52.

12. Gao X, Schwarzschild MA, Wang H, et al. Obesity and restless legs syndrome in men and women. Neurology 2009;72(14):1255–61.

13. Batool-Anwar S, Malhotra A, Forman J, et al. Restless legs syndrome and hypertension in middle-aged women. Hypertension 2011;58:791–6.

14. Koo BB, Sillau S, Dennis DA 2nd, et al. Periodic limb movements during sleep and prevalent hypertension in the multi-ethnic study of atherosclerosis. Hypertension 2015;65:70–7.

15. Siddiqui F, Strus J, Ming X, et al. Rise of blood pressure with periodic limb movements in sleep and wakefulness. Clin Neurophysiol 2007;118: 1923–30.

16. Bliwise DL, Zhang RH, Kutner NG. Medications associated with restless legs syndrome: a case-control study in the US Renal Data System (USRDS). Sleep Med 2014;15(10):1241–5.

17. Becker PM, Sharon D. Mood disorders in restless legs syndrome (Willis-Ekbom disease) [review]. J Clin Psychiatry 2014;75(7):e679–94.

18. Chopra A, Pendergrass DS, Bostwick JM. Mirtazapine-induced worsening of restless legs syndrome (RLS) and ropinirole-induced psychosis: challenges in management of depression in RLS. Psychosomatics 2011;52(1):92–4.

19. Rottach KG, Schaner BM, Kirch MH, et al. Restless legs syndrome as side effect of second generation antidepressants. J Psychiatr Res 2008;43(1):70–5.

20. Page RL 2nd, Ruscin JM, Bainbridge JL, et al. Restless legs syndrome induced by escitalopram: case report and review of the literature [review]. Pharmacotherapy 2008;28(2):271–80.

21. Perroud N, Lazignac C, Baleydier B, et al. Restless legs syndrome induced by citalopram: a psychiatric emergency? Gen Hosp Psychiatry 2007;29(1): 72–4 [Erratum appears in Gen Hosp Psychiatry 2007;29(2):177]. Nader, Perroud [corrected to Perroud, Nader]; Coralie, Lazignac [corrected to Lazignac, Coralie]; Andrei, Cicotti [corrected to Cicotti, Andrei]; Susanne, Maris [corrected to Maris, Susanne].

22. Pearson VE, Gamaldo CE, Allen RP, et al. Medication use in patients with restless legs syndrome compared with a control population. Eur J Neurol 2008;15(1):16–21.

23. Rittmannsberger H, Werl R. Restless legs syndrome induced by quetiapine: report of seven cases and review of the literature. Int J Neuropsychopharmacol 2013;16(6):1427–31.

24. Jagota P, Asawavichienjinda T, Bhidayasiri R. Prevalence of neuroleptic-induced restless legs syndrome in patients taking neuroleptic drugs. J Neurol Sci 2012;314(1–2):158–60.

25. Spencer BR, Kleinman S, Wright DJ, et al, REDS-II RISE Analysis Group. Restless legs syndrome, pica, and iron status in blood donors. Transfusion 2013;53(8):1645–52.

26. Birgegård G, Schneider K, Ulfberg J. High incidence of iron depletion and restless leg syndrome (RLS) in regular blood donors: intravenous iron sucrose substitution more effective than oral iron. Vox Sang 2010;99(4):354–61.

27. Silber MH, Richardson JW. Multiple blood donations associated with iron deficiency in patients with restless legs syndrome. Mayo Clin Proc 2003;78(1):52–4.

28. Gamaldo CE, Benbrook AR, Allen RP, et al. Childhood and adult factors associated with restless legs syndrome (RLS) diagnosis. Sleep Med 2007; 8(7–8):716–22.

29. Ulfberg J, Nyström B. Restless legs syndrome in blood donors. Sleep Med 2004;5(2):115–8.

30. Arunthari V, Kaplan J, Fredrickson PA, et al. Prevalence of restless legs syndrome in blood donors. Mov Disord 2010;25(10):1451–5.

31. Burchell BJ, Allen RP, Miller JK, et al. RLS and blood donation. Sleep Med 2009;10(8):844–9.

32. Becker PM. Bleed less than 3: RLS and blood donation. Sleep Med 2009;10(8):820–1.

33. Swanson LM, Arnedt JT, Rosekind MR, et al. Sleep disorders and work performance: findings from the 2008 National Sleep Foundation Sleep in America poll. J Sleep Res 2011;20(3):487–94.

34. Chung KT, Wong TY, Wei CI, et al. Tannins and human health: a review [review]. Crit Rev Food Sci Nutr 1998;38(6):421–64.

35. Disler PB, Lynch SR, Charlton RW, et al. The effect of tea on iron absorption. Gut 1975;16(3):193–200.

36. Rye D. The genetics and pathogenesis of restless legs syndrome: implications for the clinician. Medscape Family Medicine 2008. Available at: http://www.medscape.org. Accessed June 26, 2015.

37. Aldrich MS, Shipley JE. Alcohol use and periodic limb movements of sleep. Alcohol Clin Exp Res 1993;17(1):192–6.

38. Chavoshi F, Einollahi B, Sadeghniat Haghighi K, et al. Prevalence and sleep related disorders of restless legs syndrome in hemodialysis patients. Nephrourol Mon 2015;7(2):e24611. eCollection 2015.

39. Zhang J, Lam SP, Li SX, et al. Restless legs symptoms in adolescents: epidemiology, heritability, and pubertal effects. J Psychosom Res 2014;76(2):158–64.

40. Salman SM. Restless legs syndrome in patients on hemodialysis. Saudi J Kidney Dis Transpl 2011; 22(2):368–72.

41. Hadjigeorgiou GM, Stefanidis I, Dardiotis E, et al. Low RLS prevalence and awareness in central Greece: an epidemiological survey. Eur J Neurol 2007;14(11):1275–80.

42. Gigli GL, Adorati M, Dolso P, et al. Restless legs syndrome in end-stage renal disease [review]. Sleep Med 2004;5(3):309–15. Available at: http://www.ncbi.nlm.nih.gov/pubmed/15165541.

43. Rangarajan S, Rangarajan S, D'Souza GA. Restless legs syndrome in an Indian urban population. Sleep Med 2007;9(1):88–93.

44. Cirillo DJ, Wallace RB. Restless legs syndrome and functional limitations among American elders in the Health and Retirement Study. BMC Geriatr 2012; 12:39.

45. Lutz EG. Restless legs, anxiety and caffeinism. J Clin Psychiatry 1978;39(9):693–8.

46. Al-Jahdali HH, Al-Qadhi WA, Khogeer HA, et al. Restless legs syndrome in patients on dialysis. Saudi J Kidney Dis Transpl 2009;20(3):378–85.

47. Chen WC, Lim PS, Wu WC, et al. Sleep behavior disorders in a large cohort of Chinese (Taiwanese) patients maintained by long-term hemodialysis. Am J Kidney Dis 2006;48(2):277–84.

48. Provini F, Antelmi E, Vignatelli L, et al. Increased prevalence of nocturnal smoking in restless legs syndrome (RLS). Sleep Med 2010;11(2):218–20.

49. Mountifield JA. Restless legs syndrome relieved by cessation of smoking. CMAJ 1985;133(5):426–7.

50. Lavigne GL, Lobbezoo F, Rompré PH, et al. Cigarette smoking as a risk factor or an exacerbating factor for restless legs syndrome and sleep bruxism. Sleep 1997;20(4):290–3.

51. Oksenberg A. Alleviation of severe restless legs syndrome (RLS) symptoms by cigarette smoking. J Clin Sleep Med 2010;6(5):489–90.

52. Ishikawa A, Miyatake T. Effects of smoking in patients with early-onset Parkinson's disease. J Neurol Sci 1993;117(1–2):28–32. Available at: http://www.ncbi.nlm.nih.gov/pubmed/8410063.

53. Lahan V, Ahmad S, Gupta R. RLS relieved by tobacco chewing: paradoxical role of nicotine. Neurol Sci 2012;33(5):1209–10.

54. Quik M, Huang LZ, Parameswaran N, et al. Multiple roles for nicotine in Parkinson's disease [review]. Biochem Pharmacol 2009;78(7):677–85.

55. Keckeis M, Lattova Z, Maurovich-Horvat E, et al. Impaired glucose tolerance in sleep disorders. PLoS One 2010;5(3):e9444.

56. Bosco D, Plastino M, Fava A, et al. Role of the oral glucose tolerance test (OGGT) in the idiopathic restless legs syndrome. J Neurol Sci 2009;287(1–2):60–3.

57. de Groot S. Restless legs due to ingestion of "light" beverages containing saccharine. Results of an N-of-1 trial. Ned Tijdschr Tandheelkd 2007;114(6): 263–6 [in Dutch].

58. Allen RP, Barker PB, Horská A, et al. Thalamic glutamate/glutamine in restless legs syndrome: increased and related to disturbed sleep. Neurology 2013;80(22):2028–34.

59. Weinstock LB, Walters AS, Mullin GE, et al. Celiac disease is associated with restless legs syndrome. Dig Dis Sci 2010;55(6):1667–73.

60. Manchanda S, Davies CR, Picchietti D. Celiac disease as a possible cause for low serum ferritin in patients with restless legs syndrome. Sleep Med 2009;10(7):763–5.

61. Cikrikcioglu MA, Halac G, Hursitoglu M, et al. Prevalence of gluten sensitive enteropathy antibodies in restless legs syndrome. Acta Neurol Belg 2011; 111(4):282–6. Available at: http://www.ncbi.nlm.nih.gov/pubmed/22368967.

62. Earley CJ, Connor J, Garcia-Borreguero D, et al. Altered brain iron homeostasis and dopaminergic function in restless legs syndrome (Willis-Ekbom disease). Sleep Med 2014;15(11):1288–301.

63. Lillo-Triguero L, Del Castillo A, Morán-Jiménez MJ, et al. Brain iron accumulation in dysmetabolic iron overload syndrome with restless legs syndrome. Sleep Med 2014;15(8):1004–5.

64. Allen RP, Earley CJ. Restless legs syndrome: a review of clinical and pathophysiologic features [review]. J Clin Neurophysiol 2001;18(2):128–47.

65. Allen RP, Barker PB, Wehrl FW, et al. MRI measurement of brain iron in patients with restless legs syndrome. Neurology 2001;56(2):263–5.

66. Trotti LM, Goldstein CA, Harrod CG, et al. Quality measures for the care of adult patients with restless legs syndrome. J Clin Sleep Med 2015;11(3):311–34.

67. Picchietti DL, Hensley JG, Bainbridge JL, et al, International Restless Legs Syndrome Study Group (IRLSSG). Consensus clinical practice guidelines for the diagnosis and treatment of restless legs syndrome/Willis-Ekbom disease during pregnancy and lactation [review]. Sleep Med Rev 2015;22:64–77.

68. Lee CS, Lee SD, Kang SH, et al. Comparison of the efficacies of oral iron and pramipexole for the treatment of restless legs syndrome patients with low serum ferritin. Eur J Neurol 2014;21(2):260–6.

69. Mehmood T, Auerbach M, Earley CJ, et al. Response to intravenous iron in patients with iron deficiency anemia (IDA) and restless leg syndrome (Willis-Ekbom disease). Sleep Med 2014;15(12):1473–6.

70. Zhang X, Chen WW, Huang WJ. Efficacy of the low-dose Saccharum iron treatment of idiopathic restless legs syndrome. Panminerva Med 2015;57(3):109–13.

71. Silber MH, Becker PM, Earley C, et al, Medical Advisory Board of the Willis-Ekbom Disease Foundation. Willis-Ekbom Disease Foundation revised consensus statement on the management of restless legs syndrome. Mayo Clin Proc 2013;88(9):977–86.

72. Dosman C, Witmans M, Zwaigenbaum L. Iron's role in pediatric restless legs syndrome – a review. Paediatr Child Health 2012;17(4):193–7.

73. Aurora RN, Kristo DA, Bista SR, et al, American Academy of Sleep Medicine. The treatment of restless legs syndrome and periodic limb movement disorder in adults – an update for 2012: practice parameters with an evidenced based systematic review and meta-analyses: an American Academy of Sleep Medicine Clinical Practice Guideline [review]. Sleep 2012;35(8):1039–62.

74. Botez MI, Cadotte M, Beaulieu R, et al. Neurologic disorders responsive to folic acid therapy. Can Med Assoc J 1976;115(3):217–23.

75. Mangan D. A case report of niacin in the treatment of restless legs syndrome. Med Hypotheses 2009;73(6):1072.

76. Earley CJ, Hyland K, Allen RP. Circadian changes in CSF dopaminergic measures in restless legs syndrome. Sleep Med 2006;7(3):263–8.

77. O'Keeffe ST, Noel J, Lavan JN. Restless legs syndrome in the elderly. Postgrad Med J 1993;69:701–3.

78. Sagheb MM, Dormanesh B, Fallahzadeh MK, et al. Efficacy of vitamins C, E and their combination for treatment of restless legs syndrome in hemodialysis patients: a randomized, double-blind, placebo-controlled trial. Sleep Med 2012;13(5):542–5.

79. Çakır T, Doğan G, Subaşı V, et al. An evaluation of sleep quality and the prevalence of restless legs syndrome in vitamin D deficiency. Acta Neurol Belg 2015 [Epub ahead of print] PMID: 25904436.

80. Balaban H, Yıldız ÖK, Çil G, et al. Serum 25-hydroxyvitamin D levels in restless legs syndrome patients. Sleep Med 2012;13(7):953–7.

81. Wali S, Shukr A, Boudal A, et al. The effect of vitamin D supplements on the severity of restless legs syndrome. Sleep Breath 2015;19(2):579–83.

82. Patton SM, Cho YW, Clardy TW, et al. Proteomic analysis of the cerebrospinal fluid of patients with restless legs syndrome. Fluids Barriers CNS 2013;10(1):20.

83. Ayres S Jr, Mihan R. Leg cramps and "restless legs" syndrome. Response to vitamin E (tocopherol). Calif Med 1969;111(2):87–91.

84. Telarović S, Relja M, Trkulja V. Restless legs syndrome in hemodialysis patients: association with calcium: a preliminary report. Eur Neurol 2007;58(3):166–9.

85. Kawauchi A, Inoue Y, Hashimoto T, et al. Restless legs syndrome in hemodialysis patients: health-related quality of life and laboratory data analysis. Clin Nephrol 2006;66(6):440–6.

86. Lau A, Chan LN. Electrolytes, other minerals and trace elements. In: Lee M, editor. Basic skills in interpreting laboratory data. 4th edition. Bethesda (MD): ASHP; 2009. special publishing. p. 119–60.

87. Hornyak M, Voderholzer U, Hohagen F, et al. Magnesium therapy for periodic leg movements-related insomnia and restless legs syndrome: an open pilot study. Sleep 1998;21(5):501–5.

88. Bartell S, Zallek S. Intravenous magnesium sulphate may relieve restless legs syndrome in pregnancy. J Clin Sleep Med 2006;2(2):187–8.

89. Walters AS, Elin RJ, Cohen B, et al. Magnesium not likely to play a major role in the pathogenesis of restless legs syndrome: serum and cerebrospinal fluid studies. Sleep Med 2007;8(2):186–7. No abstract available.

90. Kunz D, Bes F. Exogenous melatonin in periodic limb movement disorder: an open clinical trial and a hypothesis. Sleep 2001;24(2):183–7.

91. Whittom S, Dumont M, Petit D, et al. Effects of melatonin and bright light administration on motor and sensory symptoms of RLS. Sleep Med 2010;11(4):351–5.

92. Michaud M, Dumont M, Selmaoui B, et al. Circadian rhythm of restless legs syndrome: relationship with biological markers. Ann Neurol 2004;55(3):372–80.

93. Duffy JF, Lowe AS, Silva EJ, et al. Periodic limb movements in sleep exhibit a circadian rhythm that is maximal in the late evening/early night. Sleep Med 2011;12(1):83–8.

94. Tribl GG, Waldhauser F, Sycha T, et al. Urinary 6-hydroxy-melatonin-sulfate excretion and circadian

rhythm in patients with restless legs syndrome. J Pineal Res 2003;35(4):295–6.

95. Cuellar NG, Ratcliffe SJ. Does valerian improve sleepiness and symptom severity in people with restless legs syndrome? Altern Ther Health Med 2009;15(2):22–8.

96. Lyon MR, Kapoor MP, Juneja LR. The effects of L-theanine (Suntheanine®) on objective sleep quality in boys with attention deficit hyperactivity disorder (ADHD): a randomized, double-blind, placebo-controlled clinical trial. Altern Med Rev 2011; 16(4):348–54.

97. Siebert U, Brach M, Sroczynski G, et al. Efficacy, routine effectiveness, and safety of horse chestnut seed extract in the treatment of chronic venous insufficiency. A meta-analysis of randomized controlled trials and large observational studies. Int Angiol 2002;21(4):305–15.

98. Vanscheidt W, Jost V, Wolna P, et al. Efficacy and safety of a Butcher's broom preparation (Ruscus aculeatus L. extract) compared to placebo in patients suffering from chronic venous insufficiency. Arzneimittelforschung 2002;52(4):243–50.

99. Pereira JC Jr, Pradella-Hallinan M, Alves RC. Saint John's wort, an herbal inducer of the cytochrome P4503A4 isoform may alleviate symptoms of Willis-Ekbom's disease. Clinics (Sao Paulo) 2013; 68(4):469–74.

100. Hazari MA, Arifuddin MS, Muzzakar S, et al. Serum calcium level in hypertension. N Am J Med Sci 2012;4(11):569–72.

101. Popoviciu L, Aşgian B, Delast-Popoviciu D, et al. Clinical, EEG, electromyographic and polysomnographic studies in restless legs syndrome caused by magnesium deficiency. Rom J Neurol Psychiatry 1993;31(1):55–61.

102. Gündüz A, Adatepe NU, Kiziltan ME, et al. Circadian changes in cortical excitability in restless legs syndrome. J Neurol Sci 2012;316(1–2):122–5.

103. Trenkwalder C, Beneš H, Grote L, et al, RELOXYN Study Group. Prolonged release oxycodone-naloxone for treatment of severe restless legs syndrome after failure of previous treatment: a double-blind, randomised, placebo-controlled trial with an open-label extension. Lancet Neurol 2013;12(12):1141–50 [Erratum appears in Lancet Neurol 2013;12(12):1133].

104. Silver N, Allen RP, Senerth J, et al. A 10-year, longitudinal assessment of dopamine agonists and methadone in the treatment of restless legs syndrome. Sleep Med 2011;12(5):440–4.

105. Ondo WG. Methadone for refractory restless legs syndrome. Mov Disord 2005;20(3):345–8.

106. Walters AS, Winkelmann J, Trenkwalder C, et al. Long-term follow-up on restless legs syndrome patients treated with opioids. Mov Disord 2001;16(6): 1105–9.

107. Martinez C, Finnern HW, Rietbrock S, et al. Patterns of treatment for restless legs syndrome in primary care in the United Kingdom. Clin Ther 2008;30(2): 405–18.

108. Knudsen K, Abrahamsson J. Epinephrine and sodium bicarbonate independently and additively increase survival in experimental amitriptyline poisoning. Crit Care Med 1997;25(4):669–74.

109. Page DH, Smailes H. Soap in bed calms restless legs. peoplespharmacy.com. 2012. Available at: www.peoplespharmacy.com/2014/11/03/soap-in-bed-calms-restless-legs/. Accessed June 26, 2015.

110. Field T, Hernandez-Reif M, Diego M, et al. Cortisol decreases and serotonin and dopamine increase following massage therapy. Int J Neurosci 2005; 115(10):1397–413.

111. Gupta R, Goel D, Ahmed S, et al. What patients do to counteract the symptoms of Willis-Ekbom disease (RLS/WED): effect of gender and severity of illness. Ann Indian Acad Neurol 2014;17(4):405–8.

112. Russell M. Massage therapy and restless legs syndrome. J Bodyw Mov Ther 2007;11(2):146–50.

113. Rozeman AD, Ottolini T, Grootendorst DC, et al. Effect of sensory stimuli on restless legs syndrome: a randomized crossover study. J Clin Sleep Med 2014;10(8):893–6.

114. Lim EC, Seet RC. Can botulinum toxin put the restless legs syndrome to rest? Med Hypotheses 2007; 69(3):497–501.

115. Rotenberg JS, Canard K, Difazio M. Successful treatment of recalcitrant restless legs syndrome with botulinum toxin type-A. J Clin Sleep Med 2006;2(3):275–8.

116. Agarwal P, Sia C, Vaish N, et al. Pilot trial of onabotulinumtoxina (Botox) in moderate to severe restless legs syndrome. Int J Neurosci 2011;121(11): 622–5.

117. Nahab FB, Peckham EL, Hallett M. Double-blind, placebo-controlled, pilot trial of botulinum toxin A in restless legs syndrome. Neurology 2008; 71(12):950–1.

118. Ghorayeb I, Bénard A, Vivot A, et al. A phase II, open label, non-comparative study of botulinum toxin in restless legs syndrome. Sleep Med 2012; 13(10):1313–6.

119. Rajaram SS, Shanahan J, Ash C, et al. Enhanced external counter pulsation (EECP) as a novel treatment for restless legs syndrome (RLS): a preliminary test of the vascular neurologic hypothesis for RLS. Sleep Med 2005;6(2):101–6.

120. Hayes CA, Kingsley JR, Hamby KR, et al. The effect of endovenous laser ablation on restless legs syndrome. Phlebology 2008;23(3):112–7.

121. Kanter AH. The effect of sclerotherapy on restless legs syndrome. Dermatol Surg 1995;21(4):328–32.

122. Jeffrey S. FDA Okays first device for restless legs syndrome [serial online]. Medscape Medical

News 2014. Available at: http://www.medscape.com/viewarticle/825971. Accessed June 10, 2014.

123. Burbank F, Buchfuhrer M, Kopjar B. Sleep improvement for restless legs syndrome patients. Part I: pooled analysis of two prospective, double-blind, sham-controlled, multi-center, randomized clinical studies of the effects of vibrating pads on RLS symptoms. Journal of Parkinsonism and Restless Legs Syndrome 2013;3:1–10.

124. Burbank F, Buchfuhrer M, Kopjar B. Improving sleep for patients with restless legs syndrome. Part II: meta-analysis of vibration therapy and drugs approved by the FDA for treatment of restless legs syndrome. Journal of Parkinsonism and Restless Legs Syndrome 2013;3:11–22.

125. Eliasson AH, Lettieri CJ. Sequential compression devices for treatment of restless legs syndrome [review]. Medicine (Baltimore) 2007;86(6):317–23.

126. Lettieri CJ, Eliasson AH. Pneumatic compression devices are an effective therapy for restless legs syndrome: a prospective, randomized, double-blinded, sham-controlled trial. Chest 2009;135(1):74–80.

127. Mitchell UH. Nondrug-related aspect of treating Ekbom disease, formerly known as restless legs syndrome. Neuropsychiatr Dis Treat 2011;7:251–7. Available at: http://www.ncbi.nlm.nih.gov/pubmed/21654870.

128. Mitchell UH, Myrer JW, Johnson AW, et al. Restless legs syndrome and near-infrared light: an alternative treatment option. Physiother Theory Pract 2011;27(5):345–51.

129. Mitchell UH, Johnson AW, Myrer B. Comparison of two infrared devices in their effectiveness in reducing symptoms associated with RLS. Physiother Theory Pract 2011;27(5):352–9.

130. Deli G, Aschermann Z, Ács P, et al. Bilateral subthalamic stimulation can improve sleep quality in Parkinson's disease. J Parkinsons Dis 2015 [Epub ahead of print]. MID: 25757828.

131. Okun MS, Fernandez HH, Foote KD. Deep brain stimulation of the GPi treats restless legs syndrome associated with dystonia. Mov Disord 2005;20(4):500–1.

132. Ondo WG, Jankovic J, Simpson R, et al. Globus pallidus deep brain stimulation for refractory idiopathic restless legs syndrome. Sleep Med 2012;13(9):1202–4.

133. Stupar M. Restless legs syndrome in a primary contact setting: a case report. J Can Chiropr Assoc 2008;52(2):81–7.

134. Pan W, Wang M, Li M, et al. Actigraph evaluation of acupuncture for treating restless legs syndrome. Evid Based Complement Alternat Med 2015;2015:343201.

135. Cui Y, Wang Y, Liu Z. Acupuncture for restless legs syndrome [review]. Cochrane Database Syst Rev 2008;(4):CD006457.

136. Wu YH, Sun CL, Wu D, et al. Observation on therapeutic effect of acupuncture on restless legs syndrome. Zhongguo Zhen Jiu 2008;28(1):27–9 [in Chinese].

137. Wang W, Fan H. Fifty cases of child restless syndrome treated with the integrated method of Chinese herbal drugs and auricular-plaster therapy. No abstract available. J Tradit Chin Med 2005;25(4):276–7.

138. Gamaldo CE, Earley CJ. Restless legs syndrome: a clinical update [review]. Chest 2006;130(5):1596–604.

139. Marin LF, Felicio AC, Prado GF. Sexual intercourse and masturbation: potential relief factors for restless legs syndrome? Sleep Med 2011;12(4):422.

140. Schiavi RC, Mandeli J, Schreiner-Engel P, et al. Aging, sleep disorders, and male sexual function. Biol Psychiatry 1991;30(1):15–24.

141. Edinger JD, Fins AI, Sullivan RJ, et al. Comparison of cognitive-behavioral therapy and clonazepam for treating periodic limb movement disorder. Sleep 1996;19(5):442–4.

142. Fulda S, Wetter TC. Where dopamine meets opioids: a meta-analysis of the placebo effect in restless legs syndrome treatment studies [review]. Brain 2008r;131(Pt 4):902–17.

143. Kjaer TW, Bertelsen C, Piccini P, et al. Increased dopamine tone during meditation-induced change of consciousness. Brain Res Cogn Brain Res 2002;13(2):255–9.

144. Iyengar PS. In yoga and the new millennium. Mumbai: YOG; 1998.

145. Crow EM, Jeannot E, Trewhela A. Effectiveness of Iyengar yoga in treating spinal (back and neck) pain: a systematic review. Int J Yoga 2015;8(1):3–14.

146. Innes KE, Selfe TK, Agarwal P, et al. Efficacy of an eight-week yoga intervention on symptoms of restless legs syndrome (RLS): a pilot study. J Altern Complement Med 2013;19(6):527–35.

Dopaminergic Therapy for Restless Legs Syndrome/Willis-Ekbom Disease

Rochelle S. Zak, MD[a],*, Arthur S. Walters, MD[b]

KEYWORDS

- Restless legs syndrome • Dopamine agonists • Treatment efficacy • Willis-Ekbom disease

KEY POINTS

- Several dopamine agonists are approved for the treatment of restless legs syndrome (RLS)/Willis-Ekbom disease (WED). Although they have similar profiles, there are specific instances that may favor one more than another.
- Sinemet can be used for short-term intermittent circumstances of forced immobilization, such as airplane flights.
- Pramipexole is useful for chronic treatment of RLS/WED in patients with good renal function and can be used in those patients who are taking medications that affect hepatic enzyme function.
- Ropinirole is useful for the chronic treatment of RLS/WED in patients with compromised renal function.
- Rotigotine is useful for the chronic treatment of RLS/WED in patients who have prominent symptoms throughout the day or who cannot take oral medications.

INTRODUCTION

Dopaminergic treatment of restless legs syndrome (RLS)/Willis-Ekbom disease (WED) has been recognized as an effective first-line treatment of this disorder.[1–3] Dopaminergic medications include levodopa, the nonergot dopamine agonists (pramipexole [Mirapex], ropinirole [Requip], rotigotine [Neupro], piribedil), and the ergot-derived dopamine agonists. The ergot-derived dopamine agonists have either been withdrawn (pergolide) or are not recommended for the usual treatment of RLS/WED (bromocriptine, cabergoline) because of reports of fibrosis and valvulopathy.[4–6] This article focuses on levodopa and the nonergot dopamine agonists, with the exception of piribedil because it is not yet US Food and Drug Administration approved and there is a paucity of data on the efficacy of this medication for RLS/WED at this time.

DOPAMINE PRECURSOR
Levodopa

The dopamine precursor levodopa combined with a dopamine carboxylase inhibitor (carbidopa/levodopa [Sinemet], carbidopa/levodopa/entacapone [Stalevo], or levodopa/benserazide [Madopar]) was one of the first documented efficacious medications for RLS and was initially reported in a small case series.[7] Since then, there have been larger clinical trials documenting the efficacy of levodopa in treating both the subjective[8,9] and objective[9,10] correlates of RLS/WED. Nausea is

[a] Sleep Disorders Center, University of California San Francisco, 2330 Post Street, San Francisco, CA 94115, USA;
[b] Department of Neurology, Vanderbilt University Medical Center, 2220 Pierce Avenue, Nashville, TN 37232, USA
* Corresponding author.
E-mail address: Rochelle.Zak@ucsf.edu

Sleep Med Clin 10 (2015) 279–285
http://dx.doi.org/10.1016/j.jsmc.2015.05.012
1556-407X/15/$ – see front matter © 2015 Elsevier Inc. All rights reserved.

the most common adverse effect.[2] The half-life of levodopa when combined with carbidopa is 1.5 hours[11] and is spread out with the continuous-release preparation.[12] It is primarily excreted in the urine.[13] However, levodopa has been shown to cause augmentation,[14] which has limited its use as a first-line agent for daily treatment of RLS/WED. Augmentation can be loosely defined as a worsening of RLS/WED symptoms secondary to treatment medication and is discussed in greater detail later.[15] Augmentation rates on L-dopa have been noted to be as high as 60%[16] to 82%.[17] However, for intermittent RLS/WED, defined as symptoms occurring only in exacerbating circumstances such as airplane flights or long drives or occurring less than twice a week, carbidopa/levodopa 25/100 (one-half to one tablet) may be a useful treatment.[18]

NONERGOT DOPAMINE AGONISTS

The nonergot dopamine agonists have become the standard of care for patients with RLS/WED for whom daily dopaminergic treatment is thought to be warranted.[1] Two oral medications, pramipexole (Mirapex) and ropinirole (Requip), and 1 transdermal medication, rotigotine (Neupro), allow clinicians to choose based on mode of metabolism (renal vs hepatic) and timing of symptoms (the transdermal route useful for significant daytime symptoms).

Pramipexole

Pharmacology
Pramipexole is a nonergot aminothiazole dopamine agonist. It is a potent agonist at the D2 subfamily of dopamine receptors with highest affinity for D3 receptors and slightly less affinity for D2 receptors,[19] having moderate affinity for the alpha2-adrenoreceptor and very low affinity for alpha1- and beta-adrenoreceptors, acetylcholine receptors, D1 receptors, and hydroxytryptamine (5-HT) receptors.[20] Pramipexole is excreted in the kidney with a half-life of 8 to 12 hours[21] in the short-acting version. The long-acting extended-release version secretes the medication consistently over 24 hours.[22]

Clinical efficacy
There is a large body of evidence supporting the efficacy of pramipexole for treating RLS/WED and its use is endorsed by both the AASM1 as well as the IRLSSG2. Scholz and colleagues[23] conducted a comprehensive meta-analysis of dopaminergic treatment of RLS/WED analyzing all available double-blind randomized placebo and actively controlled trials for the Cochrane

Collaboration. Although not every study had positive results, this analysis showed improvement in subjective parameters such as the IRLS (International RLS Severity Scale), subjective quality of sleep, and subjective disease-specific quality of life, as well as objective parameters such as a decrease in the Periodic Limb Movements of Sleep (PLMS) Index although there was no improvement in polysomnographically determined sleep efficiency.

Seven randomized placebo-controlled trials[24–30] showed a decrease in subjective RLS severity as indicated by the IRLS, with 1 having mixed results[31] (mean difference of −5.16 (95% confidence interval [CI], −6.88 to −3.43; I^2 = 76%); more negative indicates greater treatment effect). Overall, pramipexole treatment was associated with a subjective improvement in self-rated quality of sleep and disease-specific quality of life. Improvement in quality of sleep was shown by an overall increase in quality of sleep (standard mean difference, 0.44; 95% CI, 0.33–0.54; I^2 = 0%) with 5 studies showing improvement in subjective quality of sleep,[25–28,30] although 1 did not.[29] Similarly, most but not all studies showed improvement in quality of life (standard mean difference of 0.30; 95% CI, 0.13–0.47; I^2 = 60%) with 3 showing improved subjective quality of life[25,27,30] and 1 not.[32] There are 3 studies showing a decrease in PLMS Index with polysomnography (PSG) (mean difference, −30.47; 95% CI, −51.58 to −9.35; I^2 = 52%).[26,29,33] Two studies of polysomnographically demonstrated sleep efficiency did not show improvement with pramipexole (mean difference, 2.47; 95% CI, −1.60–6.55; I^2 = 0%).[26,29] As Manconi and colleagues[34] pointed out, treatment of either arousals without decreasing PLMS or decreasing PLMS without decreasing sleep instability can result in improvement of RLS symptoms. Thus, it is unclear which, if any, polysomnographic parameter is the most important for showing clinical efficacy. Nonetheless, pramipexole has shown efficacy in multiple planes.

Side effects and dosing
Commonly reported side effects include nausea, sleepiness, and insomnia.[2] Other reported side effects include headache and fatigue,[35] impulse control disorders[36] (although a more recent smaller study did not find an increased prevalence in impulse control disorders between treated and nontreated subjects with RLS and noted the prevalence to be infrequent[37]), urinary frequency,[38] postural hypotension, vivid dreams, and visual hallucinations.[39] Augmentation rate is reported as between 7% and 11%,[35,40,41] with higher rates associated with higher doses.[35] The studies of

pramipexole efficacy in RLS/WED are based on the short-acting preparation, with 1 case series showing that the long-acting preparation was efficacious for the treatment of RLS in patients who had previously experienced augmentation.[42] The recommended starting dose is 0.125 mg 2 to 3 hours before bedtime with a maximum approved dose in the United States of 0.5 mg,[43] and in Europe of 0.75 mg[44] with dosing increases every 4 to 7 days.

Ropinirole

Pharmacology

Ropinirole is also a nonergot dopamine agonist with a similar profile to pramipexole, with full agonist activity at D3 and D2 dopamine receptors, greater for D3 than D2, with lesser affinity for D4 receptors, and negligible affinity for other receptor types (D1, 5-HT1, 5-HT2, benzodiazepine, gamma-aminobutyric acid, muscarinic, alpha1-adrenoreceptors, alpha2-adrenoreceptors, and beta-adrenoreceptors).[20,45] It is primarily metabolized by the liver via the cytochrome P (CYP) 1A2 enzyme, with a lesser degree via CYP3A and, thus, is susceptible to interaction with substances that inhibit and promote those enzymes, particularly CYP1A2, such as ciprofloxacin (increased concentration) and smoking (decreased concentration).[45,46] Higher doses of estrogen, such as those used in hormone therapy, may reduce the clearance of ropinirole.[47] No dosage adjustment is necessary in patients with moderate renal impairment (creatinine clearance 30–50 mL/min), the medication has not been studied in patients with severe renal dysfunction, and it is unlikely that the drug is removed via hemodialysis.[45] The half-life of regular ropinirole is 6 hours.[45] An extended-release version of ropinirole (Requip XL) is available.

Clinical efficacy

Similarly to pramipexole, ropinirole use has been endorsed by the AASM1 and the IRLSSG2 as a treatment of chronic RLS/WED, with a meta-analysis of randomized placebo-controlled trials showing subjective improvement in symptoms and objective improvement in sleep parameters.[23] Overall, ropinirole therapy was associated with a decrease in RLS severity as measured by the IRLS with a mean difference of −4.19 (95% CI, −5.4 to −2.97; I^2 = 58%), with 9 randomized placebo-controlled trials[48–56] showing a decrease in IRLS score and 2 not.[23,57] Although the number of studies showing subjective improvement in quality of sleep was similar to the number that did not (4[50,54–56] showed improvement vs 3[57–59] that did not), the meta-analysis showed a slight

increase in sleep quality overall (standard mean difference, 0.30; 95% CI, 0.16–0.45; I^2 = 40%). Similarly, subjective assessment of quality of life improved with ropinirole (standard mean difference, 0.23; 95% CI, 0.09–0.35; I^2 = 52%) with 3 studies showing improved quality of life[50,52,55] and 4[54,56–58] not. Four studies showed a decrease in PLMS Index (1 by PSG and 3 by actigraphy)[50,55,57,58] and 1 did not (PLMS assessed by PSG),[60] with mean difference of −14.11 (95% CI, −18.79 to −9.43; I^2 = 52%). Similarly to pramipexole, sleep efficiency did not improve (mean difference, 2.19; 95% CI, −2.11–6.49; I^2 = 25%).[57,60]

Side effects and dosing

The side effect profile is similar to that of pramipexole and includes nausea, dizziness, fatigue, and headache[2] as well as other dopaminergic side effects, such as orthostatic hypotension (1%–25%) and impulse control disorders.[36,45] Augmentation rates have not been firmly established but may be as high as 24%.[41] The recommended starting dosage is 0.25 mg 1 to 3 hours before bedtime for 2 days and then increased to 0.5 mg. Dosage may be increased by 0.5 mg each week if necessary up to a maximal dosage of 4 mg per evening.[45]

Rotigotine

Pharmacology

Rotigotine has a more widespread dopaminergic agonist profile than pramipexole and ropinirole. It has greatest activity at the D3 receptor, strong affinity for D2 receptors, equal affinity for D1 and D5 receptors, and less affinity for D4 receptors.[59] For Parkinson's disease, it is thought to work through the D3/D2/D1 receptors. It also is an alpha2 antagonist and has weak agonism at 5-HT1A receptors.[59] Rotigotine is primarily excreted in the urine (71%) with a lesser amount in the feces (23%).[61] It is metabolized by multiple liver enzymes and, thus, inhibition of 1 pathway does not alter rotigotine concentrations significantly. Moderate hepatic impairment did not affect plasma concentration but there is no information on the effects of severe hepatic dysfunction. Rotigotine levels were increased in patients with severe renal impairment (creatinine clearance <30 mL/min) who were not on hemodialysis. The medication is secreted continuously over 24 hours to maintain stable concentrations,[62,63] with a terminal half-life of 5 to 7 hours.[61]

Clinical efficacy

Rotigotine is unique among RLS/WED treatments in that it is delivered transdermally at a constant rate. Thus, it is suitable for patients with prominent daytime and nighttime symptoms as well as those undergoing surgery who cannot take oral medications.[64] As with the other nonergot dopamine agonists, rotigotine results in a decrease in severity with improvement in IRLS scores. Five randomized controlled studies[65–69] all showed a significant decrease in IRLS scores (mean difference, −6.98; 95% CI, −8.99 to −4.96; I^2 = 44%). There was overall improvement in quality of sleep (standard mean difference, 0.42; 95% CI, 0.28–0.56; I^2 = 0%), with 3 randomized controlled studies[65,66,69] showing improvement and 2[67,68] not. Improvement in quality of life was noted overall (standard mean difference, 0.50; 95% CI, 0.23–0.76; I^2 = 47%) with positive findings in 2 randomized controlled studies[66,69] but not in a third.[67] One randomized controlled trial[67] showed a decrease in PLMS Index versus placebo with mean difference of −18.90 (95% CI, −27.41 to −10.39) without improvement in sleep efficiency (mean difference, 2.71; 95% CI, −3.07–8.49).

Side effects and dosing

Side effects are similar to those of the other dopaminergic medications, including most prominently nausea, headache, and fatigue, and to a lesser extent orthostatic hypotension, sleepiness, and impulse control disorders, but also include application site reactions (erythema, edema, or pruritus) and sulfite allergies.[2,61] Application site reactions represent the most common side effect, with a prevalence in a 5-year study of 37%.[70] The backing layer of the patch contains aluminum and, therefore, should be removed before patients undergo MRI or cardioversion to avoid skin burns. Although not studied with rotigotine, as a precaution, patients should avoid exposure to direct heat, such as heating pads or prolonged direct sunlight, to avoid higher than anticipated doses.[61] Clinically significant augmentation rate has been reported as 5% in the recommended dosage range and 13% overall in an open-label 5-year study with 23% meeting Max Planck Institute criteria for augmentation.[70] The recommended starting dose for the treatment of RLS/WED is 1 mg per 24 hours. The dosage may be increased by 1 mg per 24 hours weekly up to 3 mg per 24 hours.[61]

SUMMARY

Each of the dopaminergic medications (**Table 1**) is especially useful in different clinical populations. Levodopa/carbidopa is most effective with fewer side effects when used only occasionally, for patients who either need treatment only during

Table 1
Comparison of dopaminergic medications for RLS

Medication	Dosage	Half-life (h)	Metabolism/ Excretion	Degree of Augmentation (%)	Specific Indications
Carbidopa/ levodopa	25 mg/100 mg po	1.5	Primarily renal	60–82	Sporadic use (eg, airplane flights)
Pramipexole	0.125 mg po in the evening up to 0.50 mg or 0.75 mg po	8–12	Renal	7–11	Chronic therapy; can be used for patients with medications that affect hepatic enzymes
Ropinirole	0.25 mg/0.5 mg po in the evening during the first wk up to 4 mg po	6	Primarily hepatic	Up to 24	Chronic therapy; can be used for patients with moderate renal impairment
Rotigotine	1 mg/24 h to 3 mg/24 h transdermally	Secreted continuously	Primarily renal with some hepatic	5 (see above for details)	Chronic therapy; can be used for patients who have round-the-clock symptoms or who cannot take oral medications

Abbreviation: po, by mouth.

periods of prolonged forced immobilization or just on an occasional evening. For patients who require chronic therapy, either pramipexole or ropinirole is an appropriate treatment, with one potentially being chosen rather than the other based on metabolism and medication interactions, the longer-acting versions of these medications likely more helpful to patients whose symptoms begin earlier in the day. In the future, the longer-acting preparations may become preferentially prescribed as more is learned about augmentation. In addition, rotigotine is useful for patients with round-the-clock symptoms or those who would benefit from a nonoral preparation.

REFERENCES

1. Aurora RN, Kristo DA, Bista SR, et al. The treatment of restless legs syndrome and periodic limb movement disorder in adults - an update for 2012: practice parameters with an evidence-based systematic review and meta-analyses. Sleep 2012;35(8):1039–62.
2. García-Borreguero D, Kohnen R, Silber MH, et al. The long term treatment of restless legs syndrome/ Willis-Ekbom disease: evidence-based guidelines and clinical consensus best practice guidance: a report from the International Restless legs Syndrome Study Group. Sleep Med 2013;14(7):675–84.
3. Garcia-Borreguero D, Ferini-Strambi L, Kohnen R, et al. European guidelines on management of restless legs syndrome: report of a joint task force by the European Federation of Neurological Societies, the European Neurological Society and the European Sleep Research Society. Eur J Neurol 2012; 19(11):1385–96.
4. Andersohn F, Garbe E. Cardiac and noncardiac fibrotic reactions caused by ergot- and nonergotderived dopamine agonists. Mov Disord 2009;24: 129–33.
5. Schade R, Andersohn F, Suissa S, et al. Dopamine agonists and the risk of cardiac-valve regurgitation. N Engl J Med 2007;356:29–38.
6. Pritchett AM, Morrison JF, Edwards WD, et al. Valvular heart disease in patients taking pergolide. Mayo Clin Proc 2002;77:1280–6.
7. Akpinar S. Treatment of restless legs syndrome with levodopa plus benserazide. Arch Neurol 1982;39:739.
8. Trenkwalder C, Seidel V, Kazenwadel J, et al. One-year treatment with standard and sustained-release levodopa: appropriate long-term treatment of restless legs syndrome? Mov Disord 2003;18: 1184–9.
9. Saletu M, Anderer P, Hogl B, et al. Acute double-blind, placebo-controlled sleep laboratory and clinical follow-up studies with a combination treatment of rr-L-dopa and sr-L-dopa in restless legs syndrome. J Neural Transm 2003;110:611–26.
10. Polo O, Yla-Sahra R, Hirvonen K, et al. Entacapone prolongs the reduction of PLM by levodopa/carbidopa in restless legs syndrome. Clin Neuropharmacol 2007;30:335–44.
11. Available at: http://www.fda.gov/ohrms/dockets/dailys/ 01/Aug01/081701/cp00001_02_tab_01.pdf. Accessed January 3, 2015.
12. Available at: http://www.merck.ca/assets/en/pdf/ products/SINEMET_CR-PM_E.pdf. Accessed January 3, 2015.
13. Available at: http://www.micromedexsolutions. com.ucsf.idm.oclc.org/micromedex2/librarian/ND_T/ evidencexpert/ND_PR/evidencexpert/CS/EFF1CE/ ND_AppProduct/evidencexpert/DUPLICATIONSHIELD SYNC/2CCA60/ND_PG/evidencexpert/ND_B/evidenc expert/ND_P/evidencexpert/PFActionId/evidence xpert.IntermediateToDocumentLink?docId=140& contentSetId=51&title=LEVODOPA%2FCARBIDOPA& servicesTitle=LEVODOPA%2FCARBIDOPA. Accessed March 9, 2015.
14. García-Borreguero D, Williams AM. Dopaminergic augmentation of restless legs syndrome. Sleep Med Rev 2010;14(5):339–46.
15. García-Borreguero D, Allen RP, Kohnen R, et al. Diagnostic standards for dopaminergic augmentation of restless legs syndrome: report from a World Association of Sleep Medicine-International Restless Legs Syndrome Study Group consensus conference at the Max Planck Institute. Sleep Med 2007;8(5):520–30.
16. Hogl B, Garcia-Borreguero D, Kohnen R, et al. Progressive development of augmentation during long-term treatment with levodopa in restless legs syndrome: results of a prospective multi-center study. J Neurol 2010;257:230–7.
17. Allen RP, Earley CJ. Augmentation of the restless legs syndrome with carbidopa/levodopa. Sleep 1996;19:205–13.
18. Silber MH, Becker PM, Earley C, et al. Willis-Ekbom Disease Foundation revised consensus statement on the management of restless legs syndrome. Mayo Clin Proc 2013;88:977–86.
19. Bennet JP, Piercey MF. Pramipexole—a new dopamine agonist for the treatment of Parkinson's disease. J Neurol Sci 1999;163:25–31.
20. Piercey MF, Hoffmann WE, Smith MW, et al. Inhibition of dopamine neuron firing by pramipexole, a dopamine D3 receptor-preferring agonist: comparison to other dopamine receptor agonists. Eur J Pharmacol 1996;312:35–44.
21. Hubble JP, Novak P. Pramipexole: a nonergot dopamine agonist as drug therapy in Parkinson's disease. Expert Rev Neurother 2001;1:43–51.
22. Eisenreich W, Sommer B, Hartter S, et al. Pramipexole extended release: a novel treatment option in Parkinson's Disease. Parkinson's Disease 2010;1–7.

23. Scholz H, Trenkwalder C, Kohnen R, et al. Dopamine agonists for restless legs syndrome. Cochrane Database Syst Rev 2011;(3):CD006009.

24. Högl B. Efficacy and safety of pramipexole for restless legs syndrome: a 26-week, randomized, placebo-controlled, clinical trial in the European Union. AAN Congress. Seattle (WA), May 25–June 2, 2009.

25. Ferini-Strambi L, Aarskog D, Partinen M, et al. Effect of pramipexole on RLS symptoms and sleep: a randomized, double-blind, placebo-controlled trial. Sleep Med 2008;9(8):874–81.

26. Inoue Y, Hirata K, Kuroda K, et al. Efficacy and safety of pramipexole in Japanese patients with primary restless legs syndrome: a polysomnographic randomized, double-blind, placebo controlled study. Sleep Med 2010;11:11–6.

27. Montagna P, Hornyak M, Ulfberg J, et al. Randomized trial of pramipexole for patients with restless legs syndrome (RLS) and RLS-related impairment of mood. Sleep Med 2011;12(1):34–40.

28. Oertel WH, Stiasny-Kolster K, Bertholdt B, et al, Pramipexole RLS Study Group. Efficacy of pramipexole in restless legs syndrome: a six-week, multicenter, randomized, double-blind study (effect-RLS study). Mov Disord 2007;22(2):213–9.

29. Partinen M, Hirvonen K, Jama L, et al. Efficacy and safety of pramipexole in idiopathic restless legs syndrome: a polysomnographic dose-finding study–the PRELUDE study. Sleep Med 2006;7(5):407–17.

30. Winkelman JW, Sethi KD, Kushida CA, et al. Efficacy and safety of pramipexole in restless legs syndrome. Neurology 2006;67(6):1034–9.

31. Available at: http://trials.boehringer-Ingelheim.com/content/dam/internet/opu/clinicaltrial/com_EN/results/248/248.616_U08-3876.pdf. Accessed May 5, 2015.

32. Högl B, Poewe W, Garcia-Borreguero D, et al. 26-week effects of pramipexole on quality of life in restless legs syndrome. Presented at The Movement Disorder Society's 13th Annual International Congress of Parkinson's Disease and Movement Disorders. Paris, June 7–11, 2009.

33. Montplaisir J, Nicolas A, Denesle R, et al. Restless legs syndrome improved by pramipexole: a double-blind randomized trial. Neurology 1999; 52(5):938–43.

34. Manconi M, Ferri R, Zucconi M, et al. Dissociation of periodic leg movements from arousals in restless legs syndrome. Ann Neurol 2012;71:834–44.

35. Allen RP, Chen C, Garcia-Borreguero D, et al. Comparison of pregabalin with pramipexole for restless legs syndrome. N Engl J Med 2014;370:621–31.

36. Cornelius JR, Tippmann-Peikert M, Slocumb NL, et al. Impulse control disorders with the use of dopaminergic agents in restless legs syndrome: a case-control study. Sleep 2010;33:81–7.

37. Bayard S, Langenier MC, Dauvilliers Y. Decision-making, reward-seeking behaviors and dopamine agonist therapy in restless legs syndrome. Sleep 2013;36:1501–7.

38. Dooley M, Markham A. Pramipexole. A review of its use in the management of early and advanced Parkinson's disease. Drugs Aging 1998;12:495–514.

39. Pinter MM, Pogarell O, Oertel WH. Efficacy, safety, and tolerance of the non-ergoline dopamine agonist pramipexole in the treatment of advanced Parkinson's disease: a double blind, placebo controlled, randomized, multicentre study. J Neurol Neurosurg Psychiatry 1999;66:436–41.

40. Silver N, Allen RP, Senerth J, et al. A 10-year, longitudinal assessment of dopamine agonists and methadone in the treatment of restless legs syndrome. Sleep Med 2011;12:440–4.

41. Allen RP, Ondo WG, Ball E, et al. Restless legs syndrome augmentation associated with dopamine agonist and levodopa usage in a community sample. Sleep Med 2011;12:431–9.

42. Maestri M, Fulda S, Ferini-Strambi L, et al. Polysomnographic record and successful management of augmentation in restless legs syndrome/Willis-Ekbom disease. Sleep Med 2014;15:570–5.

43. Available at: http://www.accessdata.fda.gov/drugsatfda_docs/label/2008/020667s014s017s018lbl.pdf. Accessed February 27, 2015.

44. Available at: http://www.ema.europa.eu/docs/en_GB/document_library/EPAR_-_Scientific_Discussion_-_Variation/human/000134/WC500029253.pdf. Accessed February 27, 2015.

45. Available at: http://www.accessdata.fda.gov/drugsatfda_docs/label/2008/020658s018s020s021lbl.pdf. Accessed February 27, 2015.

46. Kvernmo T, Hartter S, Burger E. A review of the receptor-binding and pharmacokinetic properties of dopamine agonists. Clin Therapeu 2006;28:1065–78.

47. Available at: https://www.gsksource.com/gskprm/htdocs/documents/REQUIP-PI-PIL.PDF. Accessed February 28, 2015.

48. Adler CH, Hauser RA, Sethi K, et al. Ropinirole for restless legs syndrome: a placebo-controlled cross-over trial. Neurology 2004;62(8):1405–7.

49. Benes H, Mattern W, Peglau I, et al. Ropinirole improves depressive symptoms and restless legs syndrome severity in RLS patients: a multicentre, randomised, placebo-controlled study. J Neurol 2011;258(6):1046–54.

50. Bogan RK, Fry JM, Schmidt MH, et al, TREAT RLS US Study Group. Ropinirole in the treatment of patients with restless legs syndrome: a US-based randomized, double-blind, placebo-controlled clinical trial. Mayo Clin Proc 2006;81(1):17–27.

51. Kelly M, Mistry P. Tolerability of a forced-dose escalating regimen of ropinirole in patients with RLS. Mov Disord 2005;20(Suppl 10):S63.

52. GSK SKF-101468/205, 2007: SKF-101468/205. A 12-week, double-blind, placebo-controlled,

parallel-group study to assess the efficacy and safety of ropinirole controlled release for RLS (CR-RLS) in patients with restless legs syndrome. Available at: http://www.gsk-clinicalstudyregister.com/study/101468/205#rs. Accessed March 1, 2015.

53. GSK ROR104836, 2009: ROR 104836. A randomised, double-blind, placebo-controlled, parallel group study to evaluate the efficacy and safety of ropinirole for 26 weeks and to further evaluate the incidence of augmentation and rebound for a further 40 weeks open-label extension treatment period in subjects suffering from moderate to severe restless legs syndrome. Available at: http://www.gsk-clinical studyregister.com/study/ROR104836#ps. Accessed January 3, 2015.

54. Trenkwalder C, Garcia-Borreguero D, Montagna P, et al. Ropinirole in the treatment of restless legs syndrome: results from the TREAT RLS 1 study, a 12 week, randomised, placebo controlled study in 10 European countries. J Neurol Neurosurg Psychiatry 2004;75:92–7.

55. Kushida CA, Geyer J, Tolson JM, et al. Patient- and physician-rated measures demonstrate the effectiveness of ropinirole in the treatment of restless legs syndrome. Clin Neuropharmacol 2008;31(5):281–6.

56. Walters AS, Ondo WG, Dreykluft T, et al. Ropinirole is effective in the treatment of restless legs syndrome. TREAT RLS 2: a 12-week, double-blind, randomized, parallel-group, placebo-controlled study. Mov Disord 2004;19(12):1414–23.

57. Allen R, Becker PM, Bogan R, et al. Ropinirole decreases periodic leg movements and improves sleep parameters in patients with restless legs syndrome. Sleep 2004;27(5):907–14.

58. Available at: http://www.gsk-clinicalstudyregister.com/study/101892#rs. Accessed May 7, 2015.

59. Scheller D, Ullmer C, Berkels R, et al. The in vitro receptor profile of rotigotine: a new agent for the treatment of Parkinson's disease. Naunyn Schmiedebergs Arch Pharmacol 2009;379:73–86.

60. Available at: http://www.gsk-clinicalstudyregister.com/study/RRL103660#ps. Accessed May 7, 2015.

61. Available at: http://www.ucb.com/our-products/cns/nephro/. Accessed January 3, 2015.

62. Boroojerdi B, Wolff HM, Braun M, et al. Rotigotine transdermal patch for the treatment of Parkinson's disease and restless legs syndrome. Drugs Today (Barc) 2010;46:483–505.

63. Elshoff JP, Braun M, Andreas JO, et al. Steady-state plasma concentration profile of transdermal rotigotine: an integrated analysis of three, open-label, randomized, phase I multiple dose studies. Clin Ther 2012;34:966–78.

64. Hogl B, Oertel WH, Schollmayer E, et al. Transdermal rotigotine for the perioperative management of restless legs syndrome. BMC Neurol 2012;12:106.

65. Hening WA, Allen RP, Ondo WG, et al, The SP792 Study Group. Rotigotine improves restless legs syndrome: a 6-month randomized, double-blind, placebo-controlled trial in the United States. Mov Disord 2010;25(11):1675–83.

66. Oertel WH, Benes H, Garcia-Borreguero D, et al. Efficacy of rotigotine transdermal system in severe restless legs syndrome: a randomized, double-blind, placebo-controlled, six-week dose-finding trial in Europe. Sleep Med 2008;9(3):228–39.

67. Oertel W, Benes H, Garcia-Borreguero D, et al. Rotigotine transdermal patch in moderate to severe idiopathic restless legs syndrome. Sleep Med 2010;11(9):848–56.

68. Stiasny-Kolster K, Kohnen R, Schollmayer E, et al, Rotigotine Sp 666 Study Group. Patch application of the dopamine agonist rotigotine to patients with moderate to advanced stages of restless legs syndrome: a double-blind, placebo-controlled pilot study. Mov Disord 2004;19(12):1432–8.

69. Trenkwalder C, Benes H, Poewe W, et al. Efficacy of rotigotine for treatment of moderate-to-severe restless legs syndrome: a randomised, double-blind, placebo-controlled trial. Lancet Neurol 2008;7(7):595–604.

70. Oertel W, Trenkwalder C, Benes H, et al. Long-term safety and efficacy of rotigotine transdermal patch for moderate-to-severe idiopathic restless legs syndrome. Lancet Neurol 2011;10:710–20.

Dopaminergic Augmentation in Restless Legs Syndrome/Willis-Ekbom Disease: Identification and Management

Diego García-Borreguero, MD, PhD

KEYWORDS

- Restless legs syndrome • Augmentation • Rebound • Management • Disease progression

KEY POINTS

- Augmentation is the main clinical complication of long-term dopaminergic treatment of restless legs syndrome (RLS)/Willis-Ekbom disease and also the main reason for treatment failure of this class of drugs.
- It involves an increase in the severity of RLS symptoms during treatment.
- The incidence of augmentation increases with higher doses of dopaminergics and with longer duration of treatment.
- There is preliminary evidence showing that the incidence of augmentation is higher when short-acting dopamine agonists are used.
- Prevention strategies include managing lifestyle changes and keeping dopaminergic load as low as possible by performing in previously untreated patients, whenever feasible, a treatment trial with nondopaminergic agents.
- Treatment of augmentation might require switching to longer-acting dopaminergic agents and, in severe cases, switching to alpha-2 delta ligands (if not already tried before) or opiates.

INTRODUCTION

Since the first introduction of dopaminergic agents in 1982,[1] the overall long-term efficacy of these drugs has been well established by several retrospective studies.[2–4] Side effects are generally mild and, contrary to the observations performed during treatment with L-3,4-dihydroxyphenylalanine (L-DOPA) in Parkinson disease, cases of dyskinesia have yet to be reported.[3]

Despite the widespread use of dopaminergic drugs for restless legs syndrome (RLS)/Willis-Ekbom disease (WED), it was not until 1996 that the first clinical description of augmentation as a complication of dopaminergic treatment was made. Allen and Earley[5] described a group of 30 patients with RLS/WED who had been treated with L-DOPA, and described a condition

characterized by an earlier onset of symptoms in the afternoon along with a faster onset of symptoms when at rest, an expansion of symptoms to the upper limbs and the trunk, an overall increase in severity/frequency, and a shorter effect of the medication. Under L-DOPA, augmentation of RLS/WED symptoms occurred in 82% of the patients and was severe enough to require change of treatment in 50%.[5] The most characteristic feature of the new condition occurring during long-term treatment with L-DOPA was that there was an increase in severity beyond the one seen at baseline, a feature that differentiated it from rebound or from tolerance (ie, seen under benzodiazepines or in opiates). In other words, augmentation is a drug-induced increase in RLS/WED symptom severity beyond that experienced before

Sleep Research Institute, Paseo de la Habana 151, 28036 Madrid, Spain
E-mail address: dgb@iis.es

Sleep Med Clin 10 (2015) 287–292
http://dx.doi.org/10.1016/j.jsmc.2015.05.020

treatment was initiated, and this remains the most characteristic feature of dopaminergic augmentation, compared with pharmacologic tolerance.

CLINICAL DEFINITION

It is difficult to examine the augmentation rates for different drugs given that for a long time there was no standardized operational definition of this condition. The need to standardize clinical diagnostic criteria for augmentation was first recognized by the National Institutes of Health (NIH) who sponsored a workshop on RLS Diagnosis and Epidemiology in 2002.[6] This consensus conference generated an operational definition of augmentation, the primary feature of which was defined as a drug-induced shifting of symptoms to a period of time 2 hours earlier than was the typical period of daily onset of symptoms before pharmacologic intervention. The 2003 definition was based exclusively on clinical experience rather than on empirical data. Neither included guidelines on how to assess the severity or clinical significance of augmentation. This task was tackled several years later, in 2006, by a European

Restless Legs Syndrome Study Group–sponsored consensus conference at the Max-Planck Institute in Munich (Germany) during which, based on empirical data from clinical studies, a better operational definition for the clinical identification of augmentation was sought. These studies indicated that reliable detection of augmentation could be obtained based on a 4-hour time advance of symptoms, or a smaller (2–4 hours) advance of symptoms expressed along with other required clinical indications,[7] such as a shorter latency of symptoms at rest, a spread of symptoms to other body parts in addition to the lower limbs, or a greater intensity of symptoms. In addition, the paradoxic response to treatment, reflected by an increase in severity with increasing dose of medication, and an improvement following decreases in medication, was considered an alternative key feature for diagnosis (**Box 1**).

Several studies have been able to correlate the presence of augmentation during treatment with dopaminergic agents with the duration of treatment and with a higher medication dosage, but not with symptom severity at baseline, age or gender.[8–10] Clinical experience shows that, when

---

Box 1
Max-Planck-Institute criteria

Preamble

Augmentation is a worsening of RLS symptom severity experienced by patients undergoing treatment of RLS. The RLS symptoms in general are more severe than those experienced at baseline.

A. Basic features (all of which need to be met):

   1. The increase in symptom severity was experienced on 5 out of 7 days during the previous week.

   2. The increase in symptom severity is not accounted for by other factors, such as a change in medical status, lifestyle, or the natural progression of the disorder.

   3. It is assumed that there has been a prior positive response to treatment.

In addition, B, C, or both have to be met:

B. Persisting (although not immediate) paradoxic response to treatment: RLS symptom severity increases some time after a dose increase, and improves some time after a dose decrease.

C. Earlier onset of symptoms:

   1. An earlier onset by at least 4 hours.

   Or:

   2. An earlier onset (between 2 and 4 hours) occurs with one of the following compared with symptom status before treatment:

      a. Shorter latency to symptoms when at rest

      b. Spreading of symptoms to other body parts

      c. Intensity of symptoms is greater (or increase in periodic limb movements if measured by polysomnography or the suggested immobilization test)

      d. Duration of relief from treatment is shorter

Augmentation requires criteria A and B, A and C, or A and B and C to be met.

severe, augmentation can result in a weakening or even a loss of essential RLS/WED features; that is, symptoms spread to previously unaffected body parts, are no longer alleviated during inactivity or movement, and there is virtually no circadian pattern. In severe augmentation, RLS/WED can occur continuously during the day, can involve the entire body, and may not be noticeably affected by rest or activity, showing a remarkable similarity with neuroleptic-induced akathisia. The clinical picture obtained during dopaminergic augmentation resembles the picture obtained in severe/very severe RLS/WED. None of the clinical features of dopaminergic augmentation is specific to this condition or can be differentiated from RLS/WED.

AUGMENTATION UNDER DOPAMINERGIC AGENTS

Several problems make it particularly difficult to compare the incidence rates for the different treatments of RLS/WED. The first is the beforementioned lack of any operational definition for augmentation before 2003. Second, the estimations of the augmentation rates were performed retrospectively, used different diagnostic criteria, and were frequently based on the evaluation of clinical cases. Studies were not specifically designed to measure augmentation and frequently lacked specific information on augmentation. In addition, trials frequently were not long enough to show augmentation: augmentation is a long-term consequence of treatment, and therefore trials need to last longer than 6 months for first features of augmentation to manifest.

Some degree of augmentation has been reported with the use of all investigated dopaminergic drugs[8,11–14] and also for tramadol.[15] In the virtual absence of direct comparative studies, the incidence rate seems to be highest during treatment with levodopa and higher for shorter-acting (pramipexole, ropinirole) than longer-acting (rotigotine) dopamine-receptor agonists. However, it is unclear whether this finding is related to the masking of earlier symptom onset by the longer-acting dopaminergic agents or whether it is an augmentation-sparing effect.

Compared with dopaminergic agents, less emphasis has been placed on the performance of systematic long-term treatment with nondopaminergic agents. A recent, and probably the best-designed, study performed on augmentation so far, is a prospective double-blind comparison of 2 different doses of pramipexole (0.25 and 0.5 mg/d) with 300 mg/d of pregabalin for more than a year.[4] Although the therapeutic efficacy of

pregabalin was similar to the higher dose of pramipexole, the 1-year incidence rate of augmentation was clearly lower (2.1% vs 7.7%), and was not different from what has been observed for placebo.[16] Another recent large study reported no cases of augmentation during a 1-year treatment with prolonged-release oxycodone combined with naloxone.[17] In summary, augmentation seems to occur specifically during dopaminergic treatment.

DIFFERENTIAL DIAGNOSIS OF AUGMENTATION

Augmentation needs to be distinguished from tolerance, early morning rebound, and from the natural progression of RLS/WED or fluctuations in disease severity (**Table 1**). It is also important to ask the patient about any lifestyle changes, changes in medical factors (use of dopamine antagonists or antidepressants), or other extrinsic factors (sleep deprivation, blood loss, alcohol use) that might have an effect on the earlier onset or severity of symptoms.

Early morning rebound is characterized by the development of RLS/WED in the early morning during the declining phase of plasma levels of the drug being administered. Following rebound in the morning, there is usually a symptom-free period of time until symptoms reappear again in the afternoon or evening. In contrast, under augmentation there is an earlier onset of symptoms in the evening. However, in some cases of severe augmentation, particularly when patients experience symptoms throughout the day, it might be difficult to differentiate from rebound. Rebound is considered to be an end-of-dose effect, related to the half-life of the therapeutic agent. No correlation has been found between the occurrence of augmentation and rebound, supporting the general view that both phenomena reflect separate problems.

In contrast, distinguishing augmentation from tolerance might be more difficult from a clinical point of view. Tolerance results when the effectiveness of a medication decreases over a period of time, thereby necessitating an increase in medication to maintain the initial relief of symptoms that was seen at therapy initiation. Even in the worst case of tolerance, severity of symptoms would not strictly be expected to increase beyond the level of severity occurring without treatment. In contrast, during augmentation, the severity of symptoms might increase beyond the preexisting baseline level. This differentiation might prove to be of more theoretic than practical value in clinical practice, because most patients cannot assess the severity of their symptoms with such precision.

Table 1
Differentiating augmentation from other conditions

Augmentation	Tolerance
Additional features (symptoms spread to other body parts, shorter latency to symptoms at rest, increased intensity of symptoms)	No additional features
Increase in severity beyond baseline levels	Not worse than baseline
Augmentation	*Early Morning Rebound*
Symptom onset in afternoon or evening	Symptom onset in early morning
Anticipation of time of onset	Delayed onset of symptoms
Followed by usual course of symptoms	Followed by symptom-free interval in the morning/noon
Related to total daily dosage/severity of symptoms at baseline	Related to half-life. Occurs during the declining phase of plasma concentrations
Additional features (symptoms spread to other body parts, shorter latency to symptoms at rest, increased intensity of symptoms)	No additional features
Augmentation	*Natural Progression of RLS*
Additional features (symptoms spread to other body parts, shorter latency to symptoms at rest, increased intensity of symptoms)	Additional features
Progresses within weeks/months	Natural progression of RLS is usually slow (y)
A reduction in the dose leads ultimately to a decrease in symptoms. An increase in the dose ultimately leads to an increase in symptoms	A reduction in the dose leads to an increase in symptoms
Increase beyond baseline severity	Increase beyond baseline severity

From Garcia-Borreguero D, Williams AM. Dopaminergic augmentation of restless legs syndrome: the scope of the problem. Sleep Med 2011;12:425–6; with permission.

Furthermore, the absence of specific rating instruments for augmentation, as well as the lack of prospective studies to assess the long-term course of the different features of augmentation, makes the differentiation between these processes particularly difficult.

Another situation that needs to be differentiated from augmentation is a progressive worsening of the clinical course of RLS/WED over time. Although data on the long-term spontaneous course in untreated patients with RLS/WED are scarce and usually not well controlled, it is thought that progression is slow. However, this could be confounded with a slowly progressive, mild process of augmentation. Nevertheless, in this case a time off treatment produces opposite effects; that is, a full expression of the progressive worsening of symptoms, whereas symptoms would be reduced in augmentation.

MANAGING AUGMENTATION
Prevention

The major goal in dealing with augmentation is primarily to prevent it. For this reason, all possible known risk factors predisposing for augmentation should be avoided.

Because RLS is usually a chronic condition requiring long-term treatment, because many patients on dopaminergic treatment have gradual and insidious development of augmentation, and because of its similarity to natural progression, augmentation can be difficult to detect before it becomes a significant problem. In previously untreated patients with RLS/WED, it becomes important to keep the dopaminergic load as low as possible and consider using for initial RLS treatment medications that, although effective, have little or no risk of augmentation. Thus, a therapeutic trial with alpha-2 delta ligands (ie, gabapentin, gabapentin enacarbil, pregabalin) should be seriously considered, because these are alternative, effective first-line treatments of RLS without risk of augmentation.

If dopaminergic agents are used, their dose should be maintained as low as possible. The maximum dosage used in clinical trials should, as a general practice, not only be respected but should be avoided. Furthermore, keeping the dose within recommended limits might not be sufficient to prevent augmentation. Furthermore, low serum ferritin levels (recorded previously or in the course of treatment) and any other medical conditions or therapeutic interventions (such as adding antidopaminergic agents or selective serotonin reuptake inhibitors) that might facilitate augmentation should be excluded. An interesting area to be investigated in the future is whether drug rotation represents an effective strategy to prevent augmentation.

When to Treat Augmentation?

Clinically significant augmentation was defined by the Max-Planck Institute criteria as an increase in RLS/WED symptoms during treatment that causes[7]:

- A change in daily activities and/or behavior to accommodate the symptoms (eg, the patient stops traveling by car)
- A negative impact on quality of life (sleep, mood)
- A need to change treatment (dosage increase, dividing the dose)
- Adjustments in other medications to compensate for the increase in RLS/WED symptoms (eg, an increased intake of analgesics/hypnotics to relieve symptom intensity)

Usually, when augmentation is mild and does not interfere with a patient's daily living, no change in treatment regimen is likely to be necessary. In some cases the efficacy of dopaminergic treatment may only be slightly reduced; that is, the patient experiences mild symptoms during the day but these are not bothersome because usual daytime activities help to alleviate them. Nevertheless, it is important always to examine serum ferritin levels because low iron stores may be responsible for the mild increase in symptom severity. As a rule, when the serum ferritin level is less than 50 μg/L, additional treatment with oral iron should be considered.[18,19] An alternative possibility for managing mild augmentation is to split the dopaminergic dose by administering a first dose earlier in the afternoon, before symptom onset, and the second dose after symptoms begin; if this strategy is followed it is important to ensure that the total dose is not increased.

In more severe cases of augmentation, a change in treatment regimen may be required. When augmentation occurs with low doses of dopaminergic agents, the dosage should be reduced and divided as described earlier.[20] If augmentation occurs on levodopa, then a switch to dopamine agonists, which have lower reported rates of augmentation, can be considered.[21] Furthermore,

when augmentation occurs under treatment with a short-acting dopamine agonist, it is possible to change to longer-acting dopamine agonist (eg, rotigotine).

There is no consensus on how to cease treatment with a dopaminergic agent. The 2 options are either to slowly withdraw the drug, or abruptly stop treatment. In severe cases, intermittent (3–6 months) treatment with an alpha-2 delta ligand (gabapentin enacarbil or pregabalin) or an opiate may be necessary in order to alleviate the reappearance of symptoms (withdrawal) that may last for several days. Following 2 episodes of augmentation with dopaminergic agents, particularly if one is severe, the patient will likely need to avoid future long-term nondopaminergic treatment.

SUMMARY

Augmentation is the main clinical complication of long-term dopaminergic treatment of RLS/WED and also the main reason for treatment failure of this class of drugs. It involves an increase in the severity of RLS symptoms during treatment. The incidence of augmentation increases with higher doses of dopaminergics and with longer duration of treatment. Furthermore, there is preliminary evidence showing that the incidence of augmentation is higher when short-acting dopamine agonists are used. Prevention strategies include managing lifestyle changes and keeping dopaminergic load low. This might include, whenever feasible, to postpone any dopaminergic medication and perform a treatment trial with nondopaminergic agents (ie, alpha-2 delta ligand) first. Treatment of augmentation might require switching to longer-acting dopaminergic agents, to alpha-2 delta ligands or to opiates.

REFERENCES

1. Akpinar S. Treatment of restless legs syndrome with levodopa plus benserazide. Arch Neurol 1982; 39:739.
2. Garcia-Borreguero D, Ferini-Strambi L, Kohnen R, et al. European guidelines on management of restless legs syndrome: report of a joint task force by the European Federation of Neurological Societies, the European Neurological Society and the European Sleep Research Society. Eur J Neurol 2012; 19:1385–96.
3. Garcia-Borreguero D, Kohnen R, Silber MH, et al. The long-term treatment of restless legs syndrome/Willis-Ekbom disease: evidence-based guidelines and clinical consensus best practice guidance: a report from the International Restless Legs Syndrome Study Group. Sleep Med 2013;14:675–84.

4. Allen RP, Chen C, Garcia-Borreguero D, et al. Comparison of pregabalin with pramipexole for restless legs syndrome. N Engl J Med 2014;370:621–31.

5. Allen RP, Earley CJ. Augmentation of the restless legs syndrome with carbidopa/levodopa. Sleep 1996;19:205–13.

6. Allen RP, Picchietti D, Hening WA, et al. Restless legs syndrome: diagnostic criteria, special considerations, and epidemiology. A report from the restless Legs Syndrome Diagnosis and Epidemiology Workshop at the National Institutes of Health. Sleep Med 2003;4:101–19.

7. Garcia-Borreguero D, Allen RP, Kohnen R, et al. Diagnostic standards for dopaminergic augmentation of restless legs syndrome: report from a World Association of Sleep Medicine-International Restless Legs Syndrome Study Group consensus conference at the Max Planck Institute. Sleep Med 2007;8:520–30.

8. Oertel W, Trenkwalder C, Benes H, et al. Long-term safety and efficacy of rotigotine transdermal patch for moderate-to-severe idiopathic restless legs syndrome: a 5-year open-label extension study. Lancet Neurol 2011;10:710–20.

9. Garcia-Borreguero D, Grunstein R, Sridhar G, et al. A 52-week open-label study of the long-term safety of ropinirole in patients with restless legs syndrome. Sleep Med 2007;8:742–52.

10. Allen RP. Pregabalin versus pramipexole for restless legs syndrome. N Engl J Med 2014;370:2050–1.

11. Garcia-Borreguero D, Högl B, Ferini Strambi L, et al. Systematic evaluation of augmentation during treatment with ropinirole in restless legs syndrome: results from a prospective, multicenter study over sixty-six weeks. Mov Disord 2012;27(2):277–83.

12. Benes H, Heinrich CR, Ueberall MA, et al. Long-term safety and efficacy of cabergoline for the treatment of idiopathic restless legs syndrome: results from an open-label 6-month clinical trial. Sleep 2004;27: 674–82.

13. Winkelman JW, Johnston L. Augmentation and tolerance with long-term pramipexole treatment of restless legs syndrome (RLS). Sleep Med 2004;5:9–14.

14. Ferini-Strambi L. Restless legs syndrome augmentation and pramipexole treatment. Sleep Med 2002; 3(Suppl):S23–5.

15. Vetrugno R, La Morgia C, D'Angelo R, et al. Augmentation of restless legs syndrome with long-term tramadol treatment. Mov Disord 2007;22:424–7.

16. Giorgi L, Asgharian A, Hunter B. Ropinirole in patients with restless legs syndrome and baseline IRLS total scores ≥24: efficacy and tolerability in a 26-week, double-blind, parallel-group, placebo-controlled study followed by a 40-week open-label extension. Clin Ther 2013;35:1321–36.

17. Trenkwalder C, Benes H, Grote L, et al. Prolonged release oxycodone-naloxone for treatment of severe restless legs syndrome after failure of previous treatment: a double-blind, randomised, placebo-controlled trial with an open-label extension. Lancet Neurol 2013;12:1141–50.

18. Allen R. Dopamine and iron in the pathophysiology of restless legs syndrome (RLS). Sleep Med 2004; 5:385–91.

19. Garcia-Borreguero D. Augmentation: understanding a key feature of RLS. Sleep Med 2004;5:5–6.

20. Silber MH, Ehrenberg BL, Allen RP, et al. An algorithm for the management of restless legs syndrome. Mayo Clin Proc 2004;79:916–22.

21. Trenkwalder C, Hening WA, Montagna P, et al. Treatment of restless legs syndrome: an evidence-based review and implications for clinical practice. Mov Disord 2008;23:2267–302.

Toward a Definition of Quality Care for Patients with Restless Legs Syndrome

Lynn Marie Trotti, MD, MSc

KEYWORDS

- Restless legs syndrome • Willis-Ekbom disease • Quality • Process measure • Outcome measure

KEY POINTS

- Through a formal development process, the American Academy of Sleep Medicine (AASM) created a series of quality indicators for common sleep disorders, including restless legs syndrome.
- The AASM's restless legs syndrome quality indicators include 1 outcome measure (decreased symptom severity) and 7 process measures.
- Process measures designed to improve diagnostic accuracy are use of accepted diagnostic criteria and measurement of iron stores.
- Process measures intended to decrease symptom severity are regular measurement of severity and use of evidence-based treatments whenever appropriate.
- Process measures chosen to minimize treatment complications include counseling about side effects and regular assessment for impulse control disorders and augmentation in patients at risk.

WHY QUALITY CARE?

Quality care, defined by the Institute of Medicine as the 3-pronged quest

1. To always provide effective care to those who could benefit from it,
2. To always refrain from providing inappropriate services, and
3. To eliminate all preventable complications[1]

is not controversial; health care providers are unified in their goal of improving health and quality of life of the patients and populations they serve.

In contrast, measurement of quality, and especially the use of quality measurement in rewarding or penalizing health care providers, has received much debate.[2–5] If implemented poorly, quality improvement measures may feel like little more than an administrative burden. If implemented well, quality improvement measures have the potential to be a powerful scientific tool with which providers can evaluate, change, and reevaluate their practices to achieve the best outcomes possible for their patients.[1,4] The distinction between these 2 depends critically on design and implementation, and ensuring the latter scenario is no small challenge. A fundamental step in achieving quality improvement is defining measures of quality.

The need to improve quality of care and patient outcomes in the United States is also uncontroversial.[1,6] In response to this need and an increased societal emphasis on quality of care, the AASM commissioned a series of Workgroups to develop quality measures for common sleep disorders.[7] One of the sleep disorders they chose to focus on was restless legs syndrome (RLS), also known as Willis-Ekbom disease. In this article, the background, development process, and individual RLS quality measures that resulted from this process[8] are discussed.

Conflict of interest: Dr L.M. Trotti has no conflicts to disclose.
Department of Neurology and Sleep Center, Emory University School of Medicine, 12 Executive Park Drive Northeast, Atlanta, GA 30329, USA
E-mail address: Lbecke2@emory.edu

Sleep Med Clin 10 (2015) 293–301
http://dx.doi.org/10.1016/j.jsmc.2015.05.007
1556-407X/15/$ – see front matter

HOW CAN QUALITY CARE BE MEASURED?

There are several major types of quality measures:

1. Outcome measures (ie, how patients are meeting the overall goals of care, such as decreased mortality or increased quality of life)
2. Process measures (ie, actions taken by the provider or system in caring for an individual patient, such as disease-specific diagnostic testing)
3. Structure measures (ie, how the health care system is organized, such as patient to staff ratios)

All 3 types of measures have advantages and disadvantages (**Table 1**); for the purposes of developing sleep-specific quality metrics, AASM Workgroups were asked to develop only process and outcome measures.[7]

Key features of process measures are those that are "valid, reliable, relevant to practice, and based on the best available evidence"[3]; processes must be important determinants of outcome or they need not be measured and changed. Put in alternate terms, process measures are most useful for quality improvement if they are

1. Closely linked to the desired outcome (ie, performing the process clearly increases the likelihood of the outcome)
2. An evidence-based standard of care
3. Modifiable
4. Easily measurable[1,7]

Factors 3 and 4 are affected largely by the selection of metrics (and factor 4, in particular, represents a logistical challenge in the current health care system), whereas factors 1 and 2 are ensured by use of best available evidence for metric development.

THE DEVELOPMENT OF QUALITY MEASURES FOR RESTLESS LEGS SYNDROME

For the AASM quality metrics, the measure development process began with a broad literature search of RLS, quality care, and existing evidence-based guidelines.[8] Despite the high volume of well-conducted research into RLS pathophysiology and treatment, research into processes and quality in RLS care is much less plentiful. The literature review was followed by Workgroup proposal of outcomes and associated process measures, refinement of these measures by the Workgroup, and feedback on measures from a larger group of AASM Quality Workgroups. Following this, measures were tested in the clinics of Workgroup members and then additional

feedback was sought, now from non-AASM RLS stakeholders, and measures were further refined. To make explicit the evidence behind each process, the Workgroup rated the level of evidence linking each process measure to its associated outcome. In light of the limited body of research into RLS quality measures, most of the process measures were based on expert consensus (**Table 2**). This evidence rating reflects only the strength of the evidence directly linking the process with the outcome, not the evidence that the process is clinically important, measureable, modifiable, or standard of care. For example, augmentation is a well-recognized, clinically important treatment complication,[9] but the Workgroup was unable to find any controlled studies specifically demonstrating that assessing for augmentation reduces its impact.

The development process ultimately yielded 7 process measures, which mapped to 3 different outcomes. Outcomes were selected because they were major goals of care in patients with RLS (improve diagnostic accuracy, reduce RLS severity, and minimize treatment complications). However, only 1 of these outcomes was given an associated quantitative outcome measure (**Fig. 1**). Full details regarding each measure and its specifications can be found elsewhere.[8] All final measures were approved by the AASM Board of Directors.

RESTLESS LEGS SYNDROME QUALITY METRICS

Outcome 1: Improve Diagnostic Accuracy

The first outcome, improving accuracy of RLS diagnosis, is the least patient-oriented of the 3 outcomes. Despite this, the Workgroup thought its inclusion was important, because misdiagnosis of RLS, either through labeling non-RLS symptoms as RLS or through overlooking RLS when it is the cause of symptoms, prevents quality care.

Process 1: use approved restless legs syndrome diagnostic criteria → to improve diagnostic accuracy

This process measures how often patients with RLS are diagnosed according to accepted diagnostic criteria. Several stakeholder groups have developed diagnostic criteria for RLS (eg, the International RLS Study Group [IRLSSG], the AASM, the American Psychiatric Association), which are not identical but share core features of a circadian urge to move the legs that is worse with rest and relieved with movement. The Workgroup felt that use of any of these organizational criteria, or documentation of these 4 core features, would improve diagnostic accuracy.

Table 1
Choices of metrics for measuring quality

Measure of Quality	Example	Benefits	Limitations
Outcome measure	Decrease in severity of RLS symptoms over time	• Face validity • Patient oriented[7] • Obvious alignment with patient goals of care	• Affected by multiple factors beyond provider or health care system control[5,32] • Duration between action and outcome may be long[7] • Do not provide information about specifically how to change practice to improve outcome[5]
Process measure	Measurement of RLS severity	• Not stigmatizing[5] • Less affected by features of patient population than are outcomes[7] • Can be measured at the time of the patient encounter[7] • Most providers or systems have room for improvement on some measures[5]	• Not necessarily directly important to patients
Structure measure	Patient volume of provider caring for patients with RLS	• Generally easy to measure[7]	• Not subject to change by individual care providers[7] • Not necessarily directly important to patients

In its most recent version of RLS diagnostic criteria, the IRLSSG explicitly added a requirement to exclude RLS mimics during the diagnostic process.[10] In support of this change, the Workgroup attempted to design a process measure that captured the act of excluding mimics. Throughout the process of measure development, the Workgroup attempted to balance importance of each process with feasibility of extracting data from the medical record. Feedback regarding the process measure of excluding mimics was that the process was too complex and provider actions were likely not documented sufficiently within the medical record to move forward with such a process measure at the current time. However, exclusion of RLS mimics remains a key aspect of proper diagnosis.

Process 2: evaluate iron stores, at least serum ferritin → to improve diagnostic accuracy

This process measures how often iron stores are assessed as part of RLS diagnosis. At first glance, it seems tangentially related to the outcome of improving RLS diagnosis, if RLS diagnosis is

considered strictly as the presence or absence of the core RLS criteria. However, in acknowledgment that iron deficiency is a common comorbidity of RLS[11–13] and that treatment algorithms for RLS generally recommend testing for iron deficiency and treating with iron supplementation if deficiency is present,[14,15] the Workgroup felt that diagnosis of iron deficiency is fundamental to RLS diagnosis.

Body iron stores can be assessed with a variety of measures (**Box 1**). Hemoglobin and hematocrit can reflect severe iron deficiency but are not sufficiently sensitive to iron deficiency to be used in isolation.[16] Although ferritin measurements alone are adequate in some cases, ferritin levels may be falsely elevated in inflammation[17] and a full iron panel is often preferable.

Outcome 2: Decrease Restless Legs Syndrome Severity

Outcome 2, decrease RLS severity, is a patient-oriented goal of care. It is self-evident, in that it is the major goal driving patients to seek medical care for RLS. Because of the identified need for

Table 2
Level of evidence supporting the association between each process measure and its related outcome

Level	Definition	RLS Quality Process Measures
Level 1: Strong evidence that process measure is associated with outcome	Process given the strongest level of recommendation in AASM practice parameter or non-AASM evidence-based clinical guideline without serious bias	Process measure 4
Level 2: Moderate evidence that process measure is associated with outcome	Process given second strongest level of recommendation in AASM practice parameter, strongest or second strongest recommendation in AASM Best Practice Guide or Clinical Guideline, or moderately strong recommendation from non-AASM evidence-based clinical guideline without serious bias	N/A
Level 3: Supporting evidence that process measure is associated with outcome	Process given third strongest level of recommendation in AASM practice parameter, Best Practice Guide, or Clinical Guideline, lower level of recommendation from non-AASM evidence-based guideline without serious bias, conclusions from systematic reviews/meta-analyses, or RCTs with at least moderate effect size without serious bias	N/A
Level 4: Workgroup consensus that process measure is associated with outcome	RCTs with small effect size, observational studies, or expert consensus of the Workgroup	Process measures 1–3, 5–7

both process measures and outcome measures,[7] this outcome was chosen by the Workgroup to be an outcome measure. This outcome measure is defined as the proportion of treated patients with RLS who show a decrease in RLS severity within 12 months of being prescribed a new medication for RLS.

In early versions of this outcome measure, the Workgroup recommended that severity should be measured using the IRLSSG's severity rating scale (the IRLS).[18] However, stakeholder feedback (both through the formal AASM process and informally through presentations of early drafts at the 2014 IRLSSG and Associated Professional Sleep Societies (APSS) meetings) was sharply divided on the use of this rating scale. Some RLS experts agreed that use of the IRLS would be an effective way to quantify RLS severity in clinic, whereas others thought that the IRLS is too cumbersome in its current form (which requires the provider to be present during the administration). Efforts to validate a self-completed version of the IRLS are underway (D. Sharon, personal communication, 2014) and should substantially alleviate this concern.

A separate issue is the amount of change that should be expected when quality care is delivered. Although on the surface this seems to be an easy question to answer, the available literature provides only a guide. In randomized controlled trials (RCTs), a 4- to 6-point reduction in severity on the IRLS, compared with the reduction with placebo, seems clinically significant.[9,19,20] Clinical experience suggests that the reduction pretreatment to posttreatment should be greater than the reduction seen in RCTs, where the placebo effect is excluded by design. However, in at least 1 clinical practice, IRLS scores did not change despite guideline-based care.[21] This lack of improvement on the IRLS may reflect population characteristics, as suggested by the investigators in light of the high rates of psychiatric comorbidity, but also raises the possibility that the IRLS does not perform

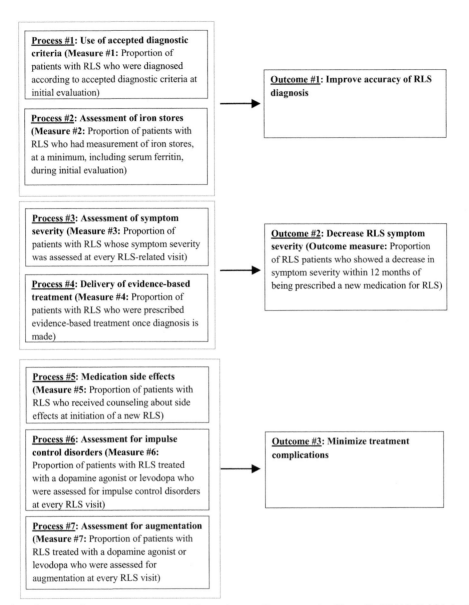

Fig. 1. Driver diagram of process measures and the outcomes they promote. (*From* Trotti LM, Goldstein CA, Harrod CG, et al. Quality measures for the care of adult patients with restless legs syndrome. J Clin Sleep Med 2015;11(3):295; with permission.)

in clinical settings the way it performs in research settings; this highlights an important caveat for this outcome measure in particular and the development of quality measures in general—expectations based on clinical and research experience may not be borne out by research into quality measures, and such research is urgently needed. Based on the above-mentioned factor, the Workgroup chose to classify decreased RLS severity as a dichotomous outcome (improved or not improved) for the purposes of this outcome measure.

Because outcomes are affected by many factors in addition to processes of care, exclusion criteria for this outcome measure (**Box 2**) were chosen to minimize the impact of known factors outside the prescriber's control.

Process 3: measure restless legs syndrome severity → to decrease restless legs syndrome severity

This process measures the proportion of patients with RLS in whom RLS severity was assessed at every visit, including both a general rating of

---

Box 1
Measures of body iron stores

- Iron
- Total iron-binding capacity
- Percent transferrin saturation
- Ferritin
- Soluble transferrin receptor

---

severity and an assessment of the severity of an associated feature of RLS (sleep quality, daytime function, daytime sleepiness, and/or mood). Measurement of RLS severity was selected as an important process to encompass several key issues regarding RLS care:

1. Frequent assessment of severity
   a. Allows identification of treatment failures
   b. Facilitates early identification of treatment complications (ie, augmentation)
   c. Provides the basis for measuring the outcome of decreased severity
2. Use of a measure of severity that also includes assessment of sleep quality, daytime function, daytime sleepiness, and/or mood
   a. Highlights the important role of RLS in worsening these features in individual patients

Process 4: use evidence-based restless legs syndrome treatment → to decrease restless legs syndrome severity

This process measures the proportion of treated patients with RLS in whom an evidence-based treatment is prescribed. The evidence linking use of evidence-based RLS treatments (eg, dopamine agonists, $\alpha2\delta$ ligands) with the outcome of reduction in RLS severity is robust, provided by multiple high-quality RCTs and codified in evidence-based treatment guidelines published by major RLS stakeholder groups (**Table 3**). Because evidence continues to accumulate, this process does not require the use of specific medications but rather use of medications that are supported by high-level evidence at the time they are prescribed.

The intention behind this measure was to encourage providers to use evidence-backed therapies whenever appropriate, with the goal of supporting the sometimes challenging transition from accumulation of RCT evidence to changed clinical practice.[22,23] In contrast, the intention of this measure was not to penalize providers who are using second- or third-line agents for specific, patient-driven reasons. In individual cases, there are at times compelling reasons to use an alternate medication, for example, in the patient who has tried and failed first-line agents, has a contraindication to first-line agents, or has another disease state that needs to be addressed before treating RLS. This measure allows exclusion of all these cases, as long as there is a documented reason for deviation from evidence-based care.

Outcome 3: Minimize Treatment Complications

Despite the wealth of data supporting the efficacy of RLS medications, there is also evidence supporting the existence of problematic medication side effects in some patients. Thus, the final outcome goal is to reduce the burden of these treatment complications.

Process 5: Counseling about medication side effects → to minimize treatment complications

This process measures the proportion of patients with RLS administered a new medication who are counseled about medication side effects. Implicit in this measure is the assumption that discussion of potential risks mitigates the impact of side effects if they develop. The Workgroup was unable to find data directly assessing this link in the RLS literature. However, in other conditions, it has been shown that patients who are counseled about side effects are less likely to experience an adverse drug event.[24–26] Further, counseling about side effects may result in earlier reporting by patients, allowing providers to respond and shorten the

---

Box 2
Exclusion criteria for measurement of outcome 2, decreased severity of RLS

- Patients refractory to 2 previous RLS medications (to avoid penalizing providers who are referred complex, refractory patients with RLS)
- Patients whose RLS symptoms are mild (who have limited opportunity for decreased severity)
- Women who are pregnant (because their RLS symptoms are expected to change during the course of pregnancy independent of treatment and because treatment options are more limited)
- Patients who are not compliant with treatment or do not follow up (to avoid penalizing providers for patient factors over which they have limited control)

Table 3
Most recent evidence-based RLS stakeholder treatment recommendations

	AASM[15]	IRLSSG[28] for Use up to 6 mo	IRLSSG[28] for 1 y or Longer	European Societies[a,33] for Use Less than 6 mo	European Societies[33] for Use at Least 6 mo	AHRQ[34]
Nonergot dopamine agonists	Level A[b]	Level A	Level B	Level A	Level A or Level C, by agent[c]	Level A
Gabapentin	Level C	Insufficient evidence	Insufficient evidence	Level A	Level C	—
Pregabalin	Level C	Leve1 A	Leve1 A	Level A	Insufficient evidence	Level A
Gabapentin enacarbil	Level B	Level B	Level B	Level A	Level B	Level A
Opiates	Level B	Insufficient evidence	Insufficient evidence	Insufficient evidence	Insufficient evidence	Insufficient evidence

Abbreviation: AHRQ, Agency for Healthcare Research and Quality.
^a European societies guidelines are a joint work of the European Federation of Neurological Societies, the European Neurological Society, and the European Sleep Research Society.
^b In the case of guidelines not rating evidence on an A to C scale, ratings were converted such that level A corresponded the highest level rating of evidence, level B the intermediate level, and level C the lowest level.
^c Level A for rotigotine and level C for pramipexole and ropinirole.

duration of the side effect.[24] The Agency of Healthcare Research and Quality recommends that patients with RLS be counseled regarding potential harms of RLS medications.[27] Therefore, this process was included to support the outcome of minimizing treatment complications.

Process 6: assessment of impulse control disorders → to minimize treatment complications

This process measures the proportion of patients with RLS treated with a dopaminergic medication who are assessed for the presence of impulse control disorders (ICDs) at every RLS-related visit. Assessment of impulsivity leads to a minimization of treatment complications if this impulsivity is

1. Caused by the medication
2. Reversible on medication discontinuation/minimization

Expert consensus, in the form of recommendations from both the IRLSSG and the Willis-Ekbom Disease Foundation, recommends the assessment of ICDs at every visit in patients at risk for this complication.[14,28]

Process 7: assessment of augmentation → to minimize treatment complications

This process measures the proportion of patients with RLS treated with a dopaminergic medication who are assessed for the presence of augmentation at every RLS-related visit. Minimizing the impact of augmentation on patients requires both assessment and a change in management strategy. Unfortunately, optimal management strategies have never been tested in RCTs. Multiple management strategies have been proposed, including changing to longer-acting medication formulations, split-dosing instead of once-daily dosing, increase in dose, decrease in dose with addition of a different agent, and cessation of offending medication.[14,29,30] Despite unanswered questions, augmentation is widely acknowledged to be a problematic side effect in patients with RLS,[9] its regular assessment is generally recommended by experts,[27,28] and so the Workgroup thought its inclusion as a process measure was warranted.

HOW SHOULD THESE MEASURES BE USED?

These measures are not a validated, final scorecard for immediate use in external benchmarking.[7] Rather, they are a first step at formally defining quality care of the adult patient with RLS, designed to present current evidence and consensus while highlighting the need for research into RLS quality care. In their present form, they could be used as part of an internal quality improvement process, an iterative process of assessment, practice change, and reassessment. Institutional, professional society, and technical support for this type of quality improvement process is clearly needed, so that individual providers can improve quality without the administrative burden of doing so detracting from their ability to care for the patient.[2,4,7,31] The process of quality measure development is also iterative; as research into quality accumulates, measures are refined over time.[1] The AASM RLS quality measures will require ongoing testing, refinement, and validation but nonetheless serve as a necessary first step in identifying which aspects of clinical care truly improve outcomes for patients with RLS.

ACKNOWLEDGMENTS

Dr L.M. Trotti thanks the members of the RLS Quality Workgroup, including Cathy A. Goldstein, MD; Christopher G. Harrod, MS; Brian B. Koo, MD; Denise Sharon, MD, PhD; Rochelle Zak, MD; and Ronald D. Chervin, MD, MS, for their dedication and unflagging efforts in developing the RLS quality measures discussed in this article. The opinions expressed in this work, with the exception of those also expressed in reference,[8] are those of Dr L.M. Trotti and do not necessarily reflect those of other Workgroup members.

REFERENCES

1. Chassin MR, Galvin RW. The urgent need to improve health care quality. Institute of Medicine National Roundtable on Health Care Quality. JAMA 1998; 280(11):1000–5.
2. Cohen RI, Jaffrey F, Bruno J, et al. Quality improvement and pay for performance: barriers to and strategies for success. Chest 2013;143(6):1542–7.
3. Kahn JM, Scales DC, Au DH, et al. An official American Thoracic Society policy statement: pay-for-performance in pulmonary, critical care, and sleep medicine. Am J Respir Crit Care Med 2010;181(7): 752–61.
4. Siegel CA, Allen JI, Melmed GY. Translating improved quality of care into an improved quality of life for patients with inflammatory bowel disease. Clin Gastroenterol Hepatol 2013;11(8):908–12.
5. Lilford RJ, Brown CA, Nicholl J. Use of process measures to monitor the quality of clinical practice. BMJ 2007;335(7621):648–50.
6. Berwick DM, Nolan TW, Whittington J. The triple aim: care, health, and cost. Health Aff (Millwood) 2008; 27(3):759–69.
7. Morgenthaler TI, Aronsky AJ, Carden KA, et al. Measurement of quality to improve care in sleep medicine. J Clin Sleep Med 2015;11(3):279–91.
8. Trotti LM, Goldstein CA, Harrod CG, et al. Quality measures for the care of adult patients with restless legs syndrome. J Clin Sleep Med 2015;11(3):311–34.
9. Hornyak M, Scholz H, Kohnen R, et al. What treatment works best for restless legs syndrome? Meta-analyses of dopaminergic and non-dopaminergic medications. Sleep Med Rev 2014;18(2):153–64.
10. Allen RP, Picchietti DL, Garcia-Borreguero D, et al. Restless legs syndrome/Willis-Ekbom disease diagnostic criteria: updated International Restless Legs Syndrome Study Group (IRLSSG) consensus criteria – history, rationale, description, and significance. Sleep Med 2014;15(8):860–73.
11. Cuellar NG, Hanlon A, Ratcliffe SJ. The relationship with iron and health outcomes in persons with restless legs syndrome. Clin Nurs Res 2011;20(2): 144–61.
12. O'Keeffe ST, Noel J, Lavan JN. Restless legs syndrome in the elderly. Postgrad Med J 1993; 69(815):701–3.
13. Ohayon MM, O'Hara R, Vitiello MV. Epidemiology of restless legs syndrome: a synthesis of the literature. Sleep Med Rev 2012;16(4):283–95.
14. Silber MH, Becker PM, Earley C, et al. Willis-Ekbom Disease Foundation revised consensus statement on the management of restless legs syndrome. Mayo Clin Proc 2013;88(9):977–86.
15. Aurora RN, Kristo DA, Bista SR, et al. The treatment of restless legs syndrome and periodic limb movement disorder in adults - an update for 2012: practice parameters with an evidence-based systematic review and meta-analyses: an American Academy of Sleep Medicine clinical practice guideline. Sleep 2012; 35(8):1039–62.
16. Silber MH, Richardson JW. Multiple blood donations associated with iron deficiency in patients with restless legs syndrome. Mayo Clin Proc 2003; 78(1):52–4.
17. Weinstock LB, Walters AS, Paueksakon P. Restless legs syndrome–theoretical roles of inflammatory and immune mechanisms. Sleep Med Rev 2012; 16(4):341–54.
18. Walters AS, LeBrocq C, Dhar A, et al. Validation of the international restless legs syndrome study group rating scale for restless legs syndrome. Sleep Med 2003;4(2):121–32.
19. Trenkwalder C, Kohnen R, Allen RP, et al. Clinical trials in restless legs syndrome–recommendations of the European RLS STUDY GROUP (EURLSSG). Mov Disord 2007;22(Suppl 18):S495–504.
20. Scholz H, Trenkwalder C, Kohnen R, et al. Dopamine agonists for restless legs syndrome. Cochrane Database Syst Rev 2011;(3):CD006009.
21. Godau J, Spinnler N, Wevers AK, et al. Poor effect of guideline based treatment of restless legs syndrome in clinical practice. J Neurol Neurosurg Psychiatry 2010;81(12):1390–5.
22. McGlynn EA, Asch SM, Adams J, et al. The quality of health care delivered to adults in the United States. N Engl J Med 2003;348(26):2635–45.

23. Grol R, Grimshaw J. From best evidence to best practice: effective implementation of change in patients' care. Lancet 2003;362(9391):1225–30.

24. Forster AJ, Murff HJ, Peterson JF, et al. Adverse drug events occurring following hospital discharge. J Gen Intern Med 2005;20(4):317–23.

25. Gandhi TK, Burstin HR, Cook EF, et al. Drug complications in outpatients. J Gen Intern Med 2000;15(3): 149–54.

26. Schnipper JL, Kirwin JL, Cotugno MC, et al. Role of pharmacist counseling in preventing adverse drug events after hospitalization. Arch Intern Med 2006; 166(5):565–71.

27. Treatment for restless legs syndrome: clinician research summary. Rockville (MD): AHRQ Publication; 2013. 12(13):EHC147-3. Available at: http://www.effectivehealthcare.ahrq.gov/search-for-guides-reviews-and-reports/?pageaction=displayProduct&productID=1674. Accessed June 6, 2015.

28. Garcia-Borreguero D, Kohnen R, Silber MH, et al. The long-term treatment of restless legs syndrome/Willis-Ekbom disease: evidence-based guidelines and clinical consensus best practice guidance: a report from the international restless legs syndrome study group. Sleep Med 2013;14(7):675–84.

29. Maestri M, Fulda S, Ferini-Strambi L, et al. Polysomnographic record and successful management of augmentation in restless legs syndrome/Willis-Ekbom disease. Sleep Med 2014;15(5):570–5.

30. Williams AM, Garcia-Borreguero D. Management of restless legs syndrome augmentation. Curr Treat Options Neurol 2009;11(5):327–32.

31. Miller RG, Brooks BR, Swain-Eng RJ, et al. Quality improvement in neurology: amyotrophic lateral sclerosis quality measures: report of the quality measurement and reporting subcommittee of the American Academy of Neurology. Neurology 2013; 81(24):2136–40.

32. Fischer C, Lingsma HF, Marang-van de Mheen PJ, et al. Is the readmission rate a valid quality indicator? A review of the evidence. PLoS One 2014; 9(11):e112282.

33. Garcia-Borreguero D, Ferini-Strambi L, Kohnen R, et al. European guidelines on management of restless legs syndrome: report of a Joint Task Force by the European Federation of Neurological Societies, the European Neurological Society and the European Sleep Research Society. Eur J Neurol 2012; 19:1385–96.

34. Wilt TJ, MacDonald R, Ouellette J, et al. Treatment for restless legs syndrome. Comparative effectiveness review no. 86. Rockville (MD): AHRQ Publication; 2012. 12(13).

Management of Restless Legs Syndrome/Willis-Ekbom Disease in Hospitalized and Perioperative Patients

CrossMark

Cathy Goldstein, MD

KEYWORDS

- Restless legs syndrome • Surgery • Perioperative • Hospitalized

KEY POINTS

- Restless legs syndrome (RLS) is chronic and associated with multiple comorbidities; therefore, it may be encountered in the inpatient or perioperative setting.
- Characteristics of the hospitalized or surgical context can exacerbate or unmask RLS and include the following: immobility, sleep deprivation and circadian disruption, blood loss and subsequent iron deficiency, withdrawal from RLS therapy, and adverse effects of medications.
- RLS and the associated discomfort and insomnia can prolong hospital stay and negatively impact outcomes.
- RLS medications should be continued during the hospital admission if possible.
- When surgery or health status precludes orally administered medications, parenteral opioids or transdermal rotigotine should be considered.
- Avoidance of excessive phlebotomy and medications known to trigger RLS may be beneficial.
- Patients should increase activity when acceptable; however other nonpharmacological interventions require further study.

INTRODUCTION

Clinical Manifestations and Epidemiology

Restless legs syndrome (RLS) is a sensorimotor neurologic disorder that also goes by the eponym Willis-Ekbom disease (WED) after the physicians who initially described the condition.[1–3] The disorder is defined by its diagnostic criteria, which include

An urge to move the legs that is usually associated with or felt to be precipitated by discomfort in the legs
The motor urgency and discomfort occur during or are worsened by rest or inactivity
The symptoms are partially or completely relieved by movement
The symptoms develop or worsen in the evening or nighttime[1]

The combination of the aforementioned symptoms is consistent with a diagnosis of RLS only when not a consequence of another medical or behavioral condition.[1] The prevalence of clinically significant RLS is 2% to 3%,[4–6] and the disorder negatively impacts sleep, daytime function, quality of life, and mood.[4,7–10] Periodic limb movements of sleep (PLMS) are involuntary, stereotyped movements of the legs seen in more than 80% of patients with RLS.[7]

Patients typically present with RLS in the third or fourth decade of life, and the condition is chronic.[11] Additionally, RLS is associated with multiple comorbidities[12]; therefore, it is not surprising that this condition is encountered in a perioperative or inpatient setting. In fact, during the 5-year open-label extension of rotigotine for

Department of Neurology, University of Michigan Sleep Disorders Center, C728 Med Inn Building, SPC 5845, 1500 E. Medical Center Drive, Ann Arbor, MI 48109-5845, USA
E-mail address: cathygo@med.umich.edu

Sleep Med Clin 10 (2015) 303–310
http://dx.doi.org/10.1016/j.jsmc.2015.05.003
1556-407X/15/$ – see front matter © 2015 Elsevier Inc. All rights reserved.

sleep.theclinics.com

moderate-to-severe RLS, nearly 20% of patients underwent a surgical intervention.[13] When hospitalized or undergoing surgery, RLS symptoms can be exacerbated in individuals with known RLS or become evident in individuals without diagnosed RLS.[14]

Pathogenesis of Restless Legs Syndrome in Hospitalized or Perioperative Patients

Multiple factors may precipitate RLS symptoms in hospitalized patients and those undergoing surgical or diagnostic procedures (**Table 1**).

Immobility

RLS is characterized by an urge to move the legs at rest. Immobility is likely the most important factor in RLS exacerbation, as both hospital admissions and surgical procedures are marked by extensive periods of immobility. Up to 83% of the hospitalization may be spent lying in bed based on accelerometer recordings.[15] This degree of immobility was seen despite the ability and willingness of the patient to ambulate.[15] Immobility worsens both sensory and motor symptoms of RLS. Individuals with RLS have marked increases in leg discomfort and periodic limb movements starting after only 10 minutes of immobility during the suggested immobility test (SIT).[16]

Sleep deprivation and circadian disruption

Sleep deprivation worsens RLS symptoms[17] and is common in hospitalized individuals. Both intensive care unit (ICU) and general ward patients display short sleep duration (4–6 hours on average), poor sleep efficiency, and frequent arousals.[18] Sleep is also reduced in postsurgical patients.[19] Noise, light, patient care interactions, mechanical ventilation, pain,[20] general anesthesia,[21] medication, and sequelae of the specific illness or procedure can contribute to disturbed sleep in hospitalized or perioperative patients.[18]

Table 1
Factors that contribute to restless legs syndrome symptoms in the perioperative or hospitalized setting

Immobility	Adverse effect of
Sleep deprivation	medications:
Blood loss	Dopamine antagonist
Cessation of RLS	antiemetics
medications	Antipsychotics
	Antihistamines
	Serotonergic
	antidepressants

Adapted from Raux M, Karroum EG, Arnulf I. Case scenario: anesthetic implications of restless legs syndrome. Anesthesiology 2010;112(6):1511–7.

The circadian rhythm is the approximately 24-hour cycle of sleep and wake,[22] as well as multiple other physiologic processes.[23] Melatonin (in the serum, saliva, or urine)[24] and core body temperature[25] are used to measure circadian phase apart from sleep. The nighttime rise in melatonin parallels the drop in core body temperature, and melatonin secretion peaks just before the core body temperature reaches its nadir 2 to 3 hours prior to habitual wake time. RLS symptoms demonstrate a circadian rhythm with maximal severity between midnight and 4 AM coinciding with the falling portion of the core body temperature rhythm.[17,26,27] RLS symptoms reach a trough between 9 AM and 1 PM Hospitalized patients have increased sleep during the daytime and reduced sleep during the night[18]; therefore, their sleep–wake behavior may be misaligned with their endogenous circadian phase, unmasking RLS symptoms (**Fig. 1**).

Alternatively, the circadian rhythm may be disturbed in critically ill and postoperative patients. The urinary metabolite of melatonin (6-sulfatoxymelatonin, aMT6s) was measured in ICU patients.[28] Nocturnal excretion of aMT6s was reduced in all ICU patients.[28] All but 2 ICU patients demonstrated a loss of the normal nocturnal peak of aMT6s.[28] Melatonin measured by both serum and urine assays demonstrated a delay of the circadian rhythm in patients after surgery.[29] Abnormal light exposure likely explains the disruption in circadian rhythms seen in hospitalized or perioperative patients.[30] Bright light is the strongest time giver that entrains the endogenous circadian rhythm to the external environment. Bright light directly suppresses melatonin and can alter circadian rhythms depending on the exposure time (a delay in circadian phase when bright light exposure occurs during the beginning of the biological night and an advance in circadian phase when the exposure occurs in the morning).[31] Individuals working nontraditional shifts are exposed to abnormal light–dark cycles and have higher prevalence of RLS compared with day shift workers.[32] Therefore, circadian disruption may have the potential to exacerbate RLS symptoms in the critically ill or postoperative patient; however, because of the confounding factors of sleep deprivation, comorbid illnesses, and smoking in shift workers, more work is needed to determine the effects of circadian disruption on RLS symptoms.[32]

Anemia

The prevalence of anemia in hospitalized patients is 30% to 40% and in most patients, iron deficiency is a significant contributor to anemia.[33]

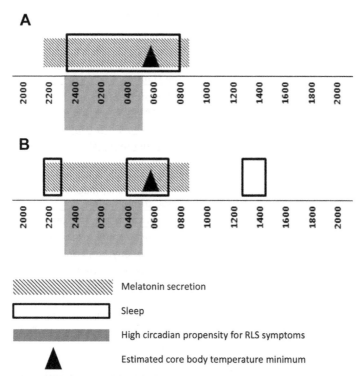

Fig. 1. Potential for sleep disruption during hospitalization to unmask RLS symptoms. Panel A represents an individual with habitual sleep time of 12 midnight to 8 AM in the outpatient setting. The highest circadian propensity for RLS symptoms overlaps with the sleep period. Upon admission to the hospital, light, noise, and patient care interactions interrupt the patient's sleep, and as seen in Panel B, the highest circadian propensity for RLS symptoms is now during the period when the patient is awake and aware of discomfort.

Iron deficiency may be chronic or acute in this population. Acute causes of iron deficiency in the inpatient or postoperative setting may be blood loss related to the acute illness (eg, gastrointestinal or other sources) or iatrogenic due to surgeries, procedures, and recurrent phlebotomy.[33]

Iron insufficiency has been implicated in the pathogenesis of RLS.[34] RLS is present in more than 20% of patients with iron deficiency anemia,[35] and low serum ferritin levels are associated with more severe symptoms in patients with RLS.[36–38] Therefore, iron deficiency is likely an important precipitant of RLS symptoms in hospitalized or postoperative patients.

Adverse medication affect

Spinal anesthesia has been implicated in multiple cases of PLMS intraoperatively[39–41] and RLS postoperatively.[42] Hogl and colleagues[42] prospectively studied 202 patients undergoing spinal anesthesia and found that 8.7% developed new-onset, self-limited RLS after their procedure. The authors considered "changes in sensorimotor spinal integration persisting after spinal anesthesia in susceptible individuals" as the etiology of RLS.[42] However, not all studies have confirmed this finding,[43] and dopamine blocking antiemetics

given with spinal anesthesia or blood loss may have been the actual precipitant of RLS.[42,43]

Other medications, either given with anesthesia[14] or apart from surgery in the inpatient setting can exacerbate RLS. The classes of medication most likely to precipitate or worsen RLS symptoms or PLMS are dopamine blocking antiemetics, antipsychotics, antihistamines, and serotonergic antidepressants[14,44–47] (Table 2).

Withdrawal from restless legs syndrome medications

RLS patients may experience an exacerbation of symptoms secondary to withdrawal from outpatient medications. Cessation of RLS medications in hospitalized or perioperative patients may be due to medication error, nothing by mouth (NPO) status, or a care provider's concern that the medication is contraindicated in the patient's current health state. Medication errors are not uncommon. The Medications at Transitions and Clinical Handoffs (MATCH) study demonstrated that more than one-third of patients are subject to medication errors upon hospital admission, and nearly half of these are due to medication omission.[48] Discontinuation of dopamine agonist or opioid medications on hospital admission or in preparation for

Table 2
Medications reported to precipitate or worsen restless legs syndrome or periodic limb movements of sleep

Class of Medication	Medication Name
Dopamine antagonist antiemetics	Droperidol, metoclopramide, domperidone, prochlorperazine
Antipsychotics	Haloperidol, olanzapine, risperidone, quetiapine
Antihistamines	Hydroxyzine, mianserin, cimetidine
Serotonergic antidepressants	
Tricyclic	Amitriptyline, clomipramine, dibenzepine, desipramine, doxepin, imipramine, maprotiline, nortriptyline, opipramol, trimipramine
Selective serotonin reuptake inhibitor	Citalopram, escitalopram, fluoxetine, paroxetine, sertraline
Mixed	Buproprion, mirtazapine, trazodone, venlafaxine
Antiepileptics	Methsuximide, phenytoin, zonisamide
Other	Lithium, levothyroxine, tramadol

Data from Refs.[14,44–47]

surgery can result in an acute rebound in RLS symptoms as the last dose is metabolized.

Special Populations

In addition to the previously described characteristics of hospitalization and surgery that can precipitate RLS, certain patient populations may be particularly vulnerable to acute worsening of RLS symptoms. The prevalence of RLS is approximately 30% to 40% in chronic obstructive pulmonary disease (COPD) patients.[49] An investigation compared COPD patients hospitalized for respiratory exacerbations with healthy volunteers and found that 54.5% of inpatients with COPD exacerbation met criteria for a diagnosis of RLS compared with 5.4% of controls ($P = .001$).[49] The mechanism linking RLS to COPD is unclear; however the previously described data suggest that patients hospitalized for COPD exacerbation may be at high risk.

RLS is common in patients with kidney disease. The prevalence in patients with end-stage renal disease (ESRD) requiring dialysis may up to 62%.[50] However, studies have been dissimilar, and the actual prevalence may be closer to 20% to 30%.[50–56] Additionally, Lee and colleagues[53] found that patients with chronic kidney disease (CKD) who do not depend on dialysis also have a high prevalence of RLS (26%). The etiology of RLS in patients with kidney disease is not well understood but may be related to both iron deficiency[50,54,57,58] and calcium, phosphorous, and parathyroid hormone metabolism abnormalities,[51,56,59,60] which are common in this population. Because of the high rate of hospitalizations[61] and increased prevalence of RLS in patients with CKD and ESRD, clinicians should be aware of the potential for worsened RLS symptoms during admission.

Complications Related to Restless Legs Syndrome in Hospitalized or Perioperative Patients

Periodic limb movements[39–41] and agitation[62] observed in individuals undergoing spinal and epidural anesthesia have the potential to disrupt the surgical procedure. Additionally, motor restlessness resulting in vigorous movement after surgery could compromise the surgical site and increase postoperative bleeding, which may require subsequent intervention.[14] Associated agitation in the setting of RLS exacerbation may also lead to vital sign instability, such as tachycardia and hypertension.[14] If RLS is not recognized and treated, unnecessary diagnostic procedures and treatments may be pursued to normalize vital signs. Marked discomfort and subsequent insomnia are likely to accompany worsened or unmasked RLS symptoms in the hospitalized or perioperative patient. This is not trivial, as insomnia and sleep deprivation can prolong hospital stay[63] and negatively impact medical outcomes.[64,65] Further, pain, fatigue, and sleep disruption reduce quality of life in hospitalized patients.[66]

MANAGEMENT GOALS

The treatment of RLS in the hospitalized or perioperative setting aims to reduce the potential for the previously described complications, reduce discomfort, decrease sleep disruption, and improve quality of life.

PHARMACOLOGIC STRATEGIES

Multiple medications have demonstrated efficacy for treating RLS. Systematic reviews suggest first-line treatment of RLS with nonergotamine dopamine agonists (eg, pramipexole, ropinirole, or transdermal rotigotine)[67,68] or calcium channel alpha-2-delta ligand medications (eg, gabapentin, pregabalin, or gabapentin encarbil).[68] In refractory cases, opioids may be used.[68] Although dosing regimens vary, most patients take their RLS medication once per day, in the evening. With the exception of transdermal rotigotine, the aforementioned medications are administered orally. Individuals who do not have a contraindication to oral medication should continue their outpatient RLS medication regimen upon hospital admission. However, NPO status is necessary during procedures that require anesthesia, as well as in multiple nonsurgical inpatient scenarios (eg, during hospital admission for pancreatitis).

Nothing by Mouth Status in the Surgical Setting

In preparation for surgery, oral RLS medications may be continued until the start of NPO status recommended by the anesthesiologist. For example, if the patient is instructed not to take anything by mouth after midnight, the evening dose of RLS medication could be taken prior to that time. The patient can resume his or her usual RLS medication regimen after surgery, once he or she can swallow safely. In individuals who take RLS medication more than once daily, parental opioids may be required, particularly if the surgery or postoperative NPO period is extensive.

Nothing by Mouth Status in the Nonsurgical, Inpatient Setting

When the duration of NPO status is prolonged, hospitalized patients will need medication administered by nonoral routes to control RLS. Intravenous opioid administration may be useful to treat RLS symptoms during this time. When oral dopamine agonist therapy can be safely reestablished, low starting doses should be used to avoid adverse effects. During the dose titration, oral opioid medication may be given on an as needed basis until the patient achieves the effective dose of dopamine agonist.

Transdermal rotigotine may also be beneficial in this situation.[13] Patients can be switched from oral dopamine agonists (with the last dose given in the afternoon or evening) to transdermal rotigotine by applying the patch the following morning. This strategy has effectively controlled motor symptoms in patients with Parkinson disease[69,70] and may be considered in hospitalized RLS patients.[13]

NONPHARMACOLOGIC STRATEGIES

Nonpharmacological measures applicable to hospitalized or perioperative RLS patients include participation in mental alerting activities,[71] increased physical activity[72] (if feasible given the patient's health state), or pneumatic compression devices.[73] One small case series demonstrated improvement in RLS symptoms in 77% of patients after traction straight leg raise was performed by a physical therapist; however, further studies are needed to evaluate the efficacy of this treatment.[74]

Blood loss and resultant iron deficiency may be unavoidable in some surgical and critical care settings. However, reducing iatrogenic causes of anemia in the hospital such as excessive phlebotomy is crucial.[33] Patients with RLS symptoms and insufficient iron stores reflected by ferritin level less than 75 µg/mL may benefit from iron supplementation.[57,75,76] However, because ferritin is an acute-phase reactant, it may not reflect inadequate iron levels, particularly in an inpatient setting.[77] Therefore, assessment with total iron-binding capacity and serum iron levels may be beneficial. Iron can be given orally as ferrous sulfate 325 mg 2 to 3 times daily with vitamin C,[78] or intravenously as iron sucrose, ferric gluconate, or ferumoxytol.[67] Iron dextran is another formulation of parental iron; however, because of the risk of anaphylaxis,[79] iron dextran should be avoided or administered carefully after an initial test dose.

Whenever possible, medications with the potential to worsen RLS (see **Table 2**) should be avoided.

The care team should devise strategies to reduce sleep deprivation and circadian disruption in the hospital such as reduction of nighttime light and noise.[18] Additionally, when acceptable, patient care activities should be clustered and take place during daytime hours.[18]

SUMMARY/DISCUSSION

RLS is a sensorimotor disorder that can cause significant discomfort, impaired quality of life, poor mood, and disturbed sleep. Because the disorder is chronic and associated with multiple comorbidities, RLS can be seen in an inpatient or perioperative setting. Certain characteristics of the hospitalized or surgical context can exacerbate or unmask RLS and include the following: immobility, sleep deprivation and circadian disruption, blood loss and subsequent iron deficiency, withdrawal from RLS therapy, and adverse effects of medications. Importantly,

RLS and the associated discomfort and insomnia can prolong hospital stay and negatively impact outcomes; therefore, treatment is crucial. RLS medications should be continued during the hospital admission when possible. If the patient is having surgery or his or her health status requires NPO status, then parenteral opioids or transdermal rotigotine should be considered. Avoidance of excessive phlebotomy and medications known to trigger RLS is also helpful. Patients should increase activity when acceptable; however other nonpharmacological interventions require further study.

REFERENCES

1. Allen RP, Picchietti DL, Garcia-Borreguero D, et al. Restless legs syndrome/Willis-Ekbom disease diagnostic criteria: updated international restless legs syndrome study group (IRLSSG) consensus criteria–history, rationale, description, and significance. Sleep Med 2014;15(8):860–73.
2. Willis T. The London practice of physick. London: Basset & Crook; 1685.
3. Ekbom K. Restless legs. Acta Med Scand 1945; 158(1):123.
4. Allen RP, Walters AS, Montplaisir J, et al. Restless legs syndrome prevalence and impact: REST general population study. Arch Intern Med 2005; 165(11):1286–92.
5. Allen RP, Stillman P, Myers AJ. Physician-diagnosed restless legs syndrome in a large sample of primary medical care patients in Western Europe: prevalence and characteristics. Sleep Med 2010;11(1):31–7.
6. Allen RP, Bharmal M, Calloway M. Prevalence and disease burden of primary restless legs syndrome: results of a general population survey in the United States. Movement Disord 2011;26(1):114–20.
7. Montplaisir J, Boucher S, Poirier G, et al. Clinical, polysomnographic, and genetic characteristics of restless legs syndrome: a study of 133 patients diagnosed with new standard criteria. Movement Disord 1997;12(1):61–5.
8. Phillips B, Hening W, Britz P, et al. Prevalence and correlates of restless legs syndrome: results from the 2005 national sleep foundation poll. Chest 2006;129(1):76–80.
9. Lee HB, Hening WA, Allen RP, et al. Restless legs syndrome is associated with DSM-IV major depressive disorder and panic disorder in the community. J Neuropsychiatry Clin Neurosci 2008;20(1):101–5.
10. Hening WA, Allen RP, Chaudhuri KR, et al. Clinical significance of RLS. Movement Disord 2007; 22(Suppl 18):S395–400.
11. Walters AS, Hickey K, Maltzman J, et al. A questionnaire study of 138 patients with restless legs syndrome: the 'Night-Walkers' survey. Neurology 1996;46(1):92–5.
12. Szentkiralyi A, Volzke H, Hoffmann W, et al. Multimorbidity and the risk of restless legs syndrome in 2 prospective cohort studies. Neurology 2014;82(22): 2026–33.
13. Hogl B, Oertel WH, Schollmayer E, et al. Transdermal rotigotine for the perioperative management of restless legs syndrome. BMC Neurol 2012;12:106.
14. Raux M, Karroum EG, Arnulf I. Case scenario: anesthetic implications of restless legs syndrome. Anesthesiology 2010;112(6):1511–7.
15. Brown CJ, Redden DT, Flood KL, et al. The underrecognized epidemic of low mobility during hospitalization of older adults. J Am Geriatr Soc 2009; 57(9):1660–5.
16. Michaud M, Lavigne G, Desautels A, et al. Effects of immobility on sensory and motor symptoms of restless legs syndrome. Movement Disord 2002;17(1): 112–5.
17. Hening WA, Walters AS, Wagner M, et al. Circadian rhythm of motor restlessness and sensory symptoms in the idiopathic restless legs syndrome. Sleep 1999;22(7):901–12.
18. Knauert MP, Malik V, Kamdar BB. Sleep and sleep disordered breathing in hospitalized patients. Semin Respir Crit Care Med 2014;35(5):582–92.
19. Madsen MT, Rosenberg J, Gogenur I. Actigraphy for measurement of sleep and sleep-wake rhythms in relation to surgery. J Clin Sleep Med 2013;9(4): 387–94.
20. Miller A, Roth T, Roehrs T, et al. Correlation between sleep disruption on postoperative pain. Otolaryngology Head Neck Surg 2015;152:964–8.
21. Lehmkuhl P, Prass D, Pichlmayr I. General anesthesia and postnarcotic sleep disorders. Neuropsychobiology 1987;18(1):37–42.
22. Czeisler CA, Weitzman E, Moore-Ede MC, et al. Human sleep: its duration and organization depend on its circadian phase. Science 1980;210(4475): 1264–7.
23. Hastings MH, Reddy AB, Maywood ES. A clockwork web: circadian timing in brain and periphery, in health and disease. Nature reviews. Neuroscience 2003;4(8):649–61.
24. Benloucif S, Burgess HJ, Klerman EB, et al. Measuring melatonin in humans. J Clin Sleep Med 2008;4(1):66–9.
25. Akerstedt T, Hume K, Minors D, et al. Experimental separation of time of day and homeostatic influences on sleep. Am J Physiol 1998;274(4 Pt 2): R1162–8.
26. Michaud M, Dumont M, Selmaoui B, et al. Circadian rhythm of restless legs syndrome: relationship with biological markers. Ann Neurol 2004;55(3):372–80.
27. Trenkwalder C, Hening WA, Walters AS, et al. Circadian rhythm of periodic limb movements and sensory symptoms of restless legs syndrome. Movement Disord 1999;14(1):102–10.

28. Shilo L, Dagan Y, Smorjik Y, et al. Patients in the intensive care unit suffer from severe lack of sleep associated with loss of normal melatonin secretion pattern. Am J Med Sci 1999;317(5):278–81.

29. Gogenur I. Postoperative circadian disturbances. Dan Med Bull 2010;57(12):B4205.

30. Missildine K. Sleep and the sleep environment of older adults in acute care settings. J Gerontol Nurs 2008;34(6):15–21.

31. Khalsa SB, Jewett ME, Cajochen C, et al. A phase response curve to single bright light pulses in human subjects. J Physiol 2003;549(Pt 3):945–52.

32. Sharifian A, Firoozeh M, Pouryaghoub G, et al. Restless legs syndrome in shift workers: a cross sectional study on male assembly workers. J circadian rhythms 2009;7:12.

33. Shander A, Goodnough LT, Javidroozi M, et al. Iron deficiency anemia–bridging the knowledge and practice gap. Transfus Med Rev 2014;28(3):156–66.

34. Garcia-Borreguero D, Williams AM. An update on restless legs syndrome (Willis-Ekbom disease): clinical features, pathogenesis and treatment. Curr Opin Neurol 2014;27(4):493–501.

35. Allen RP, Auerbach S, Bahrain H, et al. The prevalence and impact of restless legs syndrome on patients with iron deficiency anemia. Am J Hematol 2013;88(4):261–4.

36. Curgunlu A, Doventas A, Karadeniz D, et al. Prevalence and characteristics of restless legs syndrome (RLS) in the elderly and the relation of serum ferritin levels with disease severity: hospital-based study from Istanbul, Turkey. Arch Gerontol Geriatr 2012;55(1):73–6.

37. Sun ER, Chen CA, Ho G, et al. Iron and the restless legs syndrome. Sleep 1998;21(4):371–7.

38. Frauscher B, Gschliesser V, Brandauer E, et al. The severity range of restless legs syndrome (RLS) and augmentation in a prospective patient cohort: association with ferritin levels. Sleep Med 2009;10(6):611–5.

39. Watanabe S, Sakai K, Ono Y, et al. Alternating periodic leg movement induced by spinal anesthesia in an elderly male. Anesth Analg 1987;66(10):1031–2.

40. Watanabe S, Ono A, Naito H. Periodic leg movements during either epidural or spinal anesthesia in an elderly man without sleep-related (nocturnal) myoclonus. Sleep 1990;13(3):262–6.

41. Martinez LP, Koza M. Anesthesia-related periodic involuntary movement in an obstetrical patient for cesarean section under epidural anesthesia: a case report. AANA J 1997;65(2):150–3.

42. Hogl B, Frauscher B, Seppi K, et al. Transient restless legs syndrome after spinal anesthesia: a prospective study. Neurology 2002;59(11):1705–7.

43. Crozier TA, Karimdadian D, Happe S. Restless legs syndrome and spinal anesthesia. N Engl J Med 2008;359(21):2294–6.

44. Ward NG. Akathisia associated with droperidol during epidural anesthesia. Anesthesiology 1989;71(5):786–7.

45. Hoque R, Chesson AL Jr. Pharmacologically induced/exacerbated restless legs syndrome, periodic limb movements of sleep, and REM behavior disorder/REM sleep without atonia: literature review, qualitative scoring, and comparative analysis. J Clin Sleep Med 2010;6(1):79–83.

46. Drotts DL, Vinson DR. Prochlorperazine induces akathisia in emergency patients. Ann Emerg Med 1999;34(4 Pt 1):469–75.

47. Pinninti NR, Mago R, Townsend J, et al. Periodic restless legs syndrome associated with quetiapine use: a case report. J Clin Psychopharmacol 2005;25(6):617–8.

48. Gleason KM, McDaniel MR, Feinglass J, et al. Results of the medications at transitions and clinical handoffs (MATCH) study: an analysis of medication reconciliation errors and risk factors at hospital admission. J Gen Intern Med 2010;25(5):441–7.

49. Aras G, Kadakal F, Purisa S, et al. Are we aware of restless legs syndrome in COPD patients who are in an exacerbation period? Frequency and probable factors related to underlying mechanism. COPD 2011;8(6):437–43.

50. Kavanagh D, Siddiqui S, Geddes CC. Restless legs syndrome in patients on dialysis. Am J Kidney Dis 2004;43(5):763–71.

51. Gigli GL, Adorati M, Dolso P, et al. Restless legs syndrome in end-stage renal disease. Sleep Med 2004;5(3):309–15.

52. Collado-Seidel V, Kohnen R, Samtleben W, et al. Clinical and biochemical findings in uremic patients with and without restless legs syndrome. Am J kidney Dis 1998;31(2):324–8.

53. Lee J, Nicholl DD, Ahmed SB, et al. The prevalence of restless legs syndrome across the full spectrum of kidney disease. J Clin Sleep Med 2013;9(5):455–9.

54. Lin CH, Wu VC, Li WY, et al. Restless legs syndrome in end-stage renal disease: a multicenter study in Taiwan. Eur J Neurol 2013;20(7):1025–31.

55. Murtagh FE, Addington-Hall J, Higginson IJ. The prevalence of symptoms in end-stage renal disease: a systematic review. Adv Chronic Kidney Dis 2007;14(1):82–99.

56. Stefanidis I, Vainas A, Dardiotis E, et al. Restless legs syndrome in hemodialysis patients: an epidemiologic survey in Greece. Sleep Med 2013;14(12):1381–6.

57. Sloand JA, Shelly MA, Feigin A, et al. A double-blind, placebo-controlled trial of intravenous iron dextran therapy in patients with ESRD and restless legs syndrome. Am J kidney Dis 2004;43(4):663–70.

58. Merlino G, Lorenzut S, Gigli GL, et al. A case-control study on restless legs syndrome in nondialyzed

patients with chronic renal failure. Movement Disord 2010;25(8):1019–25.

59. Kawauchi A, Inoue Y, Hashimoto T, et al. Restless legs syndrome in hemodialysis patients: health-related quality of life and laboratory data analysis. Clin Nephrol 2006;66(6):440–6.

60. Takaki J, Nishi T, Nangaku M, et al. Clinical and psychological aspects of restless legs syndrome in uremic patients on hemodialysis. Am J kidney Dis 2003; 41(4):833–9.

61. Mix TC, St peter WL, Ebben J, et al. Hospitalization during advancing chronic kidney disease. Am J kidney Dis 2003;42(5):972–81.

62. Shin YK. Restless leg syndrome: unusual cause of agitation under anesthesia. South Med J 1987; 80(2):278–9.

63. Suzuki A, Kobayashi R, Okayasu S, et al. Pharmacotherapy for adverse events reduces the length of hospital stay in patients admitted to otolaryngology ward: a single arm intervention study. PLoS One 2014;9(12):e115879.

64. Arora VM, Chang KL, Fazal AZ, et al. Objective sleep duration and quality in hospitalized older adults: associations with blood pressure and mood. J Am Geriatr Soc 2011;59(11):2185–6.

65. Raymond I, Ancoli-Israel S, Choiniere M. Sleep disturbances, pain and analgesia in adults hospitalized for burn injuries. Sleep Med 2004;5(6):551–9.

66. Eyigor S, Eyigor C, Uslu R. Assessment of pain, fatigue, sleep and quality of life (QoL) in elderly hospitalized cancer patients. Arch Gerontol Geriatr 2010; 51(3):e57–61.

67. Aurora RN, Kristo DA, Bista SR, et al. The treatment of restless legs syndrome and periodic limb movement disorder in adults–an update for 2012: practice parameters with an evidence-based systematic review and meta-analyses: an American academy of sleep medicine clinical practice guideline. Sleep 2012;35(8):1039–62.

68. Garcia-Borreguero D, Kohnen R, Silber MH, et al. The long-term treatment of restless legs syndrome/Willis-Ekbom disease: evidence-based guidelines and clinical consensus best practice guidance: a report from the international restless legs syndrome study Group. Sleep Med 2013;14(7):675–84.

69. LeWitt PA, Boroojerdi B, MacMahon D, et al. Overnight switch from oral dopaminergic agonists to transdermal rotigotine patch in subjects with Parkinson disease. Clin Neuropharmacol 2007;30(5): 256–65.

70. Kim HJ, Jeon BS, Lee WY, et al. Overnight switch from ropinirole to transdermal rotigotine patch in patients with Parkinson disease. BMC Neurol 2011; 11:100.

71. Silber MH, Ehrenberg BL, Allen RP, et al. An algorithm for the management of restless legs syndrome. Mayo Clin Proc 2004;79(7):916–22.

72. Aukerman MM, Aukerman D, Bayard M, et al. Exercise and restless legs syndrome: a randomized controlled trial. J Am Board Fam Med 2006;19(5): 487–93.

73. Lettieri CJ, Eliasson AH. Pneumatic compression devices are an effective therapy for restless legs syndrome: a prospective, randomized, double-blinded, sham-controlled trial. Chest 2009;135(1): 74–80.

74. Dinkins EM, Stevens-Lapsley J. Management of symptoms of restless legs syndrome with use of a traction straight leg raise: a preliminary case series. Man Ther 2013;18(4):299–302.

75. Wang J, O'Reilly B, Venkataraman R, et al. Efficacy of oral iron in patients with restless legs syndrome and a low-normal ferritin: a randomized, double-blind, placebo-controlled study. Sleep Med 2009; 10(9):973–5.

76. Mehmood T, Auerbach M, Earley CJ, et al. Response to intravenous iron in patients with iron deficiency anemia (IDA) and restless leg syndrome (Willis-Ekbom disease). Sleep Med 2014;15(12): 1473–6.

77. Knovich MA, Storey JA, Coffman LG, et al. Ferritin for the clinician. Blood Rev 2009;23(3):95–104.

78. Silber MH, Becker PM, Earley C, et al. Willis-Ekbom disease foundation revised consensus statement on the management of restless legs syndrome. Mayo Clin Proc 2013;88(9):977–86.

79. Bailie GR, Clark JA, Lane CE, et al. Hypersensitivity reactions and deaths associated with intravenous iron preparations. Nephrol Dial Transplant 2005; 20(7):1443–9.

Restless Legs Syndrome/ Willis-Ekbom Disease and Growing Pains in Children and Adolescents

Narong Simakajornboon, MD[a],*, Thomas J. Dye, MD[a], Arthur S. Walters, MD[b]

KEYWORDS

- Pediatric restless legs syndrome (RLS) • Pediatric periodic limb movement disorder (PLMD)
- Growing pains • ADHD • Iron therapy • Dopaminergic medication

KEY POINTS

- Recent epidemiologic studies have shown that restless legs syndrome (RLS) and periodic limb movement disorder (PLMD) are common but underrecognized disorders in children and adolescents.
- There is a significant overlap between RLS and growing pains in children.
- The diagnostic criteria for pediatric RLS have recently been updated to simplify and integrate with newly revised adult RLS criteria.
- In addition to typical RLS symptoms, other clinical features such as the presence of periodic limb movements in sleep (PLMS) and family history of RLS and PLMD are useful to support the diagnosis.
- Both pharmacologic and nonpharmacologic interventions are important in the management of RLS and PLMD in children.
- Children with low iron storage are likely to benefit from iron therapy.
- Although there is limited information on pharmacologic therapy, there is emerging literature showing the effectiveness of dopaminergic medications in the management of RLS and PLMD in children.

INTRODUCTION

RLS was first described in pediatric literature in 1994.[1] Recent epidemiologic studies have shown that RLS is common in children and adolescents with prevalence of 2% to 4%.[2–4] Such figures, if confirmed by additional studies, would indicate that approximately 1 million children are affected by RLS in the United States.

The cause of pediatric RLS and PLMD is not well understood. It remains unclear as to what specific roles are played by genetic factors, dopamine dysfunction, and low iron stores in the pathophysiology of RLS and PLMD. There is significant overlap between RLS and growing pains. The diagnosis of RLS in children can be quite challenging because of their inability to verbalize RLS symptoms. The International Restless Legs Study

[a] Cincinnati Children's Hospital Medical Center, Cincinnati, OH, USA; [b] Department of Neurology, Vanderbilt University, Nashville, TN, USA
* Corresponding author. Division of Pulmonary Medicine, Department of Pediatrics, Cincinnati Children's Hospital Medical Center, 3333 Burnet Avenue, MLC 2021, Cincinnati, OH 45229.
E-mail address: narong.simakajornboon@cchmc.org

Sleep Med Clin 10 (2015) 311–322
http://dx.doi.org/10.1016/j.jsmc.2015.05.014
1556-407X/15/$ – see front matter © 2015 Elsevier Inc. All rights reserved.

Group has recently revised the pediatric RLS diagnostic criteria, which were simplified and integrated with the newly revised adult RLS criteria.[5] Special consideration and supportive clinical features have been developed to guide the application of criteria in children. The management of RLS and PLMD involves both nonpharmacologic and pharmacologic approaches. Children with evidence of low iron storage would benefit from iron therapy. Overall, there is limited experience regarding the use of dopaminergic agents in children with RLS and PLMD; other medications including benzodiazepine, anticonvulsants, as well as α-adrenergic and opioid medications have not been adequately studied in children. This article covers clinical evaluation and management of RLS and PLMD in children and the relationship with growing pains.

EPIDEMIOLOGY

RLS is common in the adult population with an estimated prevalence of 4% to 10%.[6] Approximately 25% to 40% of adult patients with RLS reported early onset of symptoms before the age of 20 years.[7,8] Several studies have evaluated the prevalence of RLS and PLMD in children in various settings. RLS was noted in 17% of children in general pediatric clinics and 5.9% of children referred to sleep clinics.[9,10] PLMD was found in 8.4% of children who were referred to sleep clinics and 7.7% to 11.9% of children from community.[11] A large-scale population study has shown that RLS is common in children and adolescents with an estimated prevalence of 1.9% in school-aged children and 2% in adolescents.[4] Another recent study in high-school students confirmed the prevalence of 2% in adolescents.[2] There is no significant difference in the prevalence of RLS among boys and girls.[4] One study has suggested that PLMD is more common in Caucasian than African American children.[12]

PATHOPHYSIOLOGY

Several causes have been proposed to play a role in the pathophysiology of RLS and PLMD including genetic factors, dopamine dysfunction, and low iron stores. Many studies have shown genetic influences in the pathogenesis of RLS and PLMD. Large population studies have shown a significant association between RLS and PLMD and a common variant in an intron of BTBD9 on chromosome 6p21.1, emphasizing the potential for both genetic predisposition and genetic susceptibility to the occurrence of RLS and PLMD.[13,14] Other genetic variants such as the homeobox gene MEIS1 on

chromosome 2p and the genes encoding MAP2K5 and the transcription factor LBXCOR1 on chromosome 15q have been reported in patients with RLS.[13] Interestingly, one study on childhood-onset RLS showed the association with MEIS1 and LBXCOR1, but not with BTBD9.[15] The role of dopamine dysfunction is discussed elsewhere.

There is emerging evidence of the role of iron in the pathophysiology of RLS and PLMD. Evidence of low iron storages have been found in cerebrospinal fluid, brain sonography, MRI, and autopsy report.[16–19] In children, low iron storage as evidenced by low ferritin and iron deficiency are found in children with RLS.[20,21] Low brain tissue iron concentration may lead to RLS and PLMD through alteration in dopaminergic system.[22]

CLINICAL MANIFESTATION

The clinical presentation of RLS and PLMD in children differs from that of RLS and PLMD in the adult population. Children with RLS and PLMD may present with nonspecific symptoms such as growing pains, restless sleep, sleep disturbances, insomnia, and daytime sleepiness.[23,24] These symptoms may go unnoticed by their parents.[4,23,25] A history of growing pains is noted in 78% to 85% of children and adolescents with RLS.[4] Sleep disturbances including sleep-onset and sleep-maintenance insomnia are common presentations in children with RLS and PLMD.[9,25] Young children may have difficulty describing symptoms of RLS and may describe these sensations with nonspecific but age-appropriate terms. Therefore, physicians and health care providers should be familiar with development-appropriate terms and descriptions. Some examples of description of sensory complaints in children are "oowies"; "boo-boos"; "tickle"; "legs need to stretch"; "ants crawling and aching feeling"; "legs hurt and feel funny"; "fidgety, restless, too much energy"; and "spider in the legs."[4,25] A family history of RLS is common in children with RLS. In fact, a positive family history of RLS and PLMD is helpful as supportive evidence in making a diagnosis of RLS in children and to raise the possibility of developing RLS over time in children who do not meet criteria for RLS.[25]

DIAGNOSIS

The diagnosis of RLS in children is challenging, particularly because young children may not be able to describe typical RLS symptoms or because these symptoms may not manifest at very young ages. The interval between the initial sleep consultation and the diagnosis of definite RLS revolves around 4.4 years.[25] In addition, the time between onset of clinical sleep disturbances and the diagnosis of definite RLS is 11.6 years.[25] RLS is underrecognized and therefore underdiagnosed, even among children whose family members seek medical advice.[4]

The International Restless Legs Syndrome Study Group has developed a set of diagnostic criteria for diagnosing RLS and PLMD in children.[6] The diagnostic criteria for pediatric RLS have recently been updated in 2013.[5] The criteria were simplified and integrated with newly revised adult RLS criteria.[26] As in adult RLS, 5 essential RLS criteria must be met in children (**Box 1**). In addition, several special features should be considered for diagnosis of pediatric RLS (**Box 2**). First, children must be able to describe RLS sensations in their own words. Therefore, adequate language development is essential to diagnose children with RLS. In fact, language and cognitive development determine the applicability of the RLS diagnostic criteria, rather than age. Physicians should be aware of the age-specific vocabulary used to describe RLS symptoms in children and adolescents. Second, it is unknown if the adult specifiers for clinical course apply to pediatric RLS. Third, as in adults, there is a significant impact on sleep,

---

Box 1
IRLSSG diagnostic criteria for RLS/WED

1. An urge to move the legs usually but not always accompanied by or thought to be caused by, uncomfortable and unpleasant sensations in the legs.[a,b]

2. The urge to move the legs and any accompanying unpleasant sensations begin or worsen during the period of rest or inactivity such as while lying down or sitting.

3. The urge to move the legs and any accompanying unpleasant sensations are partially or totally relieved by movement, such as walking or stretching, at least as long as the activity continues.[c]

4. The urge to move the legs and any accompanying unpleasant sensations during rest or inactivity only occur or are worse in the evening or night than during the day.[d]

5. The occurrence of the above-mentioned features is not solely accounted for as symptoms primary to another medical or behavioral condition (eg, myalgia, venous stasis, leg edema, arthritis, leg cramps, positional discomfort, habitual foot tapping).[e]

Specifier for clinical significance of RLS: The symptoms of RLS cause significant distress or impairment in social, occupational, educational, or other important areas of functioning by the impact on sleep, energy/vitality, daily activities, behavior, cognition, or mood.

Specifiers for clinical course of RLS[f]:

1. Chronic persistent RLS: symptoms when not treated would occur on an average at least twice weekly for the past year.

2. Intermittent RLS: symptoms when not treated would occur on an average less than 2 per week for the past year, with at least 5 lifetime events

Abbreviations: IRLSSG, International Restless Legs Syndrome Study Group; WED, Willis-Ekbom disease.
[a] Sometimes the urge to move the legs is present without the uncomfortable sensations, and sometimes the arms or other parts of the body are involved in addition to the legs.
[b] For children, the description of these symptoms should be in the child's own words.
[c] When symptoms are very severe; relief by activity may not be noticeable but must have been previously present.
[d] When symptoms are very severe; the worsening in the evening or night may not be noticeable but must have been previously present.
[e] These conditions, often referred to as RLS/WED mimics have been commonly confused with RLS/WED particularly in surveys because they produce symptoms that meet or at least come very close to meeting criteria 1 to 4 above. The list here gives some examples that have been noted as particularly significant in epidemiologic studies and clinical practice. However, RLS/WED may also occur with any of these conditions, but the RLS/WED symptoms will then be more in degree, conditions of expression, or character than those usually occurring as part of the other condition.
[f] The clinical course criteria neither apply for pediatric cases nor for some special cases of provoked RLS/WED such as pregnancy or drug-induced RLS/WED, where the frequency may be high but limited to the duration of the provocative condition.
From Picchietti DL, Bruni O, de Weerd A, et al. Pediatric restless legs syndrome diagnostic criteria: an update by the international restless legs syndrome study group. Sleep Med 2013;14:1254; and Allen RP, Picchietti DL, Garcia-Borreguero D, et al. Restless legs syndrome/Willis-Ekbom disease diagnostic criteria: updated international restless legs syndrome study group (IRLSSG) consensus criteria–history, rationale, description, and significance. Sleep Med 2014;15:860–73; with permission.

Box 2
Special considerations for the diagnosis of pediatric RLS

1. The child must describe the RLS symptoms in his or her own words.

2. The diagnostician should be aware of the typical words children and adolescents use to describe RLS.

3. Language and cognitive development determine the applicability of the RLS diagnostic criteria, rather than age.

4. It is not known if the adult specifiers for clinical course apply to pediatric RLS.

5. As in adults, a significant impact on sleep, mood, cognition, and function is found. However, impairment is manifest more often in behavioral and educational domains.

6. Simplified and updated research criteria for probable and possible pediatric RLS are available (see **Box 4**).

7. PLMD may precede the diagnosis of RLS in some cases.

From Picchietti DL, Bruni O, de Weerd A, et al. Pediatric restless legs syndrome diagnostic criteria: an update by the international restless legs syndrome study group. Sleep Med 2013;14:1255; with permission.

---

mood, cognition, and function. However, impairment is more evident in behavioral and educational domains in children. Finally, although RLS and PLMD are separate entities in adults, PLMD may precede the diagnosis of RLS in some cases.

Certain clinical features are important in supporting a diagnosis of pediatric RLS (**Box 3**). These features include the presence of more than 5 PLMS (periodic limb movements in sleep) per hour, family history of RLS or PLMD among first-degree relatives, and family history of more than 5 PLMS per hour. Because the diagnostic criteria for RLS in children are still evolving, the probable and possible RLS categories (**Box 4**) are intended for research purposes with the intent to capture the full spectrum of disease.[5,6,27] In fact, a recent retrospective study showed that some children

with RLS had previously met the research criteria for diagnosis of probable or possible RLS.[25] Therefore, probable and possible RLS may be the early manifestations of RLS in children.

The diagnostic criteria for PLMD in children are shown in **Box 5**. The PLMS index of more than 5 per hour is used as a cutoff for pediatric population. Symptoms of sleep disturbance such as sleep-onset and sleep-maintenance insomnia and daytime sleepiness are required for the diagnosis of PLMD in children. In addition, it is important to exclude limb movements associated with concurrent sleep disorders such as sleep-disordered breathing, medical or neurologic disorders, mental disorder, medications, or substance abuse. Although RLS and PLMD in adult population are separate entities, the relationship between RLS and PLMD in children is somewhat complex. The presence of PLMS is part of the supportive evidence for diagnosis of RLS in children. In addition, PLMD may be the early presentation of RLS because many children with definite RLS have been previously diagnosed with PLMD.[25]

Differential Diagnosis

The differential diagnosis for RLS includes other conditions that produce symptoms mimicking those of RLS. Careful consideration of RLS mimics is an essential component of current RLS diagnostic criteria. Therefore, clinicians should be aware of RLS mimics in children. These mimics include conditions associated with leg pain or leg discomfort such as positional discomfort, sore leg muscles, ligament sprain or tendon strain, arthritis, Osgood-Schlatter disease, chondromalacia patella, growing pains, and various types of dermatitis.[5,6,25,28] Positional discomfort or transient

---

Box 3
Clinical features supporting the diagnosis of pediatric RLS

The following features, although not essential for diagnosis, are closely associated with pediatric RLS and should be noted when present

1. PLMS more than 5 per hour

2. Family history of RLS among first-degree relatives

3. Family history of PLMS greater than or equal to 5 per hour

4. Family history of PLMD among first-degree relatives

From Picchietti DL, Bruni O, de Weerd A, et al. Pediatric restless legs syndrome diagnostic criteria: an update by the international restless legs syndrome study group. Sleep Med 2013;14:1256; with permission.

Box 4
Research diagnostic criteria for probable and possible pediatric RLS

Probable RLS

The child meets all 5 essential criteria for RLS, except criterion 4 (occurrence only or worsening in the evening or night).

Possible RLS

The child is observed to have behavior manifestation of lower extremity discomfort when sitting or lying, accompanied by motor movement of the affected limbs. The discomfort is characterized by RLS criteria 2–5 (is worse during rest and inactivity, is relieved by movement, is worse in the evening or night, and is not solely accounted for as primary to another medical or a behavioral condition).

From Picchietti DL, Bruni O, de Weerd A, et al. Pediatric restless legs syndrome diagnostic criteria: an update by the international restless legs syndrome study group. Sleep Med 2013;14:1257; with permission.

---

nerve compression can superficially meet all the criteria for RLS; these conditions are usually caused by pressure that compresses nerves and limits blood flow when lying down on one side, sitting on the legs, or crossing of the leg. The discomfort is relieved by repositioning without requiring continued movement.[27–29] Other conditions such as sore leg muscles, arthritis, ligament or tendon injury, and Osgood-Schlatter disease are usually worse with movements.[27] Less-common mimics in children include nocturnal leg cramp, peripheral neuropathy, radiculopathy, myopathy, fibromyalgia, complex regional pain syndrome, and sickle cell disease.[5,28] In addition, several medical conditions can be associated with RLS (secondary RLS) such as pregnancy, renal failure, and dialysis in children.[30]

PLMS should be differentiated from other conditions such as sleep starts or hypnic jerks, phasic movements during random eye movement (REM) sleep, fragmentary myoclonus, and myoclonic epilepsy.[29] Hypnic jerks typically occur at sleep onset or during transition from awake to sleep. Phasic movements during REM sleep are normal electromyographic (EMG) activity, which are usually associated with bursts of rapid eye movements. Fragmentary myoclonus is an EMG diagnosis, which is characterized by EMG activity that is briefer, variable in duration, and less periodic than PLMS.[29] The movements associated with myoclonic epilepsy are prominent during wakefulness.[27] PLMS can be seen in other sleep disorders such as narcolepsy, REM sleep behavior disorders, and sleep-disordered breathing.

Restless Legs Syndrome and Growing Pains

Growing pains was first described by Duchamp[31] in 1823. The prevalence of growing pains ranges from 2.6% to 49.4%.[32–36] The discrepancy

---

Box 5
Criteria for the diagnosis of pediatric PLMS

1. Polysomnography shows repetitive stereotyped limb movements that

   a. Are 0.5 to 10 seconds in duration

   b. Have a minimum amplitude of 8 μV above resting EMG value

   c. Occur in a sequence of 4 or more movements

   d. Are separated by an interval of more than 5 seconds (from onset of one limb movement to the next) and less than 90 seconds (intermovement intervals often are short and variable in children)

2. The PLMS index exceeds 5 per hour in pediatric cases

3. The PLMS causes clinically significant sleep disturbance or impairment in mental, physical, social, occupational, educational, behavioral, or other important areas of functioning

4. The PLMS are not better explained by another current sleep disorder, medical or neurologic disorder, mental disorder, medication use, or substance use disorder (eg, exclude from PLMS counts the movement at the termination of cyclically occurring apneas)

Abbreviation: EMG, electromyographic.
   From Picchietti DL, Bruni O, de Weerd A, et al. Pediatric restless legs syndrome diagnostic criteria: an update by the international restless legs syndrome study group. Sleep Med 2013;14:1257; with permission.

between prevalence among various studies may be due to different study designs, population samples, or poorly defined diagnostic criteria.[37,38] Growing pains commonly occur in children aged between 4 and 14 years,[39] with the peak prevalence at 4 to 6 years.[38] The mechanism of growing pains is not well understood. Several theories have been proposed including anatomy (postural or orthopedic defects), muscle fatigue, and psychogenic.[32,35,36] Other proposed mechanisms include lower pain threshold, decreased bone strength from overuse, changes in vascular perfusion, and joint hypermobility.[38,40–43] Peterson's[44,45] classic description of growing pains is intermittent, nonarticular pain that usually occurs in the evening and at night. The pain is generally located in both legs and thighs especially in the calf muscles, in front of the thigh and behind the knee.[44,45] The pain is not associated with local tenderness, erythema, or swelling. The results of examination are normal. The results of laboratory and imaging studies are normal.

The proposed combined diagnostic criteria for growing pains are shown in **Box 6**.[46] The criteria are modified from Evans[38] as well as Evans and Scutter[32,47] and Champion and colleagues.[48] The features described in the diagnostic criteria for growing pains are similar to those of RLS with 2 exceptions.[46] One exception is that growing pains are strictly bilateral, whereas RLS can be unilateral or bilateral. The other exception is that description of growing pains is painful, but that of RLS can be painful or nonpainful leg discomfort.[46] There are several similar features between growing pains and RLS. These overlapping features include the age of onset, nighttime predominance, location of symptoms (anterior region of the thigh, calf, and posterior part of the knee), intermittent nature of symptoms, findings on the physical examination and laboratory tests (no abnormalities), and effect on activity and well-being (no limitation of activity or effect on well-being).[46]

Several studies have been conducted to examine the relationship between growing pains and RLS. Some studies showed no relationship between growing pains and RLS,[10,49–51] whereas other studies have shown high prevalence of growing pains in children with RLS.[3,7,25,52] A recent twin family study also suggested the genetic overlap between the 2 disorders.[48] The conflicting findings from various studies are partly due to different criteria for growing pains used by various investigators. Standardized and unified diagnostic criteria for growing pains are needed to accurately define the relationship between growing pains and RLS.[46] A recent working group has been established to formulate a consensus for unified diagnostic criteria among growing pains researchers.

Diagnostic Approach

The diagnostic approach should begin with a thorough and complete clinical history. The

---

Box 6
Combined growing pains criteria

1. Pain in both legs.

2. Pain starts between the ages of 3 and 12 years.

3. Pain typically occurs at the end of the day or during the night. Pain is not a problem in the morning.

4. There is no notable limitation of activity and no limping.

5. The typical distribution of the pain is in the anterior part of the thigh, calf, and posterior part of the knees. The pain is felt in the muscle and not in the joints.

6. The pain is intermittent with some pain-free days and nights. There are periods of days, weeks, or months without leg pains.

7. Physical examination reveals no abnormalities with no evidence of orthopedic disorder, swelling, erythema, tenderness, local trauma, infection, or reduced range of motion.

8. The results of laboratory tests are within reference range with no objective findings, for example, erythrocyte sedimentation rate, radiograph, and bone scan.

9. Pain persists for at least 3 months.

10. There is no associated lack of well-being.

From Walters AS, Gabelia D, Frauscher B. Restless legs syndrome (Willis–Ekbom disease) and growing pains: are they the same thing? A side-by-side comparison of the diagnostic criteria for both and recommendations for future research. Sleep Med 2013;14:1249; with permission.

characteristic RLS symptoms include the urge to move the legs or unpleasant sensations, which are worse at night and at rest, and are partially or totally relieved by movement.[6] It is important to allow young children to give their own descriptions, not just rely on parental report. In some children, it is helpful to provide them with well-directed questions but avoid introduction of bias. The history of growing pains is common and can be used as a lead-in question for a more specific description of RLS.[4] Physicians and pediatricians should be aware of the age-specific vocabulary and try to use the languages that children understand.[28] Young children may not understand the word urge, and they may describe their symptoms with a variety of terms such as "oowies," "boo-boos," "tickle," "leg pain," "leg hurt", or "funny feeling in the leg."[28] Some children may be able to better describe their feelings by drawing, which may encourage them to talk more about their RLS symptoms.[28] It is important to ask for the typical topographic distribution of RLS symptoms in taking the history. Although true RLS can exist in almost any part of the body, the typical distribution is in the thighs and calves. The Pediatric Restless Legs Syndrome Severity Scale has recently been developed to grade the severity of RLS in children.[53] On physical examination, certain conditions such as ligament/tendon injury, orthopedic conditions, or dermatitis can be excluded. A complete neurologic examination is essential to rule out other causes of leg discomfort, such as neuropathy. For RLS, most children have normal results of examination.

Diagnosis of PLMD requires an overnight polysomnographic study to document PLMS and to exclude other coexisting sleep-disordered breathing. A previous study has shown that parental report of excessive leg movements or restless sleep is not a good predictor of PLMS in children.[54] A sleep study documenting PLMS is useful in children suspected of RLS as supportive evidence when classic RLS symptoms are absent. The presence of periodic limb movements during wakefulness (PLMW) has been shown to be a sensitive and specific tool in evaluating and grading the severity of RLS in adult patients,[55,56] but there is a lack of data on the diagnostic value of PLMW in children. Physicians should be aware of random night-to-night variability of PLMS in children.[57] Therefore, children with negative results of sleep study who have clinical features highly suspicious of RLS and PLMD may warrant a repeated sleep study. The role of other diagnostic tools such as actigraphy is limited. Although several studies have demonstrated that actigraphy is a sensitive and specific measure of PLMS in adult population,[58–60] it is insufficient in making an accurate assessment of PLMS in children.[61] Because most children with RLS and PLMD have evidence of low iron stores, it is important to obtain iron profiles including complete blood cell count, serum iron levels, and serum ferritin levels. Any child with suspected neuropathy should have additional tests including thyroid function, fasting blood sugar and insulin, and serum levels of vitamins B_6, B_9, and B_{12}.[62]

CONSEQUENCES

Recent studies have shown that RLS and PLMD can lead to both cardiovascular and neurocognitive consequences in both adults and children. The relationship between RLS and PLMD and hypertension is controversial. There are limited data on the cardiovascular consequence in children with RLS and PLMD. One study showed that the onset of leg movements of PLMS was associated with a rapidly occurring cardiac acceleration in children, suggesting evidence of vagal inhibition.[63] A recent study demonstrated the association between PLMS in children and nocturnal hypertension and higher blood pressure during the day.[64] The mechanism underlying blood pressure changes may be related to autonomic activation in the context of repeated arousals.[65] Dopamine dysfunction may also play a role in pathogenesis of hypertension in RLS and PLMD.[66,67]

Several studies have shown the association between RLS in children and neurocognitive deficits. In a population study, children reported several adverse cognitive consequences of RLS such as difficulty sitting in the late afternoon or evening, a negative effect on mood, a lack of energy, and an inability to concentrate.[4] Adolescents with RLS have been shown to have poor school performance.[68] Children with RLS are also at risk for depression and anxiety disorder.[4,25] It has been speculated that sleep disruption in children with RLS may lead to neurocognitive deficits and affective disorders.

The relationship between attention-deficit/hyperactivity disorder (ADHD) and RLS and PLMD is somewhat complex and can be explained by several possibilities.[69] First, sleep disruption associated with RLS and PLMD may lead to inattentiveness and hyperactivity. Second, RLS and PLMD may be comorbidities of ADHD. Third, RLS and PLMD and subset of ADHD may share common dopamine dysfunction.[70–73] In fact, improvement and even resolution of ADHD symptoms was noted after dopaminergic therapy in children with ADHD and RLS.[74,75] Fourth, diurnal manifestations of RLS and PLMD may mimic

ADHD.[69] Finally, iron deficiency may be a shared pathophysiologic finding in children with RLS, PLMD, and ADHD.[76] Iron deficiency has been shown to contribute to the severity of ADHD symptoms in children with coexisting ADHD and RLS.[76]

Another comorbidity of RLS and PLMD is common parasomnias, such as confusional arousals, night terrors, sleepwalking, and nightmares. Several studies have shown that there is an increased frequency of parasomnias in children with RLS and PLMD.[23,77] The coexistence of RLS and PLMD and parasomnias and the resolution of parasomnias after treatment of RLS and PLMD suggest that sleep disruption associated with RLS and PLMD may trigger or facilitate the appearance of parasomnias.[78]

MANAGEMENT
Nonpharmacologic

Many factors including medications, sleep deprivation, nicotine, and alcohol have been shown to precipitate or aggravate RLS and PLMD.[27,62] Therefore, it is essential to identify and examine ways of avoiding these factors. Several medications, such as selective serotonin reuptake inhibitors, metoclopramide, diphenhydramine, and dopamine antagonists have been shown to aggravate RLS and PLMD.[27,62] Parents should be advised to avoid caffeine in their children. Adolescent patients should avoid smoking and drinking alcohol. Regular sleep routine and good sleep hygiene are essential for the management of RLS in children.[27,62] Regular exercise is beneficial and has been shown to improve RLS symptoms.[79,80] Light exercise is recommended and can be used as an adjunctive therapy in children.

Pharmacologic

At present, there is no medication approved by the US Food and Drug Administration (FDA) for RLS and PLMD in children. Although there is emerging literature supporting medical therapy in children with RLS and PLMD, the experience on the use of these medications in children is still limited. The guideline from the Standard of Practice Committee of the American Academy of Sleep Medicine states that no specific recommendations can be made regarding the use of dopaminergic medication in children with RLS or PLMD.[81] A recent population survey has shown that only 6.2% of children and 6.4% of adolescents with definite RLS received ongoing prescription medications. Furthermore, only 1.5% of patients received appropriate and specific medications for RLS treatment.[4]

Iron Treatment

Iron deficiency and low iron stores play important roles in the pathophysiology or RLS and PLMD. Several studies have shown the benefit of iron therapy in reducing RLS symptoms.[20,21,82,83] Other studies have suggested the benefit of raising serum ferritin levels above 50 ng/mL.[20,21] The dose of iron therapy is 3 mg of elemental iron/kg/d corresponding to the dose used for iron deficiency anemia. Some children may benefit from vitamin C to improve iron absorption. The most common side effect is constipation. Other side effects are dark stool, nausea, and epigastric pain. Iron treatment should be avoided in children with hemolytic anemia and hemochromatosis. The duration of treatment used in the authors' previous study was 3 months followed by slow tapering for 1 year.[20] The preliminary long-term follow-up of these children treated with iron therapy showed sustained clinical improvements 1 to 2 years after iron therapy, with serum iron and ferritin levels remaining adequate.[84,85] Iron therapy seems to lead to long-lasting improvement in clinical symptoms and should be considered as the initial option, when serum ferritin levels are less than 50 μg/L. It is important to periodically check serum iron and ferritin levels after iron treatment and adjust the iron dose accordingly.

Medications

There is increasing literature on the use of dopaminergic mediations in children. Although ropinirole and pramipexole are FDA-approved medications in adults with RLS and PLMD, there is no approved medication in children. Published case reports show the effectiveness of levodopa,[75] ropinirole,[74] pramipexole,[78] and pergolide[75] in young children and adolescents. The use of dopaminergic medication was associated with clinical improvement of RLS symptoms and reduction of PLMS index and associated arousals.[75,78] L-Dopa and dopamine agonists resulted in long-term improvements in children with RLS and PLMD.[25,75,86] In children with RLS and ADHD, improvement and even resolution of ADHD symptoms was noted after dopaminergic therapy.[74,75] In addition, resolution of parasomnia was reported in children with RLS and parasomnia following treatment with dopaminergic medications.[78] One study has shown that clinical efficacy of ropinirole in patients with RLS is not affected by the age of onset, suggesting that the early- and late-onset phenotypes of RLS share a common responsiveness to dopamine agonists.[87] Side effects of dopaminergic medications include nasal congestion, nausea, vomiting, insomnia, daytime sleepiness, fluid retention, hallucination, obsessive compulsive behavior, and augmentation. Because the development of augmentation is dependent on the duration of treatment with dopaminergic medication, there is a particular concern in children who are likely to be treated for long term.

Other medications including benzodiazepines, anticonvulsants, as well as α-adrenergic and opioid medications have not been adequately studied in children. Clonidine is commonly used for children with sleep-onset problems and can be effective in children with RLS and PLMD.[88] Clonazepam is commonly used for the treatment of RLS and PLMD in children. However, it may aggravate hyperactivity in children with ADHD.[27] Gabapentin has been shown to reduce RLS symptoms and improve sleep quality.[89,90]

It is important for children with RLS and PLMD to have regular follow-up visits to monitor clinical symptoms and side effects and to adjust the dose of medication as needed. A wide range of optimal doses for dopaminergic medications has been reported.[27] Children receiving iron therapy should be periodically reassessed for their serum iron and ferritin levels, and the dose of iron supplement should be gradually adjusted to achieve the desired normalization of serum ferritin and iron levels. Repeated sleep study may be needed in children with PLMD who do not respond to iron before starting other medications. As genetic factors play an important role in RLS and PLMD, parents may be affected and should be referred for further evaluation and treatment.

PROGNOSIS

At present, there is limited information on the long-term outcomes associated with RLS and PLMD in children. In adults with early-onset RLS, there is a slow progression of the disease along with long periods of stability. A small percentage of patients can have a period of remission.[7,24,91] In children, the same pattern of slow progression has been reported.[25]

REFERENCES

1. Walters AS, Picchietti DL, Ehrenberg BL, et al. Restless legs syndrome in childhood and adolescence. Pediatr Neurol 1994;11:241–5.
2. Yilmaz K, Kilincaslan A, Aydin N, et al. Prevalence and correlates of restless legs syndrome in adolescents. Dev Med Child Neurol 2011;53:40–7.
3. Turkdogan D, Bekiroglu N, Zaimoglu S. A prevalence study of restless legs syndrome in Turkish children and adolescents. Sleep Med 2011; 12:315–21.
4. Picchietti D, Allen RP, Walters AS, et al. Restless legs syndrome: prevalence and impact in children and adolescents–the Peds REST study. Pediatrics 2007;120:253–66.
5. Picchietti DL, Bruni O, de Weerd A, et al. Pediatric restless legs syndrome diagnostic criteria: an update by the international restless legs syndrome study group. Sleep Med 2013;14:1253–9.
6. Allen RP, Picchietti D, Hening WA, et al. Restless legs syndrome: diagnostic criteria, special considerations, and epidemiology. A report from the restless legs syndrome diagnosis and epidemiology workshop at the national institutes of health. Sleep Med 2003;4:101–19.
7. Bassetti CL, Mauerhofer D, Gugger M, et al. Restless legs syndrome: a clinical study of 55 patients. Eur Neurol 2001;45:67–74.
8. Montplaisir J, Boucher S, Poirier G, et al. Clinical, polysomnographic, and genetic characteristics of restless legs syndrome: a study of 133 patients diagnosed with new standard criteria. Mov Disord 1997;12:61–5.
9. Kotagal S, Silber MH. Childhood-onset restless legs syndrome. Ann Neurol 2004;56:803–7.
10. Chervin RD, Archbold KH, Dillon JE, et al. Associations between symptoms of inattention, hyperactivity, restless legs, and periodic leg movements. Sleep 2002;25:213–8.
11. Crabtree VM, Ivanenko A, O'Brien LM, et al. Periodic limb movement disorder of sleep in children. J Sleep Res 2003;12:73–81.
12. O'Brien LM, Holbrook CR, Faye Jones V, et al. Ethnic difference in periodic limb movements in children. Sleep Med 2007;8:240–6.
13. Winkelmann J, Schormair B, Lichtner P, et al. Genome-wide association study of restless legs syndrome identifies common variants in three genomic regions. Nat Genet 2007;39:1000–6.
14. Stefansson H, Rye DB, Hicks A, et al. A genetic risk factor for periodic limb movements in sleep. N Engl J Med 2007;357:639–47.
15. Muhle H, Neumann A, Lohmann-Hedrich K, et al. Childhood-onset restless legs syndrome: clinical and genetic features of 22 families. Mov Disord 2008;23:1113–21 [quiz: 1203].
16. Godau J, Wevers AK, Gaenslen A, et al. Sonographic abnormalities of brainstem structures in restless legs syndrome. Sleep Med 2008;9:782–9.
17. Godau J, Klose U, Di Santo A, et al. Multiregional brain iron deficiency in restless legs syndrome. Mov Disord 2008;23:1184–7.
18. Earley CJ, Connor JR, Beard JL, et al. Ferritin levels in the cerebrospinal fluid and restless legs syndrome: effects of different clinical phenotypes. Sleep 2005;28:1069–75.
19. Allen RP, Barker PB, Wehrl F, et al. MRI measurement of brain iron in patients with restless legs syndrome. Neurology 2001;56:263–5.

20. Simakajornboon N, Gozal D, Vlasic V, et al. Periodic limb movements in sleep and iron status in children. Sleep 2003;26:735–8.

21. Kryger MH, Otake K, Foerster J. Low body stores of iron and restless legs syndrome: a correctable cause of insomnia in adolescents and teenagers. Sleep Med 2002;3:127–32.

22. Earley CJ, Connor JR, Beard JL, et al. Abnormalities in CSF concentrations of ferritin and transferrin in restless legs syndrome. Neurology 2000;54:1698–700.

23. Picchietti DL, Walters AS. Moderate to severe periodic limb movement disorder in childhood and adolescence. Sleep 1999;22:297–300.

24. Walters AS, Hickey K, Maltzman J, et al. A questionnaire study of 138 patients with restless legs syndrome: the 'Night-Walkers' survey. Neurology 1996;46:92–5.

25. Picchietti DL, Stevens HE. Early manifestations of restless legs syndrome in childhood and adolescence. Sleep Med 2008;9:770–81.

26. Allen RP, Picchietti DL, Garcia-Borreguero D, et al. Restless legs syndrome/Willis-Ekbom disease diagnostic criteria: updated international restless legs syndrome study group (IRLSSG) consensus criteria–history, rationale, description, and significance. Sleep Med 2014;15:860–73.

27. Picchietti MA, Picchietti DL. Restless legs syndrome and periodic limb movement disorder in children and adolescents. Semin Pediatr Neurol 2008;15: 91–9.

28. Picchietti MA, Picchietti DL. Advances in pediatric restless legs syndrome: Iron, genetics, diagnosis and treatment. Sleep Med 2010;11:643–51.

29. American Academy of Sleep Medicine. Restless leg syndrome and periodic limb movement disorder. In: American Academy of Sleep Medicine, editor. The international classification of sleep disorders: diagnostic and coding manual. Westchester (IL): American Academy of Sleep Medicine; 2005. p. 178–86.

30. Davis ID, Baron J, O'Riordan MA, et al. Sleep disturbances in pediatric dialysis patients. Pediatr Nephrol 2005;20:69–75.

31. Duchamp R-G. Maladies de la croissance. Paris: Fain; 1823.

32. Evans AM, Scutter SD. Prevalence of "growing pains" in young children. J Pediatr 2004;145:255–8.

33. Abu-Arafeh I, Russell G. Recurrent limb pain in schoolchildren. Arch Dis Child 1996;74:336–9.

34. Williams MF. Rheumatic conditions in schoolchildren: an investigation into growing pains and nodules (GRAINS). Lancet 1928;211:720–1.

35. Naish JM, Apley J. 'Growing pains': a clinical study of non-arthritic limb pains in children. Arch Dis Child 1951;26:134.

36. Oberklaid F, Amos D, Liu C, et al. "Growing pains": clinical and behavioral correlates in a community sample. J Dev Behav Pediatr 1997;18:102–6.

37. Alcantara J, Davis J. The chiropractic care of children with "growing pains": a case series and systematic review of the literature. Complement Ther Clin Pract 2011;17:28–32.

38. Evans AM. Growing pains: contemporary knowledge and recommended practice. J Foot Ankle Res 2008;1:4.

39. Simon MW. Growing pains in children solved and resolved. Clin Pediatr 2015;54(7):706.

40. Hashkes PJ, Friedland O, Jaber L, et al. Decreased pain threshold in children with growing pains. J Rheumatol 2004;31:610–3.

41. Friedland O, Hashkes PJ, Jaber L, et al. Decreased bone speed of sound in children with growing pains measured by quantitative ultrasound. J Rheumatol 2005;32:1354–7.

42. Aromaa M, Sillanpaa M, Rautava P, et al. Pain experience of children with headache and their families: a controlled study. Pediatrics 2000;106:270–5.

43. Gedalia A, Press J, Klein M, et al. Joint hypermobility and fibromyalgia in schoolchildren. Ann Rheum Dis 1993;52:494–6.

44. Peterson H. Growing pains. Pediatr Clin North Am 1986;33:1365–72.

45. Peterson H. Leg aches. Pediatr Clin North Am 1977; 24:731–6.

46. Walters AS, Gabelia D, Frauscher B. Restless legs syndrome (Willis–Ekbom disease) and growing pains: are they the same thing? A side-by-side comparison of the diagnostic criteria for both and recommendations for future research. Sleep Med 2013;14: 1247–52.

47. Evans AM, Scutter SD. Development of a questionnaire for parental rating of leg pain in young children: internal validity and reliability testing following triangulation. Foot 2004;14:42–8.

48. Champion D, Pathirana S, Flynn C, et al. Growing pains: twin family study evidence for genetic susceptibility and a genetic relationship with restless legs syndrome. Eur J Pain 2012;16:1224–31.

49. Gamaldo CE, Benbrook AR, Allen RP, et al. Childhood and adult factors associated with restless legs syndrome (RLS) diagnosis. Sleep Med 2007;8:716–22.

50. Rajaram S-S, Walters AS, England SJ, et al. Some children with growing pains may actually have restless legs syndrome. Sleep 2004;27:767–73.

51. EKBOM KA. Growing pains and restless legs. Acta Paediatr 1975;64:264–6.

52. Balendran J, Champion D, Jaaniste T, et al. A common sleep disorder in pregnancy: restless legs syndrome and its predictors. Aust N Z J Obstet Gynaecol 2011;51:262–4.

53. Arbuckle R, Abetz L, Durmer JS, et al. Development of the Pediatric Restless Legs Syndrome Severity Scale (P-RLS-SS): a patient-reported outcome measure of pediatric RLS symptoms and impact. Sleep Med 2010;11:897–906.

54. Martin BT, Williamson BD, Edwards N, et al. Parental symptom report and periodic limb movements of sleep in children. J Clin Sleep Med 2008;4:57–61.

55. Allen RP, Dean T, Earley CJ. Effects of rest-duration, time-of-day and their interaction on periodic leg movements while awake in restless legs syndrome. Sleep Med 2005;6:429–34.

56. Michaud M, Paquet J, Lavigne G, et al. Sleep laboratory diagnosis of restless legs syndrome. Eur Neurol 2002;48:108–13.

57. Picchietti MA, Picchietti DL, England SJ, et al. Children show individual night-to-night variability of periodic limb movements in sleep. Sleep 2009;32: 530–5.

58. King MA, Jaffre MO, Morrish E, et al. The validation of a new actigraphy system for the measurement of periodic leg movements in sleep. Sleep Med 2005; 6:507–13.

59. Morrish E, King MA, Pilsworth SN, et al. Periodic limb movement in a community population detected by a new actigraphy technique. Sleep Med 2002;3:489–95.

60. Kazenwadel J, Pollmacher T, Trenkwalder C, et al. New actigraphic assessment method for periodic leg movements (PLM). Sleep 1995;18:689–97.

61. Montgomery-Downs HE, Crabtree VM, Gozal D. Actigraphic recordings in quantification of periodic leg movements during sleep in children. Sleep Med 2005;6:325–32.

62. Gamaldo CE, Earley CJ. Restless legs syndrome: a clinical update. Chest 2006;130:1596–604.

63. Walter LM, Foster AM, Patterson RR, et al. Cardiovascular variability during periodic leg movements in sleep in children. Sleep 2009;32:1093–9.

64. Wing YK, Zhang J, Ho CK, et al. Periodic limb movement during sleep is associated with nocturnal hypertension in children. Sleep 2010;33:759–65.

65. Siddiqui F, Strus J, Ming X, et al. Rise of blood pressure with periodic limb movements in sleep and wakefulness. Clin Neurophysiol 2007;118:1923–30.

66. Walters AS, Rye DB. Review of the relationship of restless legs syndrome and periodic limb movements in sleep to hypertension, heart disease, and stroke. Sleep 2009;32:589.

67. Hussain T, Lokhandwala MF. Renal dopamine receptors and hypertension. Exp Biol Med (Maywood) 2003;228:134–42.

68. Pagel JF, Forister N, Kwiatkowki C. Adolescent sleep disturbance and school performance: the confounding variable of socioeconomics. J Clin Sleep Med 2007;3:19–23.

69. Cortese S, Konofal E, Lecendreux M, et al. Restless legs syndrome and attention-deficit/hyperactivity disorder: a review of the literature. Sleep 2005;28: 1007–13.

70. Oner P, Oner O. Relationship of ferritin to symptom ratings children with attention deficit hyperactivity disorder: effect of comorbidity. Child Psychiatry Hum Dev 2008;39:323–30.

71. Cortese S, Lecendreux M, Bernardina BD, et al. Attention-deficit/hyperactivity disorder, Tourette's syndrome, and restless legs syndrome: the iron hypothesis. Med Hypotheses 2008;70:1128–32.

72. Konofal E, Lecendreux M, Arnulf I, et al. Iron deficiency in children with attention-deficit/hyperactivity disorder. Arch Pediatr Adolesc Med 2004;158: 1113–5.

73. Sever Y, Ashkenazi A, Tyano S, et al. Iron treatment in children with attention deficit hyperactivity disorder. A preliminary report. Neuropsychobiology 1997;35:178–80.

74. Konofal E, Arnulf I, Lecendreux M, et al. Ropinirole in a child with attention-deficit hyperactivity disorder and restless legs syndrome. Pediatr Neurol 2005; 32:350–1.

75. Walters AS, Mandelbaum DE, Lewin DS, et al. Dopaminergic therapy in children with restless legs/periodic limb movements in sleep and ADHD. Dopaminergic therapy study group. Pediatr Neurol 2000;22:182–6.

76. Konofal E, Cortese S, Marchand M, et al. Impact of restless legs syndrome and iron deficiency on attention-deficit/hyperactivity disorder in children. Sleep Med 2007;8:711–5.

77. Picchietti DL, England SJ, Walters AS, et al. Periodic limb movement disorder and restless legs syndrome in children with attention-deficit hyperactivity disorder. J Child Neurol 1998;13:588–94.

78. Guilleminault C, Palombini L, Pelayo R, et al. Sleepwalking and sleep terrors in prepubertal children: what triggers them? Pediatrics 2003;111:e17–25.

79. Mortazavi M, Vahdatpour B, Ghasempour A, et al. Aerobic exercise improves signs of restless leg syndrome in end stage renal disease patients suffering chronic hemodialysis. ScientificWorldJournal 2013; 2013:628142.

80. Aukerman MM, Aukerman D, Bayard M, et al. Exercise and restless legs syndrome: a randomized controlled trial. J Am Board Fam Med 2006;19:487–93.

81. Littner MR, Kushida C, Anderson WM, et al. Practice parameters for the dopaminergic treatment of restless legs syndrome and periodic limb movement disorder. Sleep 2004;27:557–9.

82. Starn AL, Udall JN Jr. Iron deficiency anemia, pica, and restless legs syndrome in a teenage girl. Clin Pediatr 2008;47:83–5.

83. Mohri I, Kato-Nishimura K, Tachibana N, et al. Restless legs syndrome (RLS): an unrecognized cause for bedtime problems and insomnia in children. Sleep Med 2008;9:701–2.

84. Simakajornboon N, Kheirandish-Gozal L, Sharon D, et al. A long-term follow-up study of periodic limb movement disorders in children after iron therapy. Sleep 2006;29:A76–7.

85. Dye TJ, Simakajornboon N. Long term treatment outcomes of iron supplementation in Pediatric RLS and PLMD. Sleep 2014. The 28th Annual Meeting of the Associated Professional Sleep Societies, LLC; 2014; Minneapolis, MN: American Academy Sleep Medicine One Westbrook Corporate Center ste 920. Westchester, IL 60154 USA.

86. Martinez S, Guilleminault C. Periodic leg movements in prepubertal children with sleep disturbance. Dev Med Child Neurol 2004;46:765–70.

87. Allen RP, Ritchie SY. Clinical efficacy of ropinirole for restless legs syndrome is not affected by age at symptom onset. Sleep Med 2008;9:899–902.

88. Newcorn JH, Schulz K, Harrison M, et al. Alpha 2 adrenergic agonists. Neurochemistry, efficacy, and clinical guidelines for use in children. Pediatr Clin North Am 1998;45:1099–122, viii.

89. Happe S, Sauter C, Klosch G, et al. Gabapentin versus ropinirole in the treatment of idiopathic restless legs syndrome. Neuropsychobiology 2003;48: 82–6.

90. Garcia-Borreguero D, Larrosa O, de la Llave Y, et al. Treatment of restless legs syndrome with gabapentin: a double-blind, cross-over study. Neurology 2002;59:1573–9.

91. Winkelmann J, Wetter TC, Collado-Seidel V, et al. Clinical characteristics and frequency of the hereditary restless legs syndrome in a population of 300 patients. Sleep 2000;23:597–602.

Restless Legs Syndrome/ Willis-Ekbom Disease and Pregnancy

Chiara Prosperetti, MD, Mauro Manconi, MD, PhD*

KEYWORDS

- Restless legs syndrome • Willis-Ekbom disease • Pregnancy • Sleep

KEY POINTS

- Restless legs syndrome (RLS)/Willis-Ekbom disease is around 3-fold more prevalent in pregnant than in non-pregnant women.
- Symptoms are particularly strong and frequent during the third trimester of pregnancy and disappear around delivery.
- A pre-existing form of RLS tends to worsen during pregnancy. Women who experience RLS during pregnancy have a higher risk of symptoms in further pregnancies and of developing a primary form of RLS later in life, than women free of symptoms during pregnancy.
- Possible causes behind this association are still unknown, but hormonal, metabolic (complex B vitamins and iron), and motor behavioral changes have been mentioned as possible pathogenetic hypotheses, whereas a genetic predisposition might explain the individual vulnerability of women.
- This article discusses the pregnancy-related RLS, with particular attention to its epidemiology, course, possible mechanisms, management and the impact of symptoms.

INTRODUCTION

In 1940 Mussio-Fournier and Rawak[1] described the clinical features of a family in which a few members were affected by "pruritus, urticaria and paresthesias" in the lower limbs; the syndrome resembled what Karl Axel Ekbom[2] 5 years later named as restless legs syndrome (RLS). One woman belonging to that family reported that symptoms worsened during pregnancy. A few years later, Ekbom[2] observed that this disturbance was more prevalent in women compared with men and was particularly frequent during pregnancy. Since then, the association between RLS and pregnancy has been further confirmed by several other epidemiological studies.[3–5] RLS is around 3-fold more prevalent during pregnancy than in the general non-pregnant population, affecting about 15% to 25% of gestations in Western countries. Most pregnant women develop symptoms in late pregnancy, with a recovery around delivery.[5] This article reviews the epidemiology, underlying mechanisms, impact, and management of pregnancy-related RLS.

PREVALENCE

Karl Axel Ekbom[2] performed the first structured epidemiological study on the prevalence of RLS during pregnancy, finding a rate of 11.3% among 486 pregnant women. Since then, several investigations have been conducted on this topic and all of them confirmed the high prevalence of RLS during pregnancy. However, the rate of prevalence among the studies ranges between 11% and 29%, with a variability that probably depended on the different methodologies used. The main source of variability of the studies published before 1995

Sleep Center, Neurocenter of Southern Switzerland, Civic Hospital of Lugano, Via Tesserete 46, 6900 Lugano, Switzerland
* Corresponding author.
E-mail address: mauro.manconi@eoc.ch

Sleep Med Clin 10 (2015) 323–329
http://dx.doi.org/10.1016/j.jsmc.2015.05.016
1556-407X/15/$ – see front matter © 2015 Elsevier Inc. All rights reserved.

was probably the absence of standard diagnostic criteria for RLS. A second source of variability is the type of assessment of the diagnostic criteria. Although the use of self-administered questionnaires or telephone interviews enlarged the studies populations, it reduced the specificity of the results; the method of face-to-face interview guaranteed a higher certainty of diagnosis but investigated smaller populations. Manconi and colleagues[4] used the standard diagnostic criteria to ascertain RLS by a face-to-face interview in a population of 606 pregnant women living in the middle-east of Italy. Twenty-six percent of women interviewed within a few days after delivery reported having experienced RLS symptoms in their pregnancies, with a clear peak of prevalence during the third trimester. In the same cohort, around 9% to 10% of women had already experienced RLS symptoms before pregnancy, whereas in the remaining 16% of them the symptoms appeared for the first time during pregnancy. Most women reported a recovery of RLS around the time of delivery. Another source of prevalence variability is represented by the ethnicity or geography explored and by the type of protocol; cross-sectional investigations usually reported a lower prevalence compared with studies that assessed the whole cumulative rate during pregnancy. In 2004 a German population study[6] confirmed that RLS is more prevalent in women than in men, and, according to age, is more prevalent in multiparous women than in nulliparous women. The prevalence of the disease in nulliparous women up to 64 years of age did not differ from the prevalence in men of the same age. This observation suggested that pregnancy and child bearing might be the main promoting factors for the female predominance of RLS in the general population. These results were confirmed by a second German cross-sectional primary care study, analyzing the association between the offspring and RLS in 9.278 women. The reported prevalence increased proportionally according to the number of children up to 3 and then reached a plateau.[7] So far, only few prospective cohort studies have been performed. In a cohort of 501 pregnant Swiss women, Hubner and colleagues[5] found that 58 (12%) were affected by RLS according to the International RLS Study Group criteria. The incidence of the symptoms was greater during the third trimester, whereas the severity of the symptoms according to the International RLS Rating Scale was worse during the second trimester. No differences were found in age, ethnicity, pregnancy duration, education, and weight; however, a role was played by family and previous pregnancy history. Symptoms did not increase in the course of

pregnancy and tended to ameliorate in the weeks before delivery.

PATHOGENESIS

The reason why pregnancy causes or worsens RLS is still unknown. So far, a few hypotheses have been generated but are being supported by extensive evidence.

The Hormonal Hypothesis

Data regarding the prevalence of RLS in non-pregnant and in pregnant women strongly suggest a role of hormonal exposure in the mechanism of the disease. The hormone that plays the principal role within the endocrinologic storm of pregnancy is still unknown. Both progesterone and estrogens act as neurosteroids and exert a complex, poorly understood modulation at the central nervous system. An epilepsy study showed a proconvulsive action of estrogens and a protective role of progesterone against seizures.[8] For RLS outside of pregnancy, it has been observed that women using estrogen-based therapies are more prone to develop the disease than non–estrogen users.[9] Another interesting observation comes from the study of Dzaja and colleagues,[10] which compared levels of estrogens, progesterone, prolactin, testosterone, follicle-stimulating hormone, luteinizing hormone, iron, ferritin, magnesium, and hemoglobin in pregnant women who did and did not develop pregnancy-related RLS and in a control group. Although all these parameters, as expected, were significantly higher during pregnancy compared to the control nonpregnant group, women developing RLS showed increased estradiol levels compared with the pregnant non-RLS group, whereas other hormonal parameters did not differ between these two groups.[10] The estrogenic theory also might correlate with the high incidence of symptoms during the third trimester, when the plasmatic levels are the highest. However, prolactin and progesterone levels also reached their highest values in the same period of pregnancy, and levels of all of these hormones dramatically decreased around delivery, except for prolactin, which follows a pulsatile trend of secretion during the breastfeeding period.

The Metabolic Hypothesis

Iron and folate requirements are much higher during pregnancy than in the non-pregnant state. Because of either fetal needs or hemodilution, the hematological levels of both decrease across pregnancy. Together with the protective effect of folate in preventing neurotube malformations, this explains why gynecologists commonly suggest oral supplementation of iron and folate during pregnancy. The role of iron in non-pregnant RLS is well known. A single study suggested that folate supplementation before pregnancy might help in reducing the incidence of pregnancy-related RLS.[11] Lee and colleagues,[12] in a small cohort of pregnant women, showed that iron and folate levels, although within the normal range, were lower in those presenting RLS than in pregnant women without RLS. The results from a recent Czech study that investigated 300 women at their third trimester of pregnancy are similar. By using a self-administered questionnaire, exploring the presence of the standard criteria, there were significantly lower hemoglobin levels and less hypochromic anemia in the RLS group[13] compared with the non-RLS group. Previous studies[3,4] did not find significant differences in iron, ferritin, and folate serum levels in pregnancy-related RLS compared with healthy pregnant women. Cerebrospinal fluid values of iron and folate have never been measured during pregnancy and this might be an interesting research topic to consider for the future.

Psychomotor Behavioral Hypothesis

Insomnia, fatigue, and stress often affect women during the last trimester of pregnancy. It has been postulated that these factors might be contributors for the development of RLS in late pregnancy.[3] Although interesting, this hypothesis is not yet supported by evidence. Phillips and colleagues[14] studied the motor habits during late pregnancy in women with and without RLS. There was no voluntary or enforced reduction of activity and stress during the last days of pregnancy, which would be expected based on the amelioration of the symptoms in the last days before delivery.

PREGNANCY-RELATED RISK FACTORS FOR RESTLESS LEGS SYNDROME

Pregnancy is one of the main risk factors for RLS; even stronger in multiparous than in primiparous women. Those women who had experienced RLS during pregnancy are more likely to develop an idiopathic RLS form later in life, with a 3-fold to 4-fold increase compared with women who did not experienced RLS during pregnancy. Moreover, women with pregnancy-related RLS have a much higher risk of reappearance of RLS symptoms in a new pregnancy.[15] The major incriminated (but still not confirmed) risk factors for pregnancy-related RLS are represented by low iron and folate levels during pregnancy.[16] A study conducted in Pakistan interviewed women at the hospital admission for delivery and showed using a multivariate analysis that family history of RLS, history of RLS in prior pregnancies, and history of RLS even when nonpregnant, associated or not with hemoglobin values of 11 g/dL or less, were independent predictors of RLS during pregnancy. Subgroup analysis revealed that family history of RLS and anemia were associated with de novo RLS, whereas family history of RLS and multiparity were predictors of preexisting RLS.[17] A reliable risk factor for RLS during pregnancy was represented by an episode of RLS in a previous pregnancy. Another risk factor for pregnancy-related RLS has been identified in sleep respiratory disturbances. A Swedish study showed that snoring in the first trimester was correlated with increased prevalence of RLS in all 3 trimesters.[18] Sleep apnea, which is highly prevalent in late pregnancy, is also known to exacerbate and trigger RLS.[19] Fetal growth and consequent stretch/compression of the nerve roots have been suggested as a potential contributing factor for RLS during pregnancy. In addition, water retention in the legs was postulated to be a trigger for the symptoms. However, neither of the two previously mentioned hypotheses was supported.[5] Mother weight of more than 79 kg showed a significant association with appearance of the disturbance in an Italian cohort.[4] Prepregnancy depression has been linked to RLS development during pregnancy and patients with RLS have been more prone to develop postpartum depression.[20] The idea that pregnancy acts by unidentified factors in women already genetically predisposed to RLS is suggestive and is supported by the positive family history of RLS in these women; however, the allelic variants linked to primary RLS have never been tested in pregnancy-related RLS.

IMPACT AND OUTCOMES

Prospective studies showed that, within the first month after delivery, RLS symptoms tend to disappear (prevalence of 6.8% at 1 month and 5%–6% at 6 months).[4] However, most of the implications of pregnancy-related RLS are the consequences of chronic sleep loss during gestation. A recent meta-analysis regarding the effects of sleep loss during pregnancy showed evidence linking it with perinatal depression, gestational diabetes, hypertension and preeclampsia, length of labor and caesarean delivery, preterm birth, and fetal growth.[21] However, none of these correlations is supported by strong evidence and they have yet to be confirmed. The hypothesis by which an alteration of sleep could lead to an adverse pregnancy outcome might be related to the activation of the hypothalamus-pituitary-adrenal axis and proinflammatory system alteration.[22] Studies on sleep deprivation and sleep restriction models have shown a mild, temporary increase in the activity of the major neuroendocrine stress systems (the autonomic sympathoadrenal system and the hypothalamic-pituitary-adrenal axis).[23]

Postnatal depression is also linked to poor sleep during pregnancy, and specifically with RLS during pregnancy. Therefore, treating severe pregnancy-related RLS might be considered in order to prevent postpartum depression, especially when there is a history of a preexisting mood disorder.[20]

MANAGEMENT AND TREATMENT

A recent consensus on the management of RLS during pregnancy and lactation[24] presented a flow chart for the diagnosis and the management of the disorder. As in epilepsy, prepregnancy counseling is recommended in women with preexisting RLS. In these cases it is indicated to assess ferritin values and to discuss potential treatments during pregnancy, including their risks and benefits.

During pregnancy, the diagnosis must reflect the same standard diagnostic criteria used for non-gestational cases. Mimics of the disease during pregnancy include leg cramps, positional discomfort, and leg/ankle edema. The severity of the disease (determined by the frequency of the disturbance and its impact) is fundamental to decide whether or not it is worth discussing a treatment. The first-line treatments are mostly behavioral/non-pharmacological. For severe cases, a few pharmacologic options might be considered if used cautiously, although no drugs currently have a specific indication for RLS during pregnancy.

Nonpharmacologic Treatments

These mainly consist of measures to contain symptoms and avoid aggravating factors. Apart from the well-known iron deficiency, prolonged immobility (eg, while traveling) and the use of serotonergic antidepressants should be limited, or preferably avoided. It might be also recommended to avoid alcohol and tobacco use in the presence of RLS symptoms.[25] Moderate to intense exercise,[26] and avoiding activities that may expose individuals to the risk of abdominal trauma (eg, horse-riding, soccer, basketball) should be encouraged, but not in close to bedtime because strenuous activities might worsen the symptoms and interfere with sleep. Similarly, moderate and relaxing exercises like yoga may be beneficial for RLS. Massage[27] and pneumatic compressions[28] also seem to be beneficial and not harmful,

whereas near-infrared therapy, although possibly effective in nonpregnant RLS, is not recommended during gestation because it generates nitric oxide, the effects of which are not well established during pregnancy and lactation.[29]

Pharmacologic/Supplementation Treatments

Iron supplementation
For nonpregnancy RLS, recent treatment guidelines recommend oral iron supplements if serum ferritin level is less than 50 to 75 µg/L.[30,31] During pregnancy, iron supplementation is prescribed when ferritin values decrease to less than 30 µg/L.[32] It is also established that iron supplementation it acceptably safe, and is possibly beneficial for both mother and fetus.[33] Therefore, the consensus guidelines[24] recommend to consider iron supplementation in RLS-affected pregnant women if ferritin levels are less than 75 µg/L. Iron assessment should include hemoglobin, serum ferritin, iron saturation and iron binding capacity. If needed, oral ferrous sulfate at 65 mg once or twice per day should be prescribed. Intravenous iron supplementation should be taken into account if the serum ferritin levels are less than 30 µg/L, but only during the second or third trimester of pregnancy or in the postpartum period. Intravenous iron administration has been shown to be effective in nonpregnancy RLS[34–36] and in small open-label studies during pregnancy.[32,37,38] The main risk in administering intravenous iron is a possible anaphylactic reaction, which should be taken into account and discussed with the patient. In patients with an overload of iron, such as in hemochromatosis, iron supplementation should be avoided.

Dopaminergics
The use of dopamine agonists (pramipexole, ropinirole, and rotigotine) has not been studied enough during pregnancy. The scant literature available for dopamine agonists used during pregnancy mainly concerns patients with the juvenile form of Parkinson disease. Some data exist regarding the use of levodopa during pregnancy in women with dystonia or RLS.[39–41] The use of the combination levodopa/benserazide should be avoided because of the possibility of bone alterations in the fetus.[42] In cases of refractory RLS during pregnancy (defined as an inadequate response to at least 1 nonpharmacologic intervention and iron),[24] guidelines recommend the use of carbidopa/levodopa in the extended-release formulation (to avoid the risk of augmentation) at the daily dose of 20/100 mg up to 50/200 mg. Although dopaminergics naturally inhibit lactation (through prolactin inhibition), the effect is rapidly reversible at discontinuation of the therapy.

Alpha-2-delta ligands

Gabapentin and pregabalin are considered first-line medications in the treatment of non–pregnancy-related RLS.[31,43] Data regarding their use during pregnancy are controversial. Therefore the consensus guidelines state that these medications have insufficient evidence to be recommended. Although there is some experience in the use of gabapentin in pregnant epileptic women,[44–46] in animal models receiving high doses of gabapentin during late pregnancy an impairment of synaptogenic processes[47] was reported. Gabapentin passes through breast milk, but it has been calculated that the infant receives about 1% to 4% of the maternal weight-adjusted dose, without any apparent specific effect.[48]

Clonazepam

The use of benzodiazepines during pregnancy is controversial for different reasons: low risk of orofacial malformations during early pregnancy[49] and risk of maternal and fetus sedation at term.[50] There is enough literature to assure that at low dosages (0.25–1 mg once daily) the use of clonazepam during the second and third trimesters of pregnancy and lactation is acceptably safe, if not combined with other anticonvulsants or diphenhydramine.[51–53] The consensus guidelines[24] allow this therapy to be considered for selected cases at the dosage reported.

Opioids

The efficacy of opioids, and in particular of oxycodone, in nonpregnancy RLS is well known and opioids are usually considered in severe refractory cases.[31] The use of opioid-based therapy during pregnancy has been extensively studied in cases of chronic pain and drug addiction.[54–56] However, antenatal exposure to opioids during the first semester increases the risk of congenital heart disease,[54] and later in pregnancy exposes the newborn to the risk of sudden infant death syndrome[57] or neonatal abstinence syndrome/neonatal opioid withdrawal syndrome.[58] Taking all this in consideration, a low dosage of oxycodone is recommended only in severe cases and only during the second and third trimesters.[24] To note that few Asians, 3% to 10% of Europeans, and up to 30% of Arabians and Africans may carry the CYP2D6 variant, producing ultrafast opioid metabolism, which may cause overdose-like reactions at standard doses.[59]

REFERENCES

1. Mussio-Fournier JD, Rawak F. Familiäres Auftreten von Pruritus, Urticaria un parästhetischer Hyperkinese der unteren Extremitäten. Confin Neurol 1940;3:110–4.
2. Ekbom KA. Restless legs syndrome. Acta Med Scand 1945;158(S):1–123.
3. Goodman JD, Brodie C, Ayida GA. Restless legs syndrome in pregnancy. BMJ 1988;297:1101–2.
4. Manconi M, Govoni V, De Vito A, et al. Restless legs syndrome and pregnancy. Neurology 2004;63: 1065–9.
5. Hubner A, Krafft A, Gadient S, et al. Characteristics and determinants of restless legs syndrome in pregnancy: a prospective study. Neurology 2013;80: 738–42.
6. Berger K, Luedemann J, Trenkwalder C, et al. Sex and the risk of restless legs syndrome in the general population. Arch Intern Med 2004;164(2):196–202.
7. Rettig K, Trenkwalder C, Berger K. Die Häufigkeit des restless legs syndroms in der primärärztlichen versorgung. Nervenheilkunde 2008;27:334.e8.
8. Alam MN, Ahmad A, Al-Abbasi FA, et al. Female ovarian steroids in epilepsy: a cause or remedy. Pharmacol Rep 2013;65(4):802–12.
9. Budhiraja P, Budhiraja R, Goodwin JL. Incidence of restless legs syndrome and its correlates. J Clin Sleep Med 2012;8(2):119–24.
10. Dzaja A, Wehrle R, Lancel M, et al. Elevated estradiol plasma levels in women with restless legs during pregnancy. Sleep 2009;32(2):169–74.
11. Botez MI, Lambert B. Folate deficiency and restless legs syndrome in pregnancy. N Engl J Med 1977; 297:670.
12. Lee KA, Zaffke ME, Baratte-Beebe K. Restless legs syndrome and sleep disturbance during pregnancy: the role of folate and iron. J Womens Health Gend Based Med 2001;10:335–41.
13. Minár M, Košutzká Z, Habánová H, et al. Restless legs syndrome in pregnancy is connected with iron deficiency. Sleep Med 2015;16(5):589–92.
14. Phillips B, Young T, Finn L, et al. Epidemiology of restless legs syndrome in adults. Arch Intern Med 2000;160(14):2137–41.
15. Cesnik E, Casetta I, Turri M, et al. Transient RLS during pregnancy is a risk factor for the chronic idiopathic form. Neurology 2010;75(23):2117–20.
16. Manconi M, Ulfberg J, Berger K, et al. When gender matters: restless legs syndrome. Report of the "RLS and Woman" workshop endorsed by the European RLS Study Group. Sleep Med Rev 2012;16:297–307.
17. Sikandar R, Khealani BA, Wasay M. Predictors of restless legs syndrome in pregnancy: a hospital based cross sectional survey from Pakistan. Sleep Med 2009;10(6):676–8.
18. Sarberg M, Josefsson A, Wiréhn AB, et al. Restless legs syndrome during and after pregnancy and its relation to snoring. Acta Obstet Gynecol Scand 2012;91(7):850–5.

19. Rodrigues RN, Abreu e Silva Rodrigues A, Pratesi R, et al. Outcome of restless legs severity after continuous positive air pressure (CPAP) treatment in patients affected by the association of RLS and obstructive sleep apneas. Sleep Med 2006;7:235–9.

20. Wesstrom J, Skalkidou A, Manconi M, et al. Prepregnancy restless legs syndrome (Willis-Ekbom disease) is associated with perinatal depression. J Clin Sleep Med 2014;10:527–33.

21. Palagini L, Bruno RM, Gemignani A, et al. Sleep loss and hypertension: a systematic review. Curr Pharm Des 2013;19:2409–19.

22. Wright KP Jr, Drake AL, Frey DJ, et al. Influence of sleep deprivation and circadian misalignment on cortisol, inflammatory markers, and cytokine balance. Brain Behav Immun 2015;47:24–34.

23. Meerlo P, Sgoifo A, Suchecki D. Restricted and disrupted sleep: effects on autonomic function, neuroendocrine stress systems and stress responsivity. Sleep Med Rev 2008;12:197–210.

24. Picchietti DL, Hensley JG, Bainbridge JL, et al. Consensus clinical practice guidelines for the diagnosis and treatment of restless legs syndrome/Willis Ekbom disease during pregnancy and lactation. Sleep Med Rev 2014;22:64–77.

25. Schlesinger I, Erikh I, Avizohar O, et al. Cardiovascular risk factors in restless legs syndrome. Mov Disord 2009;24:1587–92.

26. Giannaki CD, Sakkas GK, Karatzaferi C, et al. Effect of exercise training and dopamine agonists in patients with uremic restless legs syndrome: a six-months randomized, partially double blind, placebo controlled comparative study. BMC Nephrol 2013; 14:194.

27. Russel M. Massage therapy and restless legs syndrome. J Bodyw Mov Ther 2007;11:146–50.

28. Lettieri CJ, Eliasson AH. Pneumatic compression devices are an effective therapy for restless legs syndrome: a prospective, randomized, double blinded, sham controlled, trial. Chest 2009;135: 74–80.

29. Mitchell UH, Myrer JW, Johnson AW, et al. Restless legs syndrome and near infra-red light: an alternative treatment option. Physiother Theory Pract 2011;27:345–51.

30. Garcia-Borreguero D, Ferini-Strambi L, Kohnen R, et al. European guidelines on management of restless legs syndrome: report of a joint task force by the European Federation of Neurological Societies, the European Neurological Society and the European Sleep Research Society. Eur J Neurol 2012; 19:1385–96.

31. Aurora RN, Kristo DA, Bista SR, et al. The treatment of restless legs syndrome and periodic limb movement disorder in Adults - an update for 2012: practice parameters with an evidence based systematic review and meta-analyses. Sleep 2012; 35:1039–62.

32. Pavord S, Myers B, Robinson S, et al. UK guidelines on the management of iron deficiency in pregnancy. Br J Haematol 2012;156:588–600.

33. Bothwell TH. Iron requirements in pregnancy and strategies to meet them. Am J Clin Nutr 2000;72: 257S–64S.

34. Grote L, Leissner L, Hedner J, et al. A randomized, double-blind, placebo controlled, multi-center study of intravenous iron sucrose and placebo in the treatment of restless legs syndrome. Mov Disord 2009; 24:1445–52.

35. Ondo WG. Intravenous iron dextran for severe refractory restless legs syndrome. Sleep Med 2010; 11:494–6.

36. Allen RP, Adler CH, Du W, et al. Clinical efficacy and safety of IV ferric carboxymaltose (FCM) treatment of RLS: a multi-centred, placebo-controlled preliminary clinical trial. Sleep Med 2011;12:906–13.

37. Christoph P, Schuller C, Studer H, et al. Intravenous iron treatment in pregnancy: comparison of high dose ferric carboxymaltose vs iron sucrose. J Perinat Med 2012;40:469–74.

38. Schrier SL, Auerbach M. Treatment of the adult with iron deficiency anemia. In: Basow DS, editor. Upto-Date. Waltham (MA): UpToDate; 2013. Available at: http://www.uptodate.com/home/help-manual-citing. Accessed June 11, 2015.

39. Serikawa T, Shimohata T, Akashi M, et al. Successful twin pregnancy in a patient with parkin-associated autosomal recessive juvenile parkinsonism. BMC Neurol 2011;11:72.

40. Watanabe T, Matsubara S, Baba Y, et al. Successful management of pregnancy in a patient with Segawa disease: case report and literature review. J Obstet Gynaecol Res 2009;35:562–4.

41. Dostal M, Weber-Schoendorfer C, Sobesky J, et al. Pregnancy outcome following use of levodopa, pramipexole, ropinirole, and rotigotine for restless legs syndrome during pregnancy: a case series. Eur J Neurol 2013;20(9):1241–6.

42. Briggs GG, Freeman RK, Yaffe SJ, et al. Drugs in pregnancy and lactation. 9th edition. Philadelphia: Lippincott Williams & Wilkins; 2011.

43. Allen RP, Picchietti DL, Garcia-Borreguero D, et al, International Restless Legs Syndrome Study Group. Restless legs syndrome/Willis-Ekbom disease diagnostic criteria: updated International Restless Legs Syndrome Study Group (IRLSSG) consensus criteria–history, rationale, description, and significance. Sleep Med 2014;15(8):860–73.

44. Montorius G. Gabapentin exposure in human pregnancy: results from the Gabapentin Pregnancy Registry. Epilepsy Behav 2003;4:310–7.

45. Almgren M, Källén B, Lavebratt C. Population-based study of antiepileptic drug exposure in

utero–influence on head circumference in newborns. Seizure 2009;18(10):672–5.

46. Hernandez Diaz S, Smith CS, Shen A, et al. Comparative safety of antiepileptic drugs during pregnancy. Neurology 2012;78:1692–9.

47. Eroglu C, Allen NJ, Susman MW, et al. Gabapentin receptor $\alpha2\delta$-1 is a neuronal thrombospondin receptor responsible for excitatory CNS synaptogenesis. Cell 2009;139:380–92.

48. Ohman I, Thomson T. Gabapentin kinetics during delivery, in the neonatal period and during lactation. Epilepsia 2009;50(Suppl 10):108.

49. Lin AE, Peller AJ, Westgate MN, et al. Clonazepam use in pregnancy and the risk of malformations. Birth Defects Res A Clin Mol Teratol 2004;70(8):534–6.

50. Fisher JB, Edgren BE, Mammel MC, et al. Neonatal apnea associated with maternal clonazepam therapy: a case report. Obstet Gynecol 1985;66: 34S–5S.

51. Kargas GA, Kargas SA, Bruyere HJ Jr, et al. Perinatal mortality due to interaction of diphenhydramine and temazepam. N Engl J Med 1985;313:1417–8.

52. Weinstock L, Cohen LS, Bailey JW, et al. Obstetrical and neonatal outcome following clonazepam use during pregnancy: a case series. Psychother Psychosom 2001;70:158–62.

53. Kelly LE, Poon S, Madadi P, et al. Neonatal benzodiazepine exposure during breast-feeding. J Pediatr 2012;161:448–51.

54. Broussard CS, Rasmussen SA, Reefhuis J, et al. Maternal treatment with opioids analgesics and risks for birth defects. Am J Obstet Gynecol 2011;204: 314.e1–11.

55. Brennan MC, Rayburn WF. Counselling about risks of congenital anomalies from prescription opioids. Birth Defects Res A Clin Mol Teratol 2012;94:620–5.

56. Jong GW, Koren G. Maternal treatment with opioids analgesics and risk for birth defects. Am J Obstet Gynecol 2011;205:e10.

57. Burns L, Conroy E, Mattick RP. Infant mortality among women on a methadone program during pregnancy. Drug Alcohol Rev 2010;29:551–6.

58. Hudak ML, Tan RC. Neonatal drug withdrawal. Pediatrics 2012;129:e540–60.

59. Smith HS. Opioid metabolism. Mayo Clin Proc 2009; 84:213–24.

Restless Legs Syndrome/ Willis–Ekbom Disease and Periodic Limb Movements in Sleep in the Elderly with and without Dementia

Michela Figorilli, MD[a], Monica Puligheddu, MD[a],
Raffaele Ferri, MD[b],*

KEYWORDS

- Restless legs syndrome • Willis–Ekbom disease • Elderly • Sleep

KEY POINTS

- Restless legs syndrome/Willis–Ekbom disease (RLS/WED; primary or comorbid) goes often unrecognized in the elderly, with or without dementia.
- RLS/WED is a predictor for lower physical function.
- RLS/WED in demented patients: a challenge within a challenge.
- Treatment in seniors has to be tailored taking into account comorbidities, cotherapies, and the burden of adverse drug events.

INTRODUCTION

Restless legs syndrome/Willis–Ekbom disease (RLS/WED) increases in prevalence with age up to 60 to 70 years, except in the Asian population, where an age-related increase has not been found and is greater in women than in men.[1] An increasing prevalence of RLS/WED with age may also occur in association with the increasing presence of risk factors or comorbid conditions in the elderly, such as iron deficiency and renal failure[2] (**Box 1**).

Anemia is among the most common conditions in the elderly, and in general it is sideropenic. Iron deficiency anemia in seniors may be caused by several individual or combined factors, such

as poor diet, reduced iron absorption, occult blood loss, medications (eg, aspirin, nonsteroidal antiinflammatory drugs), and chronic disease.[3]

Allen and colleagues,[1] in the REST general population study, have demonstrated a prevalence of RLS/WED of up to 8% in the elderly. Beaulieu-Bonneau and Hudon[4] showed a prevalence of sleep disturbances between 14% and 59% in mild cognitively impaired patients and, in the same population, RLS/WED was found in 30.8% and PLMD was observed in 36.9%. A multicenter, Italian, clinical, cross-sectional study[5] showed an RLS/WED prevalence of 6.1% in degenerative and vascular dementia, which is not different from that found in the healthy elderly population.

Funding Sources: Dr M. Figorilli and Dr M. Puligheddu: Nil; Dr R. Ferri: Italian Ministry of Health ("Ricerca Corrente").
Conflict of Interest: Nil.
[a] Neurophysiology Unit, Sleep Disorder Center, University of Cagliari, SS554 Bivio Sestu, Monserrato, Cagliari 09042, Italy; [b] Department of Neurology I.C., Sleep Research Centre, Oasi Institute for Research on Mental Retardation and Brain Aging (IRCCS), Via C. Ruggero, 73, Troina 94018, Italy
* Corresponding author.
E-mail address: rferri@oasi.en.it

Sleep Med Clin 10 (2015) 331–342
http://dx.doi.org/10.1016/j.jsmc.2015.05.011

Box 1
Medical disorders and conditions associated with restless legs syndrome/Willis–Ekbom disease

1. Low serum ferritin level: anemia is one of the most frequent diseases among the elderly
2. Sleep disorders: narcolepsy, obstructive sleep apnea, insomnia, RBD
3. Heart failure
4. Diabetes
5. Rheumatologic disorder: rheumatoid arthritis, fibromyalgia, and spondyloarthropathy
6. Renal failure
7. Chronic obstructive pulmonary disease
8. Neurologic disorders: neurodegenerative (PD, MSA, ALS), MS, myotonic dystrophy, migraine.
9. Radiculopathy and spinal cord injury
10. Polyneuropathies
11. Stroke
12. Psychiatric disorders: anxiety and depression
13. Chronic liver disease
14. Certain medications (selective serotonin reuptake inhibitors, selective norepinephrine reuptake inhibitors, lithium, dopamine antagonists, neuroleptics, antipsychotics, tricyclic antidepressants, tramadol, lithium, L-thyroxine, sodium-oxibate, zonisamide, clebopride, anterferon-alpha)

Abbreviations: ALS, atrophic lateral sclerosis; MS, multiple sclerosis; MSA, multiple system atrophy; PD, Parkinson's disease; RBD, REM sleep behavior disorder.

In particular, the prevalence and risk of RLS/WED was higher in patients affected by Alzheimer disease and mild cognitively impaired than in vascular dementia, frontotemporal dementia, Lewy body dementia, and Parkinson's disease dementia. A recent study has not found an increased prevalence and risk for RLS/WED in Lewy body dementia/Parkinson's disease dementia.[6]

In this review, we have analyzed the features of 3 main types of RLS/WED: (1) primary or idiopathic RLS/WED (often called here simply RLS/WED), (2) comorbid RLS/WED, and (3) RLS/WED in cognitively impaired patients. In this review, we prefer to use the term "comorbid" RLS/WED because it is often impossible to establish if the other condition (ie, iron deficiency, chronic renal failure, use of antidepressant or neuroleptics, neuropathy, or neurologic disease) is an aggravating or a causal factor; sometimes, it cannot be excluded that the coexistence of the 2 conditions is merely casual and owing to essentially epidemiologic reasons.

PRIMARY RESTLESS LEGS SYNDROME/WILLIS–EKBOM DISEASE IN THE ELDERLY

The definition of primary RLS/WED may be challenged in the elderly because of the high frequency of the cumulating comorbidities in this population, among which iron deficiency and renal failure are the most frequent. Indeed, a familiar distribution can subtend a genetic predisposition.[7]

Early-Onset Restless Legs Syndrome/Willis–Ekbom Disease

The early onset of RLS/WED has been defined when the disease appears before the age of 45 years.[7] Early-onset RLS/WED has a high level of familiarity with 40% to 90% of patients reporting an affected first-degree relative.[7,8]

Patient age per se likely plays a fundamental role in the severity of RLS/WED. The symptoms of RLS/WED generally become significant later in life, with an average age at diagnosis of about 53 years.[7,9] Therefore, an early onset might lead to a slowly progressive disorder and to an intermittent course. In addition, iron status seems to be less effective in early-onset RLS than in the late-onset type; nevertheless, Earley and colleagues[10] showed low cerebrospinal fluid ferritin levels as well in patients with idiopathic RLS/WED.

Late-Onset Restless Legs Syndrome/Willis–Ekbom Disease

In late-onset disease (after age 45), RLS/WED seems to have less familiarity and stronger relations to serum iron status than the early-onset variation (≤45 years); moreover, the symptoms often occur more suddenly, with rapid progression to a continuous syndrome. Aggravating factors are common.[7]

Clinical picture

Essential features The essential clinical features of RLS/WED in the elderly are similar to those of the younger population.[11–14] Among the elderly, jumping off the bed at night, in search of relief from the unpleasant sensations, may lead to an increased risk of falls and consequent loss of autonomy.[13] Patients report their discomfort in different ways and often show difficulties in explaining their sensations. Bassetti and colleagues[15] reported that more than 50% of their RLS/WED patients described their symptom as pain. In contrast, some patients complain only about the urge to move without the sensory symptoms.

The worsening of RLS/WED and associated periodic limb movements in sleep (PLMS) with aging[16] suggests that this syndrome might be associated with other conditions known to be common in older populations, such as iron deficiency, use of substances such as antidepressants, selective serotonin reuptake inhibitors, lithium, and antipsychotics.[17] In addition, several social or lifestyle factors seem to contribute to RLS/WED symptoms, such as increased body mass index and caffeine intake, sedentary lifestyle or prolonged immobility, tobacco use, and lower income.[17] These conditions and social factors are frequent in all seniors (healthy, dependent, or frail), with different degrees of associated comorbidities and consequences in the management of the disease.

Associated features

In the elderly, RLS/WED is highly associated with severe sleep disturbance, impaired quality of life, lesser physical functioning,[18] decreased daytime cognitive performance[19,20] and frequent mood and anxiety disorders.[21]

Sleep complaints In the general population, up to 90% of patients suffering from RLS/WED complain of severe difficulties in initiating and maintaining sleep. The disturbed sleep is often the main reason for seeking medical attention. Daytime fatigue and daytime sleepiness are also common complaints.[22] However, some studies have reported a relatively low degree of daytime sleepiness in RLS/WED patients with respect to their degree of sleep loss,[15] perhaps owing to a hyperarousal background that minimizes the amount of sleepiness. According to the physiologic modifications in sleep with aging, the burden of RLS/WED on sleep quality seems to be prominent.[2]

Periodic limb movements PLMS (with or without RLS) have been correlated with cortical and autonomic arousal, with an increased sympathetic activity and, probably, cardiovascular consequences.[23–25] The increased sympathetic activity, with changes in heart rate[23] and even in blood pressure, might contribute to the risk of cardiovascular disease in patients with RLS, especially in the elderly.[26,27] However, the relationship of cause and effect between PLMS and cerebrovascular risk has yet to be established in the elderly.[25] In the elderly, independent of RLS, periodicity and circadian distribution of PLMS might help to differentiate the proportions of the phenomenon owing to the movement disorder or to the aging process per se, with possible speculations for treatment.[16]

Mood and anxiety disorders Some studies have shown an increased prevalence of mood and anxiety disorders in patients suffering from RLS/WED[21,28] in both the general population and the elderly. The presence of clinically relevant depressive symptoms may have a role for new-onset RLS/WED and, similarly, untreated RLS/WED is associated with depression and anxiety. Furthermore, the severity of RLS/WED correlates positively with depression/anxiety symptoms and the treatment of RLS/WED improves depressive features. In the elderly population, it is important to recognize and treat depression and anxiety, because of their relationship with worse quality of life and other comorbidities.

Cognitive Implications of Restless Legs Syndrome/Willis–Ekbom Disease

There are several studies in the literature on cognitive performance in RLS/WED patients with inconsistent findings,[29–32] both in the adult population as well as in the elderly. It has been suggested that patients suffering from RLS/WED may show deficits in prefrontal cortex function as a result of chronic sleep loss, because cognitive tasks depending on the prefrontal cortex function are particularly sensitive to sleep loss.[30,32–34]

The Diagnosis of Restless Legs Syndrome/Willis–Ekbom Disease

The diagnosis of RLS/WED is by definition based on clinical data, using an in-depth medical history and a physical examination assessing the presence of the essential diagnostic criteria and the absence of mimics.[11] Physical and neurologic examination of the limbs should be normal, with no evidence of vascular insufficiency, arthritis, decreased osteotendinous reflexes, altered sensibility or strength, or impaired balance and walk. Sometimes, the examination shows static hyperalgesia as well as vibratory hyperesthesia.[29,30] Especially in the elderly population, the clinician should be careful to rule out possible signs or symptoms of myelopathy, radiculopathy, and neuropathy. Moreover, it is important to assess the presence of predisposing and precipitating factors, such as familiarity of RLS/WED, gender (female sex), and iron deficiency, certain medications (sedating antihistamines, dopamine receptor antagonists, and antidepressants), chronic renal failure, and prolonged immobility.

Supportive features

There are supportive features that could help the clinician in the diagnosis of RLS/WED, such as family history of RLS/WED, PLM, improvement of symptoms with dopaminergic therapy, and a relative lack of expected daytime sleepiness. There are no specific laboratory tests for the diagnosis of RLS/WED. However, considering that iron deficiency is often associated with RLS/WED, serum ferritin should be assessed, as well as renal function, because of the relationship between RLS/WED and uremia, and serum glucose (diabetes).

Periodic leg movements In doubtful cases, a polysomnography study (laboratory or ambulatory), in untreated RLS/WED patients, might support the diagnosis if demonstrates (a) PLMW before sleep onset and during nocturnal awakenings, (b) PLMS, and/or (c) altered sleep parameters (increased sleep latency, high arousal index, and decreased sleep efficiency).

PLMS during sleep show a clear age-related increase in RLS/WED[16]; the PLMS index increases with age also in healthy individuals, and PLMS can be found particularly after the age of 40 years,[31] for this reason some authors considered cutoff values as high as greater than 15 per hour. More recent measures of the time structure of LM activity during sleep (periodicity and distribution through the night)[16,32,33] offer additional information in the elderly. LM activity periodicity (periodicity index) shows age-related changes clearly different from those seen for the PLMS index because it increases progressively up to the age of 35 years and then remains stable up to the age of 85 years and in the oldest individuals, the characteristic decreasing trend of PLMS through the night is often lost.[16]

However, it must be mentioned that some dependent or frail seniors might be unable to undergo an ambulatory or laboratory polysomnography; in these cases, the detection of PLM might be done using an ankle actigraphy.

Differential Diagnosis of Restless Legs Syndrome/Willis–Ekbom Disease: The Mimics

Up to 40% of patients without RLS/WED report some urge or desire to move the legs while at rest; for this reason, a differential diagnosis is needed to carefully rule out these cases.[34] The most frequent mimics of RLS, from the more to the less common, are leg cramps, positional discomfort, local leg injury, arthralgia/arthritis, leg edema, venous stasis, peripheral neuropathy, radiculopathy, habitual foot tapping, anxiety, myalgia, drug-induced akathisia, myelopathy, myopathy, vascular or neurogenic claudication, hypotensive akathisia, orthostatic tremor, painful legs, and moving toes.[11,34,35] Several of these conditions are frequently encountered in the elderly population[14,36] and an accurate semistructured history interview and examination are essential to rule them out. The pain caused by arthritis, vascular problems, sports/orthopedic injuries, and neuropathy may have a nocturnal presentation and might be worse at rest, but generally is not improved by movement. However, in the general population, about 50% of patients with RLS/WED report pain as their main symptom[15]; moreover, it is possible that any of these mimics might occur in a patient at the same time as RLS. When the diagnosis of RLS/WED is doubtful, the assessment of the presence of the supportive features might be helpful.

Treatment: The Importance of Tailoring

Nonpharmacologic approach

Nonpharmacologic treatments (**Box 2**) should be preferred in milder cases of RLS/WED and might be used as add-on therapy for patients with more severe RLS/WED to improve their outcome and reduce the dependence on medications and prevent or delay augmentation. In case of iron

---

Box 2
Nonpharmacologic treatment of restless legs syndrome/Willis–Ekbom disease

1. Education: performing sedentary tasks in the morning instead of in the evening

2. Optimized sleep hygiene

3. Practice moderate exercise during daytime

4. Smoking cessation, alcohol avoidance, caffeine reduction or elimination

5. Discontinuation of precipitating medications if appropriate[2]

deficiency (ferritin concentration of <50 μg/L), patients should receive iron substitution therapy.

Pharmacologic therapy

The pharmacologic therapy in the elderly population has to be tailored taking into account comorbidities, other therapies, and the burden of adverse drug events (**Fig. 1**). Drug treatment for RLS/WED can be carried out with several substances: non–ergot-derived dopaminergic agents, opioids, benzodiazepines (such as clonazepam), and antiepileptic drugs (such as gabapentin and pregabalin, alpha2-ligands). All of these medications have been demonstrated to have several adverse events in the elderly, especially in the dependent and in frail seniors. However, the details of the drug therapy for RLS/WED are reported in Dopaminergic Therapy for Restless Legs Syndrome/Willis-Ekbom Disease by Zak elsewhere in this issue, and we only focus briefly on aspects related to the elderly population here.

Although the majority of the adverse events of non–ergot-derived dopaminergic agents are mild or moderate in severity,[37,38] side effects, such as sleepiness, hypotension, hallucinations, and others psychotic adverse events (**Box 3**), should be managed carefully because of their related increased risk of falls in the elderly,[2] both healthy and dependent or frail seniors. Dopaminergic agents do not shown particular interaction with other drugs, an important aspect especially in the elderly, with the exception of other medications that affect vigilance and central nervous system, such as sedatives, hypnotics, and neuroleptics.

Dopaminergic agents are known to induce often augmentation, an increase of RLS/WED symptom severity: earlier onset (≥2 hours earlier), more severe, spread of symptoms to other body parts, and resistance to higher doses of medication.[39] Aging per se is associated with decreasing dopaminergic function that may increase the risk of augmentation.[39] Augmentation in the elderly should be approached as in the other patients and more details are reported in Dopaminergic Augmentation in Restless Legs Syndrome/Willis Ekbom Disease (RLS/WED): Differential Diagnosis Between Disease Progression, End-of-Dose Rebound and Augmentation by Garcia-Borreguero elsewhere in this issue.

Alpha-2-ligands should be used carefully in the elderly population with impaired renal function (**Box 4**). In addition, they have shown an addictive effect with oxycodone, compromising cognitive function and motor function. Clonazepam should be used with attention in all elderly patients—healthy, dependent, or frail—and should be avoided in renal failure, chronic liver disease, glaucoma, chronic respiratory disease, sleep-related breathing disorders, and dysphagia. The more frequent adverse events of clonazepam are sleepiness, ataxia, and behavioral disorders (**Box 5**). Opioids should be used carefully in elderly patients with impaired renal and hepatic function[40] (**Box 6**). Clinicians should start low and titrate slow the opioids in the elderly, taking into account polytherapy and multiple comorbidities.[40]

COMORBID RESTLESS LEGS SYNDROME/WILLIS–EKBOM DISEASE IN THE ELDERLY

The International Classification of Sleep Disorders-3[41] uses the term "secondary" RLS/WED when the condition occurs in association with iron deficiency, pregnancy, or chronic renal failure. Several other conditions have been associated with RLS, such as diabetes neuropathies, small fibers neuropathies,[29] radiculopathy, hypothyroidism, hyperthyroidism, folic deficiency, rheumatoid arthritis, chronic liver disease,[42] and chronic obstructive pulmonary disease.[43] Nevertheless, it is unclear whether RLS/WED is truly a secondary form or the conditions listed represent just comorbidities; moreover, RLS/WED may be worsened or triggered by medications, both directly and indirectly, such as nonsteroidal antiinflammatory drugs that increase risk of iron deficiency.[44] For these reasons, we refer to all these forms with the term "comorbid" RLS/WED, which has been more associated with a later disease and requires special consideration in the elderly. Different from primary RLS/WED, some comorbid form may remit once the comorbidity (iron deficiency, chronic renal disease) is treated.[45]

Diagnosis of Comorbid Restless Legs Syndrome/Willis–Ekbom Disease

The diagnosis of comorbid RLS/WED requires an accurate clinical and pharmacologic history, in-depth physical and neurologic examinations, laboratory testing, and in doubtful cases second-line tests to rule out possible mimics that may worsen restless legs symptoms[45] (**Box 7**).

Iron deficiency in the elderly

This type of RLS/WED typically shows a late onset and a strong relationship with iron deficiency.[46] Serum ferritin levels of less than 50 μg/L have been documented in 58% of patients with onset after 64 years.[47] Altered iron metabolism represents a condition associated with RLS/WED deserving a special note for the elderly, because low or normal low serum ferritin levels are common among the aged population, with the cutoff for serum ferritin of 50 μg/L.[48] Even though, in the

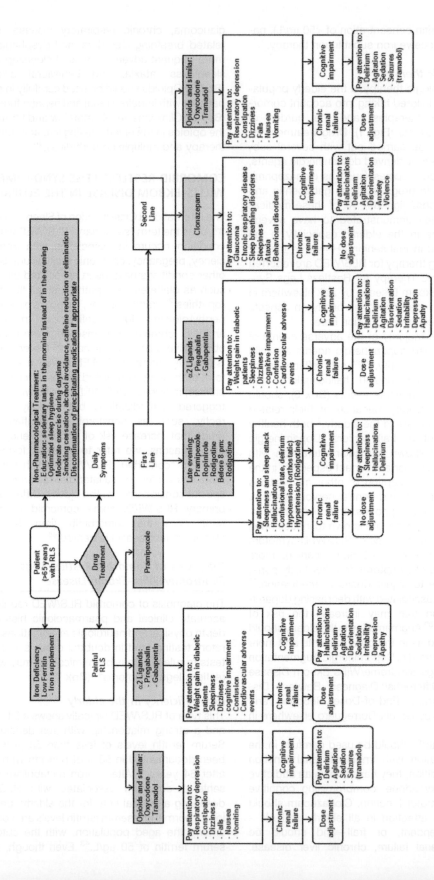

Fig. 1. Treatment algorithm. RLS, restless leg syndrome.

Box 3
Dopaminergic agents: side effects
1. Hallucinations (mainly visual)
2. Dyskinesia
3. Sleepiness and sleep attack
4. Impulsive compulsive disorder
5. Confusional state, delirium
6. Headache
7. Dizziness
8. Hypotension (mainly orthostatic) or hypertension (rotigotine)
9. Nausea, constipation, and vomiting
10. Fatigue
11. Peripheral edema
12. Skin irritation reaction (rotigotine)

case of chronic inflammatory conditions, habitual in older people, a cutoff of 70 µg/L should be considered.[49] The elderly population, with or without dementia has plausible risk factors for iron deficiency, such as malnutrition and poor diet, treatment with aspirin, nonsteroidal antiinflammatory drugs, and a chronic inflammatory condition[50] (**Box 8**). Nevertheless, there are some cases with serum ferritin levels within the conventional normal range,[10] although this does not exclude the possibility of iron deficiency because of the presence of individuals at risk for iron depletion. Therefore, it is important to take into account the personal clinical features in the interpretation of serum ferritin levels in elderly RLS/WED patients.[51]

Chronic renal failure

RLS/WED has a high prevalence (from 12% to 62%) among patients with chronic renal failure, mostly on hemodialysis; however, nondialyzed patients with chronic renal failure are older than those under dialysis, and have several comorbidities, such as hypertension, anemia, diabetes, and thyroid disease.[52–54] In patients with chronic renal failure, it is important to treat RLS/WED both pharmacologically and nonpharmacologically, avoiding the administration of medications with renal toxicity (such as alpha-2-ligands and opioids) and optimizing the management of chronic kidney disease[55] (see **Fig. 1**).

RESTLESS LEGS SYNDROME/WILLIS–EKBOM DISEASE IN THE COGNITIVELY IMPAIRED ELDERLY

RLS/WED has been reported to show a prevalence of between 6% and 12% in cognitively impaired seniors.[5,56] RLS/WED in demented patients is associated with neuropsychiatric symptoms, poor cognitive and physical outcomes, and increased disability. Further studies are needed to assess the impact or RLS/WED in mild cognitive impairment and to what extent sleep disruption contributes to the progression of dementia in this population.[4,5,57] However, the diagnosis of RLS/WED in demented patients represents a challenge within a challenge; the sensory features of RLS/WED might be hard to be explained by cognitively impaired elderly. No specific suggestions for this special population are available currently.[11] One of the latest workshops of the International Restless Legs Syndrome Study Group (IRLSSG) has

Box 4
Alpha-2-ligand: side effects
1. Increased appetite with weight gain
2. Neurologic: sleepiness, dizziness; common: ataxia, tremors, dysarthria, cognitive impairment (memory and attention), sedation, paresthesia, balance impairment, headache, diplopia, blurred vision; uncommon: syncope, stupor, myoclonus, psychomotor hyperactivity, intentional tremor, nystagmus, cognitive deficits, language disturbance
3. Psychiatric: euphoria, confusion, irritability, disorientation, insomnia; Uncommon: hallucinations, panic attack, agitation, depression, and apathy; suicidal ideation (frequency not determined)
4. Cardiovascular: tachycardia, first-degree atrioventricular block, peripheral edema (gabapentin); uncommon: hypertension, hypotension; rare: arrhythmia, congestive heart failure and prolonged QT interval (frequency not determined)
5. Breathing disorder: dyspnea, uncommon; pulmonary edema (frequency not determined)
6. Constipation, vomiting
7. Renal failure, incontinence
8. Leukopenia (gabapentin)

Box 5
Clonazepam: side effects

1. Neurologic: sleepiness, delayed reaction, tremors, ataxia, dizziness, dysarthria; rare: headache
2. Psychiatric: impaired concentration, memory deficits, hallucinations, agitation, confusional state, and disorientation; paradox reaction, irritability, agitation, anxiety, sleep disturbances, nightmare, restlessness, aggressiveness
3. Diplopia, nystagmus
4. Cardiovascular: tachycardia, congestive heart failure (frequency not determined)
5. Breathing disorder: depressed respiratory drive, hypersecretion in the upper airways
6. Rarely: nausea, epigastric pain, hypersalivation, gastritis, constipation
7. Hepatomegaly, transitory augmentation of transaminase and alcaline phosphatase
8. Anemia, leukopenia, thrombocytopenia and eosinophilia
9. Rare: incontinence

---

highlighted the lack of diagnostic criteria for the cognitively impaired population.[11]

Diagnosis of Restless Legs Syndrome/Willis–Ekbom Disease in Cognitively Impaired Seniors

The clinical diagnosis of RLS/WED can be made by clinician interaction with the patient and assessment by the clinician of the patient's subjective reports of the essential features of RLS/WED. Cognitively impaired elderly patients often present communication problems that might distort the description of the core RLS/WED symptoms.[11] However, a validated method for the diagnosis of RLS/WED in this population is not available. RLS/WED can be suspected in cognitively impaired seniors when they present low or low-normal serum iron status combined with high rates of PLMW or PLMS. These patients might deserve specific attention because of the possible benefit from iron therapy, as nondemented elderly do.[13,47,48,51]

Special considerations for the assessment of RLS/WED in the cognitively impaired have been proposed by the IRLSSG[12] (**Box 9**). Adapting these special considerations to the latest diagnostic criteria, we should rule out mimics and other potential causes of the symptoms.

Other supportive criteria for the diagnosis of RLS/WED in the cognitively impaired elderly should be considered[12] (**Box 10**). The differential diagnosis of RLS/WED in this population should be carried out with respect to painful neuropathy,

---

Box 6
Opioids: side effects

1. Neurologic: sleepiness, dizziness, sedation, cognitive impairment, seizure (tramadol)
2. Psychiatric: mood disorders, confusion, amnesia; uncommon: hallucinations
3. Cardiovascular: hypotension
4. Breathing disorder: depressed respiratory drive, dyspnea
5. Gastrointestinal: constipation, nausea, vomiting, xerostomia, abdominal pain, dyspepsia
6. Skin: pruritus, rash, hyperhidrosis
7. Urinary retention
8. Tolerance and addiction

Box 7
Comorbid restless legs syndrome/Willis–Ekbom disease: laboratory tests

1. Iron studies
2. Full blood count
3. Serum vitamin B_{12} and folate
4. Serum glucose and HbA1C
5. Urea and electrolytes
6. Serum creatinine
7. Albumin levels
8. Thyroids hormones
9. Neurophysiologic examination: nerve conduction velocity (neuropathy)

Box 8
Causes of iron-deficiency anemia in the elderly

1. Malnutrition
2. Reduced efficiency of iron absorption
3. Occult blood loss: gastrointestinal neoplasm, peptic ulcer, hiatus hernia, colonic vascular ecstasy, Crohn's disease
4. Chronic inflammatory disease
5. Gastrointestinal disease not associated with bleeding: atrophic gastritis, celiac disease, and *Helicobacter pylori* infection
6. Institutionalization
7. Medications: aspirin, nonsteroidal antiinflammatory drugs

Box 10
Supportive features for the diagnosis of probable RLS/WED in the cognitively impaired elderly

1. Response to dopaminergic therapy
2. Patient's past history suggestive of RLS/WED, as reported by caregiver (or family member)
3. Positive family history of RLS/WED
4. Observed PLM, or recorded by polysomnography or actigraphy
5. Significant sleep-onset problems
6. Better sleep quality in the day than in the night
7. Use of restraints at night (for institutionalized patients)
8. Low serum ferritin level
9. End-stage renal disease
10. Diabetes
11. Peripheral neuropathy or radiculopathy confirmed clinically or by electromyograghic or nerve conduction evidence

Abbreviations: PLM, periodic leg movements; RLS/WED, restless legs syndrome/Willis–Ekbom disease

---

arthritis, neuroleptic-induced akathisia, nonspecific pacing or sleep disturbance associated with dementia, pruritus, leg cramps, vascular insufficiency, anxiety disorder, and agitated depression.

RLS/WED in demented patients seems to be associated with nocturnal agitation behavior.[58] Sometimes, wandering might represent an unrecognized RLS/WED phenotype; notably, wandering has long been recognized as one of the most difficult and intractable components of dementia. There is now increasing attention about at least some cases of wandering, especially in the early evening hours, that might underline RLS/WED symptoms.[12] Several studies have shown a correlation between apathy and RLS/WED in Alzheimer disease; the two conditions might have a common pathophysiologic basis consisting in a dysfunction of the central dopaminergic system.[59–61] Neuroleptic-induced akathisia has been recognized as a mimic of RLS/WED and seems to be common among the cognitively impaired treated with neuroleptics.[62] Motor restlessness induced by neuroleptics is usually generalized, generally without sensory discomfort, and often it has no relief by movement.

Management of Restless Legs Syndrome/Willis–Ekbom Disease in Cognitively Impaired Seniors

The treatment and management of RLS/WED have mandatory importance in patients with dementia to prevent institutionalization and poor outcome and reduced quality of life of these patients and

---

Box 9
Diagnostic consideration for cognitively impaired elderly

1. Signs of legs discomfort: rubbing or kneading the legs and/or groaning while holding the lower extremities.
2. Excessive motor activity in the lower limbs: pacing, fidgeting, repetitive movements of legs, repetitive foot tapping, rubbing the feet together, and the inability to remain seated.
3. Signs of leg discomfort exclusively present or worse during periods of inactivity.
4. Signs of leg discomfort are diminished with activity.
5. Criteria 1 and 2 occur only in the evening or at night, or are worse at those times during the day.

Box 11

Medications associated with RLS/WED, often used as treatment of cognitively impaired patients

1. Antidepressants: escitalopram, citalopram, fluoxetine, paroxetine, sertraline, venlafaxine, duloxetine, mianserine, mirtazapine, amitriptyline, imipramine

2. Neuroleptics: thioridazine, loxapine, olanzapine, risperidone, aripripazaole, clozapine, quietapine

3. Lithium

their caregivers.[63] All suggestions for the management of RLS/WED in the elderly without cognitive impairment are relevant also for this population (see **Fig. 1**). All the associated comorbidities and secondary causes have to be investigated and treated. Nevertheless, several medications used in the management of dementia often worsen symptoms of RLS/WED (**Box 11**).

Furthermore, the medications of RLS/WED have several adverse events, such as hallucinations, indirect risk of falls, and agitation, that must be carefully investigated and managed in the demented patients, because they can be associated with important complications and a reduced quality of life for patients and caregivers (**Box 12**). The nonpharmacologic strategies should be optimized and added to the pharmacologic treatment to improve the management of RLS/WED also in demented patients.

Box 12

Adverse events of RLS/WED treatment and dementia

1. Dopamine agonist: hallucinations, confusional state, delirium, and sleepiness

2. Alpha-2-ligands: hallucinations, confusional state, agitation, disorientation, sedation, irritability, cognitive impairment (domain of memory and attention), depression, apathy, suicidal ideation, panic attacks

3. Clonazepam: hallucination, confusional state, agitation, disorientation, impairment of memory and concentration, anxiety, and aggressiveness

4. Opioids: confusional state, agitation, sedation, cognitive impairment, seizures (tramadol)

SUMMARY

RLS/WED is associated with lower physical functioning[18,64] and untreated RLS/WED is associated with depression.[65] Furthermore, the presence of clinically relevant depressive symptoms may be a risk factor for new-onset RLS/WED and RLS/WED also predicts incident depressive symptoms.[66] The consequences of untreated RLS/WED include fragmented sleep, often resulting in falls, reduced quality of life, and institutionalization.[67] For all these reasons, research should focus on the assessment of the impact of RLS/WED in the frail elderly and in patients with dementia. This strategy has not yet been established, but it is easy to foresee a dramatic impact in the management of these patients and on the associated caregiver burden. RLS/WED might represent a treatable stressor and its recognition and effective treatment would definitely create a better quality of life.

REFERENCES

1. Allen RP, Walters AS, Montplaisir J, et al. Restless legs syndrome prevalence and impact: REST general population study. Arch Intern Med 2005;165(11): 1286–92.

2. Bloom HG, Ahmed I, Alessi CA, et al. Evidence-based recommendations for the assessment and management of sleep disorders in older persons. J Am Geriatr Soc 2009;57(5):761–89.

3. Lopez-Contreras MJ, Zamora-Portero S, Lopez MA, et al. Dietary intake and iron status of institutionalized elderly people: relationship with different factors. J Nutr Health Aging 2010;14(10):816–21.

4. Beaulieu-Bonneau S, Hudon C. Sleep disturbances in older adults with mild cognitive impairment. Int Psychogeriatr 2009;21(4):654.

5. Guarnieri B, Adorni F, Musicco M, et al. Prevalence of sleep disturbances in mild cognitive impairment and dementing disorders: a multicenter Italian clinical cross-sectional study on 431 patients. Dement Geriatr Cogn Disord 2012;33(1):50–8.

6. Puligheddu M, Figorilli M, Aricò D, et al. Time structure of leg movement activity during sleep in untreated Parkinson disease and effects of dopaminergic treatment. Sleep Med 2014;15(7):816–24.

7. Allen RP, Earley CJ. Defining the phenotype of the restless legs syndrome (RLS) using age-of-symptom-onset. Sleep Med 2000;1(1):11–9.

8. Allen RP. Controversies and challenges in defining the etiology and pathophysiology of restless legs syndrome. Am J Med 2007;120(1 Suppl 1):S13–21.

9. Walters AS, Hickey K, Maltzman J, et al. A questionnaire study of 138 patients with restless legs syndrome: the "night-walkers" survey. Neurology 1996; 46(1):92–5.

10. Earley CJ, Connor JR, Beard JL, et al. Abnormalities in CSF concentrations of ferritin and transferrin in restless legs syndrome. Neurology 2000;54(8): 1698–700.

11. Allen RP, Picchietti DL, Garcia-Borreguero D, et al. Restless legs syndrome/Willis–Ekbom disease diagnostic criteria: updated International Restless Legs Syndrome Study Group (IRLSSG) consensus criteria – history, rationale, description, and significance. Sleep Med 2014;15(8):860–73.

12. Allen RP, Picchietti D, Hening WA, et al. Restless legs syndrome: diagnostic criteria, special considerations, and epidemiology. A report from the restless legs syndrome diagnosis and epidemiology workshop at the National Institutes of Health. Sleep Med 2003;4(2):101–19.

13. O'keeffe ST, Noel J, Lavan JN. Restless legs syndrome in the elderly. Postgrad Med J 1993; 69(815):701–3.

14. Rothdach AJ, Trenkwalder C, Haberstock J, et al. Prevalence and risk factors of RLS in an elderly population the MEMO study. Neurology 2000;54(5):1064–8.

15. Bassetti CL, Mauerhofer D, Gugger M, et al. Restless legs syndrome: a clinical study of 55 patients. Eur Neurol 2001;45(2):67–74.

16. Ferri R, Manconi M, Lanuzza B, et al. Age-related changes in periodic leg movements during sleep in patients with restless legs syndrome. Sleep Med 2008;9(7):790–8.

17. Phillips B, Young T, Finn L, et al. Epidemiology of restless legs symptoms in adults. Arch Intern Med 2000;160(14):2137–41.

18. Zhang C, Li Y, Malhotra A, et al. Restless legs syndrome status as a predictor for lower physical function. Neurology 2014;82(14):1212–8.

19. Richards KC, Roberson PK, Simpson K, et al. Periodic leg movements predict total sleep time in persons with cognitive impairment and sleep disturbance. Sleep 2008;31(2):224.

20. Allen RP, Earley CJ. Restless legs syndrome: a review of clinical and pathophysiologic features. J Clin Neurophysiol 2001;18(2):128–47.

21. Winkelmann J, Prager M, Lieb R, et al. "Anxietas tibiarum". Depression and anxiety disorders in patients with restless legs syndrome. J Neurol 2005; 252(1):67–71.

22. Fulda S, Wetter TC. Is daytime sleepiness a neglected problem in patients with restless legs syndrome? Mov Disord 2007;22(Suppl 18):S409–13.

23. Ferri R, Zucconi M, Rundo F, et al. Heart rate and spectral EEG changes accompanying periodic and non-periodic leg movements during sleep. Clin Neurophysiol 2007;118(2):438–48.

24. Winkelman JW, Shahar E, Sharief I, et al. Association of restless legs syndrome and cardiovascular disease in the sleep heart health study. Neurology 2008;70(1):35–42.

25. Koo BB, Blackwell T, Ancoli-Israel S, et al. Association of incident cardiovascular disease with periodic limb movements during sleep in older men: outcomes of Sleep Disorders in Older Men (MrOS) study. Circulation 2011;124(11):1223–31.

26. Ferrillo F, Beelke M, Canovaro P, et al. Changes in cerebral and autonomic activity heralding periodic limb movements in sleep. Sleep Med 2004;5(4): 407–12.

27. Pennestri MH, Montplaisir J, Colombo R, et al. Nocturnal blood pressure changes in patients with restless legs syndrome. Neurology 2007;68(15): 1213–8.

28. Li Y, Mirzaei F, O'Reilly EJ, et al. Prospective study of restless legs syndrome and risk of depression in women. Am J Epidemiol 2012;176(4):279–88.

29. Bachmann CG, Rolke R, Scheidt U, et al. Thermal hypoaesthesia differentiates secondary restless legs syndrome associated with small fibre neuropathy from primary restless legs syndrome. Brain 2010;133(Pt 3):762–70.

30. Stiasny-Kolster K, Magerl W, Oertel WH, et al. Static mechanical hyperalgesia without dynamic tactile allodynia in patients with restless legs syndrome. Brain 2004;127(Pt 4):773–82.

31. Pennestri M-H, Whittom S, Adam B, et al. PLMS and PLMW in healthy subjects as a function of age: prevalence and interval distribution. Sleep 2006;29(9): 1183–7.

32. Ferri R, Zucconi M, Manconi M, et al. Computer-assisted detection of nocturnal leg motor activity in patients with restless legs syndrome and periodic leg movements during sleep. Sleep 2005;28(8): 998–1004.

33. Ferri R, Zucconi M, Manconi M, et al. New approaches to the study of periodic leg movements during sleep in restless legs syndrome. Sleep 2006;29(6):759–69.

34. Hening WA, Allen RP, Washburn M, et al. The four diagnostic criteria for restless legs syndrome are unable to exclude confounding conditions ("mimics"). Sleep Med 2009;10(9):976–81.

35. Möller C, Wetter TC, Köster J, et al. Differential diagnosis of unpleasant sensations in the legs: prevalence of restless legs syndrome in a primary care population. Sleep Med 2010;11(2):161–6.

36. Celle S, Roche F, Kerleroux J, et al. Prevalence and clinical correlates of restless legs syndrome in an elderly French population: the Synapse study. J Gerontol A Biol Sci Med Sci 2010;65(2):167–73.

37. Allen RP, Chen C, Garcia-Borreguero D, et al. Comparison of pregabalin with pramipexole for restless legs syndrome. N Engl J Med 2014; 370(7):621–31.

38. Winkelman JW, Sethi KD, Kushida CA, et al. Efficacy and safety of pramipexole in restless legs syndrome. Neurology 2006;67(6):1034–9.

39. Allen RP, Ondo WG, Ball E, et al. Restless legs syndrome (RLS) augmentation associated with dopamine agonist and levodopa usage in a community sample. Sleep Med 2011;12(5):431–9.

40. Chau DL, Walker V, Pai L, et al. Opiates and elderly: use and side effects. Clin Interv Aging 2008;3(2):273.

41. American Academy of Sleep Medicine. International classification of sleep disorders. 3rd edition. Darien, IL: American Academy of Sleep Medicine; 2014.

42. Franco RA, Ashwathnarayan R, Deshpandee A, et al. The high prevalence of restless legs syndrome symptoms in liver disease in an academic-based hepatology practice. J Clin Sleep Med 2008;4(1):45.

43. Kaplan Y, Inonu H, Yilmaz A, et al. Restless legs syndrome in patients with chronic obstructive pulmonary disease. Can J Neurol Sci 2008;35(3):352–7.

44. Taylor-Gjevre RM, Gjevre JA, Nair B, et al. Hypersomnolence and sleep disorders in a rheumatic disease patient population. J Clin Rheumatol 2010; 16(6):255–61.

45. Klingelhoefer L, Cova I, Gupta S, et al. A review of current treatment strategies for restless legs syndrome (Willis–Ekbom disease). Clin Med 2014; 14(5):520–4.

46. Milligan SA, Chesson AL Jr. Restless legs syndrome in the older adult. Drugs Aging 2002;19(10):741–51.

47. O'Keeffe ST. Secondary causes of restless legs syndrome in older people. Age Ageing 2005;34(4): 349–52.

48. O'Keeffe ST, Gavin K, Lavan JN. Iron status and restless legs syndrome in the elderly. Age Ageing 1994; 23(3):200–3.

49. Quinn C, Uzbeck M, Saleem I, et al. Iron status and chronic kidney disease predict restless legs syndrome in an older hospital population. Sleep Med 2011;12(3):295–301.

50. Fairweather-Tait SJ, Wawer AA, Gillings R, et al. Iron status in the elderly. Mech Ageing Dev 2014;136–137:22–8.

51. O'Keeffe ST. Iron deficiency with normal ferritin levels in restless legs syndrome. Sleep Med 2005; 6(3):281–2.

52. Araujo SM, de Bruin VM, Nepomuceno LA, et al. Restless legs syndrome in end-stage renal disease: clinical characteristics and associated comorbidities. Sleep Med 2010;11(8):785–90.

53. Gigli G. Restless legs syndrome in end-stage renal disease. Sleep Med 2004;5(3):309–15.

54. Mucsi I, Molnar MZ, Ambrus C, et al. Restless legs syndrome, insomnia and quality of life in patients on maintenance dialysis. Nephrol Dial Transplant 2005;20(3):571–7.

55. Giannaki CD, Hadjigeorgiou GM, Karatzaferi C, et al. Epidemiology, impact, and treatment options of restless legs syndrome in end-stage renal disease patients: an evidence-based review. Kidney Int 2014;85(6):1275–82.

56. Pistacchi M, Gioulis M, Contin F, et al. Sleep disturbance and cognitive disorder: epidemiological analysis in a cohort of 263 patients. Neurol Sci 2014; 35(12):1955–62.

57. Vos SJB, Verhey F, Frölich L, et al. Prevalence and prognosis of Alzheimer's disease at the mild cognitive impairment stage. Brain 2015;138(Pt 5): 1327–38.

58. Kim S-S, Oh KM, Richards K. Sleep disturbance, nocturnal agitation behaviors, and medical comorbidity in older adults with dementia: relationship to reported caregiver burden. Res Gerontol Nurs 2014;7(5):206–14.

59. Talarico G, Canevelli M, Tosto G, et al. Restless legs syndrome in a group of patients with Alzheimer's disease. Am J Alzheimers Dis Other Demen 2013; 28(2):165–70.

60. Mitchell RA, Herrmann N, Lanctôt KL. The role of dopamine in symptoms and treatment of apathy in Alzheimer's disease. CNS Neurosci Ther 2011; 17(5):411–27.

61. Pritchard AL, Pritchard CW, Bentham P, et al. Investigation of the role of the dopamine transporter in susceptibility to behavioural and psychological symptoms of patients with probable Alzheimer's disease. Dement Geriatr Cogn Disord 2008;26(3): 257–60.

62. Brindani F, Vitetta F, Gemignani F. Restless legs syndrome: differential diagnosis and management with pramipexole. Clin Interv Aging 2009;4:305.

63. Rose KM, Beck C, Tsai P-F, et al. Sleep disturbances and nocturnal agitation behaviors in older adults with dementia. Sleep 2011;34(6):779–86.

64. Allen RP, Bharmal M, Calloway M. Prevalence and disease burden of primary restless legs syndrome: results of a general population survey in the United States. Mov Disord 2011;26(1):114–20.

65. Lee HB, Ramsey CM, Spira AP, et al. Comparison of cognitive functioning among individuals with treated restless legs syndrome (RLS), untreated RLS, and no RLS. J Neuropsychiatry Clin Neurosci 2014; 26(1):87–91.

66. Szentkiralyi A, Völzke H, Hoffmann W, et al. The relationship between depressive symptoms and restless legs syndrome in two prospective cohort studies. Psychosom Med 2013;75(4):359–65.

67. Richards K, Shue VM, Beck CK, et al. Restless legs syndrome risk factors, behaviors, and diagnoses in persons with early to moderate dementia and sleep disturbance. Behav Sleep Med 2010;8(1):48–61.

Restless Leg Syndrome in Neurologic and Medical Disorders

 CrossMark

Nadir Askenasy, MD, PhD[a], Jean-Jacques Askenasy, MD, PhD[b],*

KEYWORDS

- Restless leg syndrome • Leg quietness homeostasis • Neurotransmitters • Motor unit potentials
- Flip-flop switch

KEY POINTS

- RLS is caused by imbalanced activity of neurotransmitters associated with a variety of physiologic and pathologic conditions.
- Leg quiescence homeostasis (LQH) reflects variable conditions of sustained muscle inactivity during sleep and wakefulness.
- Perturbed neurotransmitter activity occurs under variable LQH steady states.
- Flip-flop switch model of the sleep-wake cycle may be applied to rest and restless situations.

INTRODUCTION

Thomas Willis originally described in the seventeenth century "the diseased are no more able to sleep, than if they were in a place of the greatest torture." This description was rediscovered and termed restless leg syndrome (RLS) in the mid-twentieth century by Ekbom.[1] Diagnostic criteria for this prevalent syndrome elaborated in a consensus meeting in 2002[2] are being continuously revised considering that RLS is persistently underdiagnosed.[3,4] RLS is associated with general risk factors including female gender, pregnancy, lower socioeconomic status, poor health, elderly age, and positive family history of RLS.[5–9]

Primary RLS includes idiopathic disease of unknown cause and familial disease with genetic predisposition often associated with mutations in chromosomes 2p, 9p, 12q, 14q, 16p, and 20p.[10,11] The association of RLS with a variety of diseases and disorders is evidence of involvement of multiple factors in the pathophysiology of this syndrome. Outstanding is the interesting incidence of RLS in the last trimester of pregnancy persisting for several months after delivery, which is not a pathologic condition.[4]

ASSOCIATED DISORDERS

RLS is associated with a variety of neurologic disorders of various etiologies,[12,13] including peripheral neuropathy[14,15]; cerebrovascular disorders, headaches and particularly migraine[16]; persistent anxiety[17]; autoimmune disorders affecting the nervous system; radiculopathies[18]; movement disorders; and psychiatric disorders.[7–9] Despite the association between RLS and Parkinson disease,[8,19–21] a clear causal association has not yet been determined,[21] as with other neurodegenerative disorders.[22] Although a summary of 32 epidemiologic studies found that idiopathic RLS is often associated with comorbid factors, such as mood disorders and insomnia,[23] there is no apparent relationship between the incidence and severity of RLS and comorbid factors, such as anxiety, depression, and pain in Parkinson disease.[24]

The authors have no conflict of interest to declare.
[a] Frankel Laboratory, Petach Tikva, Israel; [b] Department of Neurology, Sackler Medical School, Tel-Aviv University, Tel Aviv 69978, Israel
* Corresponding author.
E-mail address: ajean@post.tau.ac.il

Obstructive sleep apnea is often associated with increased incidence of periodic limb movements (PLM)[25] and RLS; however, the latter does not correlate with hypersomnia characteristic of sleep-related breathing disorders.[26] RLS is variably responsive to obstructive sleep apnea treatment by continuous positive air pressure.[27] Other sleep disorders including hypersomnia, narcolepsy, and disrupted sleep are associated with increased RLS incidence, and are usually accompanied by elevated markers of inflammation.[9] The association of RLS with sleep deprivation and/or fragmentation may be caused by reduction in pain thresholds, modulated by a variety of neurotransmitters, particularly dysfunction of monoaminergic circuits.[28]

The association of RLS with autoimmune disorders has been long recognized[29] with significant comorbidity of inflammation, intestinal bacterial overgrowth, iron deficiency, and peripheral neuropathy, suggesting an immunologic basis of secondary RLS.[30] Some studies found elevated inflammatory cytokines, most prominent interleukin-6 and tumor necrosis factor-α,[30] although other studies failed to observe such a correlation.[31] Autoimmune and inflammatory disorders include celiac[32]; Sjögren syndrome; rheumatoid arthritis[33,34]; systemic lupus erythematosus[30]; inflammatory bowel disease[35]; fibromyalgia[36]; and several less defined disorders often classified as musculoskeletal system and connective tissue disorders, such as osteoarthritis, polyarthropathies, disorders of muscle, ligament and fasciae, disorders of joints, and disorders of synovium, tendons, and bursa.[31,37,38] Noteworthy is the four-fold higher incidence of RLS in patients with multiple sclerosis than in the general population,[31,39] which is often associated with higher scores of disability,[40] primary progressive disease, and cervical spine lesions.[41]

The initial disorder associated with RLS has been anemia, particularly iron deficiency anemia,[1] although it is frequently encountered in other element deficiencies, such as folic acid.[42] It is possible that anemia *per se* is a predisposing factor, because RLS appears at increased incidence in patients with hereditary hemolytic anemias.[8,43] Likewise, anemia as a common symptom of iron and folate deficiencies may underlie the higher incidence of RLS in pregnancy.[44] However, the proposed mechanism predisposing to RLS is a decrease in cerebral iron concentrations,[45] which serves as a cofactor of tyrosine hydroxylase required for dopamine synthesis.[46] Relative iron deficiency in the brain may be caused by excessive hepatic synthesis of hepcidin under conditions of systemic inflammation.[31]

RLS is associated with several disorders causing decreased cerebral, spinal (cervical and lumbar), and peripheral blood flow.[47] These conditions are caused by several respiratory, cardiac, and vascular pathologies responsible for inadequate oxygenation or compromised peripheral circulation. Indeed, peripheral hypoxia and low oxygen pressure in resting and immobilized subjects is associated with the appearance of RLS symptoms.[48] First, RLS is prevalent in various respiratory conditions including asthma, emphysema, bronchiolitis,[38] and recipients of lung transplants,[49] and the incidence is as high as 50% during acute exacerbations of chronic obstructive lung disease.[50,51] Second, patients suffering from coronary artery disease and heart failure often experience RLS,[52] with questionable participation of sympathetic hyperactivity in PLM.[53] Third, peripheral vascular disease precipitates RLS. Afferent vascular insufficiency has been treated with external counterpulsation, achieving sustained amelioration of symptoms.[54] Peripheral vascular insufficiency may also be caused by impaired venous return, and RLS has been successfully treated in some cases by endovenous laser ablation.[55]

Acute and chronic renal failure[56] and various causes of uremia[13] are conditions associated with high incidence of neuromuscular disorders. Patients with uremia often experience RLS in association with sleep disorders, excessive daytime sleepiness, anxiety, and depression, although it is difficult to determine which are the primary causes and which are the secondary consequences.[57] Although persisting throughout extended periods of dialysis, RLS disappearance within several months after successful renal transplantation establishes a causal relationship to renal disorders and uremia.[58,59] Notably, uremia-associated RLS is rather refractory to treatment with dopamine agonists.[60]

Additional metabolic disorders associated with increased RLS incidence include diabetes,[7] obesity,[5] and variations in thyroid function (thyrotoxicosis and hypothyroidism) possibly by modulation of dopamine levels.[61]

Antidepressants provoke PLM[62] and case reposts disclose exacerbation or induction of RLS including tricyclic antidepressants, selective serotonin reuptake inhibitors, antihistamines, and lithium, along antipsychotic and antiepileptic agents.[63]

A HYPOTHESIS ON THE MECHANISM OF RESTLESS LEG SYNDROME

Interpretation of the multiple disorders associated with RLS points to iron deficiency and chronic inflammation as two major causes of decreased dopamine synthesis and function. Although increasing dopamine levels is one of the efficient treatments of RLS, dopamine analogues can also augment RLS.[63–65] As in most other disorders associated with impaired neurotransmiter activity, it is difficult to envision that steady state variations in dopamine concentrations and other signaling agents is the primary cause of this disorder. It is questioned, therefore, what is the pathophysiologic basis of this motor-sensory syndrome.

The hypothesis presented here states that RLS is triggered by sudden changes in the activities of one or several neurotransmitters at selected sites within the brain superposed on disturbed neural circuits. A better-defined physiologic situation of such neuromodulation is a coordinated hypothalamic switch in neurotransmitter activities during arousal: a group of neurotransmitters found at lowest levels (nadir) suddenly rise to highest levels (zenith) within circuits linking the brainstem reticular formation and basal ganglia.[66] Reciprocal connections between these sites act as a flip-flop switch of activation through removal of inhibition as a positive feedback loop. Most prominent modulation of neurotransmitters during arousal includes norepinephrine, dopamine, hypocretin, and glutamate in the thalamus and sriatum.[66]

The flip-flop model relates to the interplay between neurotransmitters as an explanation of the sudden change in phase between sleep and wakefulness, extended to provide a basis for transition to rapid eye movement sleep (**Fig. 1**).[67] Variations include catecholamines, acetylcholine, histamine, metabotropic glutamate receptor, adenosine receptor, corticotropin-releasing hormone, thyrotropin-releasing hormone, neuropeptide Y, ghrelin, leptin, glucose, melanin-concentrating hormone, cortistatin, and hypocretin. These systems operate simultaneously at multiple topographic areas in the brainstem, hypothalamus, limbic system, and cortical activator system (**Fig. 2**). The delicate interplay between cholinergic and monoaminergic components of the brainstem and basal forebrain nuclei provoke sudden arousal. Such synchronized activity along projections to selected cortical areas may elicit motor activity and the sensory "urge to move."

Muscle activity is suppressed during sleep and wakeful relaxation, independent of tonus and the number of sporadic motor unit potentials that can be detected by high speed electromyography.[68] The conceived way to describe this phenomenon is leg (limb) quietness homeostasis (LQH), the last term relating to the relative state of quietness in reference to tonus, spontaneous motor unit

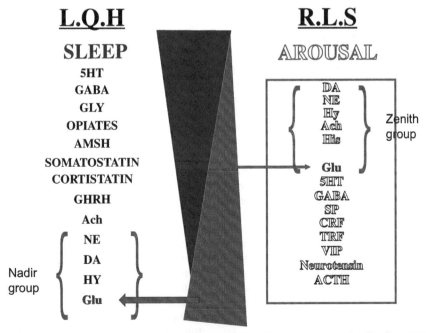

Fig. 1. Arousal is a complex phenomenon involving neurotransmitters common to the flip-flop switch of wake-sleep. 5HT, 5-hydroxytryptamine; Ach, acetylcholine; ACTH, adrenocorticotropic hormone; AMSH, associated molecule with SH3 domain; CRF, corticotropin-releasing factor; DA, dopamine; GABA, γ-aminobutyric acid; GHRH, growth hormone–releasing hormone; Glu, glutamate; GLY, glycine; His, histamine; Hy, hypocretine; LQH, leg quietness homeostasis; NE, norepinephrine; RLS, restless leg syndrome; SP, substance P; TRF, thyrotropin-releasing factor; VIP, vasoactive intestinal polypeptide.

Hypothesis

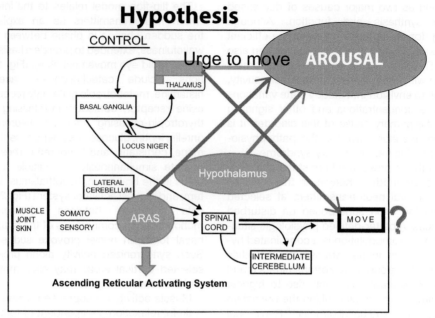

Fig. 2. Hypothesized initiation of RLS as a conscious event of uncontrolled urge to move. The zenith constellation of neurotransmitters provokes arousal, the thalamic sensation of "urge to move," and the activation of the thalamobasal ganglia circuits responsible for waking.

activity, the stages of sleep, and the degrees of wakeful relaxation. LQH is in fact terminated by arousal, with transition of several neurotransmitters from nadir to zenith activities. Possibly, a similar delicate balance in constellation of neurotransmitters that modulates LQH during arousal also provokes RLS. This flip-flop model suggests analogy in equilibrium of rest-restless leg and the sleep-wakefulness switch. Basically, sudden changes in neurotransmitters may trigger RLS and/or associated PLM phenomena, depending on the ascending reticular system, thalamus, and muscle activity during wakefulness and sleep. The mathematical interpretation of the switch model assumes exponential variations in function of monoaminergic cells, although it is not fully accounted for as the cause of these variations.[69,70] In the case of neuromuscular activity it is easier to adopt models of spontaneous excitation caused by spontaneous changes in gradients to reach activity thresholds, as detected in sleep electromyography.[68] However, the analogy of a flip-flop switch in LQH may involve complex circuits of several neurotransmitters operating at distinct sites and synchronized through positive feedback disinhibition.

INTERPRETATION OF THE PROPOSED MECHANISM

There are several considerations supporting the proposed model of RLS. First, RLS is closely associated with PLM at a comorbidity rate of 80%,[2,71,72] which is also present during daytime in patients with severe RLS.[73] PML involves synchronized motor activity of one limb, predominantly legs,[74] associated with a variety of sleep disorders that partially overlap with RLS. Notably, RLS correlates best with PLM-associated arousals rather than PLM severity[75,76] consistent with the relationship of this disorder to sleep fragmentation and deprivation.[28]

Second, the morphology of basal nuclei revealed no gross abnormalities in structure, no degenerative features, and quite stable dopamine activities in patients with RLS.[77] Severity of both RLS and PLM relate to higher γ-aminobutyric acid levels in the thalamus and lower levels in the cerebellum, as determined by localized magnetic resonance spectroscopy.[78] Similar reduced γ-aminobutyric acid levels were observed by PET measurements in patients suffering from Tourette syndrome, a compulsive movement disorder.[79] Other studies detected high thalamic levels of glutamate[80] and reduced N-acetyl aspartate in medial thalamus[81] in patients with RLS.

Third, the levels of neurotransmitters are not the only determinant of pathologic motion. For example, reduced levels of dopamine[34,46] are compensated by elevated levels of the cognate receptors.[82] Imaging studies showed decreased striatal dopamine-binding capacity, which may be caused either by lower numbers and/or affinity of the D_2 receptors, or rather increased synaptic dopamine levels and concurrent feedback reduction in receptor propensity.[83] Other studies found no significant variations in D_2 receptors in patients with RLS with and without dopamine therapy, emphasizing again the limitations of modulation of dopamine within the striatum by exogenous supplementation.[84]

Fourth, communication between the reticular nuclei in the brainstem with the thalamus, striatum, and cortical projections during arousal are in connotation with the conscious nature of RLS, as exemplified by enhanced neural activity in the anterior cingulate cortex.[77] The circadian variations with peak occurrence in late evening[85,86] and the disturbed circadian rhythms of dopamine metabolism and activity associated with RLS[72] point to a functional rather than a structural or morphologic basis for RLS pathology. Even if the primary pathology causing RLS is at the peripheral level (ie, radiculopathy, impaired blood flow and oxygenation), retrograde projection of neural circuits must be involved to create the extreme discomfort accompanying this disorder. Accordingly, RLS is often associated with mechanical and functional disturbance of the proprioceptive tracts.[87]

Fifth, dopamine and dopamine receptor analogues generally alleviate symptoms to the extent that these agents can be used to test the RLS diagnosis.[88] In addition, symptomatic relief may be achieved with antiepileptic agents, opioids, and benzodiazepines.[89–91] Augmentation of RLS by dopaminergic and other agents[63–65] occurs usually after prolonged administration,[89] suggesting that pathogenic imbalance persists in new steady state activities of these neurotransmitters. Muscle quietness is similarly disturbed either by administration or withdrawal of antidopaminergic, antihistaminic, antidepressant, antipsychotic, and anticonvulsant agents, consistent with the concept that oscillations in neuromodulation are in fact involved in the mechanism of RLS.

SUMMARY

Adopting the flip-flop switch model of sleep-wake states, RLS is proposed to be mediated by sudden changes in neurotransmitter activities in key ganglia, which may be the primary cause triggering RLS or involve secondary circuits. Such neuromodulatory variations may occur in health and disease, under a variety of steady state configurations of activities of neurotransmitters, their receptors, and the baseline activity of the involved nuclei. Therefore, it is proposed to use the term LQH to integrate the overall baseline conditions

of the system, which may be perturbed in many ways to elicit conscious urge and motor activity. RLS is therefore a functional perturbation without structural and morphologic abnormalities, which is transient, reversible, and recurrent under a variety of steady states.

REFERENCES

1. Ekbom KA. Restless legs: a clinical study. Acta Med Scand 1945;158(Suppl):121–2.
2. Allen RP, Picchiettib D, Heningc WA, et al. Restless legs syndrome: diagnostic criteria, special considerations, and epidemiology. Sleep Med 2003;4:101–19.
3. Allen RP, Picchietti RP, Garcia-Borreguero D, et al, International Restless Legs Syndrome Study Group. Restless legs syndrome/Willis-Ekbom disease diagnostic criteria: updated International Restless Legs Syndrome Study Group (IRLSSG) consensus criteria—history, rationale, description, and significance. Sleep Med 2014;15:860–73.
4. Picchietti DL, Hensley JG, Bainbridge JL, et al, International Restless Legs Syndrome Study Group (IRLSSG). Consensus clinical practice guidelines for the diagnosis and treatment of restless legs syndrome/Willis-Ekbom disease during pregnancy and lactation. Sleep Med Rev 2015;22:64–77.
5. Phillips B, Young T, Finn L, et al. Epidemiology of restless legs symptoms in adults. Arch Intern Med 2000;160:2137–41.
6. Barrière G, Cazalets JR, Bioulac B, et al. The restless legs syndrome. Prog Neurobiol 2005;77:139–65.
7. Ohayon MM, O'Hara R, Vitiello MV. Epidemiology of restless legs syndrome: a synthesis of the literature. Sleep Med Rev 2012;16:283–95.
8. Yeh P, Walters AS, Tsuang JW. Restless legs syndrome: a comprehensive overview on its epidemiology, risk factors, and treatment. Sleep Breath 2012;16:987–1007.
9. Becker PM, Novak M. Diagnosis, comorbidities, and management of restless legs syndrome. Curr Med Res Opin 2014;30:1441–60.
10. Winkelmann J, Muller-Myhsok B, Wittchen HU, et al. Complex segregation analysis of restless legs syndrome provides evidence for an autosomal dominant mode of inheritance in early age at onset families. Ann Neurol 2002;52:297–302.
11. Stefansson H, Rye DB, Hicks A, et al. A genetic risk factor for periodic limb movements in sleep. N Engl J Med 2007;357:639–47.
12. Odin P, Mrowka M, Shing M. Restless legs syndrome. Eur J Neurol 2002;9(Suppl 3):59–67.
13. Sethi KD, Mehta SH. A clinical primer on restless legs syndrome: what we know, and what we don't know. Am J Manag Care 2012;18(Suppl 5):S83–8.

14. Rutkove SB, Matheson JK, Logigian EL. Restless legs syndrome in patients with polyneuropathy. Muscle Nerve 1996;19:670–2.

15. Jacome DE. Blepharoclonus, pseudoasterixis, and restless feet. Am J Med Sci 2001;322:137–40.

16. Schürks M, Winter A, Berger K, et al. Migraine and restless legs syndrome: a systematic review. Cephalalgia 2014;34:777–94.

17. d'Onofrio F, Bussone G, Cologno D, et al. Restless legs syndrome and primary headaches: a clinical study. Neurol Sci 2008;29(Suppl 1):S169–72.

18. Walters AS, Wagner M, Hening WA. Periodic limb movements as the initial manifestation of restless legs syndrome triggered by lumbosacral radiculopathy. Sleep 1996;19:825–6.

19. Askenasy JJ. Approaching disturbed sleep in late Parkinson's disease: first step toward a proposal for a revised UPDRS. Parkinsonism Relat Disord 2001;8:123–31.

20. Gao X, Schwarzschild MA, O'Reilly EJ, et al. Restless legs syndrome and Parkinson's disease in men. Mov Disord 2010;25:2654–7.

21. Möller JC, Unger M, Stiasny-Kolster K, et al. Restless legs syndrome (RLS) and Parkinson's disease (PD)-related disorders or different entities? J Neurol Sci 2010;289:135–7.

22. Iranzo A, Comella CL, Santamaria J, et al. Restless legs syndrome in Parkinson's disease and other neurodegenerative diseases of the central nervous system. Mov Disord 2007;22(Suppl 18):S424–30.

23. Becker PM, Sharon D. Mood disorders in restless legs syndrome (Willis-Ekbom disease). J Clin Psychiatry 2014l;75:e679–94.

24. Rana AQ, Qureshi AR, Rahman L, et al. Association of restless legs syndrome, pain, and mood disorders in Parkinson's disease. Int J Neurosci 2014;3:1–13.

25. Warnes H, Dinner DS, Kotagal P, et al. Periodic limb movements and sleep apnoea. J Sleep Res 1993;2:38–44.

26. Roux FJ. Restless legs syndrome: impact on sleep-related breathing disorders. Respirology 2013;18:238–45.

27. Gharagozlou P, Seyffert M, Santos R, et al. Rhythmic movement disorder associated with respiratory arousals and improved by CPAP titration in a patient with restless legs syndrome and sleep apnea. Sleep Med 2009;10:501–3.

28. Goulart LI, Delgado Rodrigues RN, Prieto Peres MF. Restless legs syndrome and pain disorders: what's in common? Curr Pain Headache Rep 2014;18:461.

29. Devins GM, Edworthy SM, Paul LC, et al. Restless sleep, illness intrusiveness, and depressive symptoms in three chronic illness conditions: rheumatoid arthritis, end-stage renal disease, and multiple sclerosis. J Psychosom Res 1993;37:163–70.

30. Hassan N, Pineau CA, Clarke AE, et al. Systemic lupus and risk of restless legs syndrome. J Rheumatol 2011;38:874–6.

31. Weinstock LB, Walters AS, Paueksakon P. Restless legs syndrome: theoretical roles of inflammatory and immune mechanisms. Sleep Med Rev 2012;16:341–54.

32. Moccia M, Pellecchia MT, Erro R, et al. Restless legs syndrome is a common feature of adult celiac disease. Mov Disord 2010;25:877–81.

33. Reynolds G, Blake DR, Pall HS, et al. Restless leg syndrome and rheumatoid arthritis. Br Med J (Clin Res Ed) 1986;292:659–60.

34. Hening WA, Caivano CK. Restless legs syndrome: a common disorder in patients with rheumatologic conditions. Semin Arthritis Rheum 2008;38:55–62.

35. Ohman L, Simren M. Pathogenesis of IBS: role of inflammation, immunity and neuroimmune interactions. Nat Rev Gastroenterol Hepatol 2010;7:163–73.

36. Stehlik R, Arvidsson L, Ulfberg J. Restless legs syndrome is common among female patients with fibromyalgia. Eur Neurol 2009;61:107–11.

37. Taylor-Gjevre RM, Gjevre JA, Skomro R, et al. Restless legs syndrome in a rheumatoid arthritis patient cohort. J Clin Rheumatol 2009;15:12–5.

38. Banno K, Delaive K, Walld R, et al. Restless legs syndrome in 218 patients: associated disorders. Sleep Med 2000;1:221–9.

39. Schürks M, Bussfeld P. Multiple sclerosis and restless legs syndrome: a systematic review and meta-analysis. Eur J Neurol 2013;20:605–15.

40. Sieminski M, Losy J, Partinen M. Restless legs syndrome in multiple sclerosis. Sleep Med Rev 2015;22:15–22.

41. Manconi M, Rocca MA, Ferini-Strambi L, et al. Restless legs syndrome is a common finding in multiple sclerosis and correlates with cervical cord damage. Mult Scler 2008;14:86–93.

42. Patrick LR. Restless legs syndrome: pathophysiology and the role of iron and folate. Altern Med Rev 2007;12:101–12.

43. Salas RE, Gamaldo CE, Allen RP. Update in restless legs syndrome. Curr Opin Neurol 2010;23:401–6.

44. Lee KA, Zaffke ME, Baratte-Beebe K. Restless legs syndrome and sleep disturbance during pregnancy: the role of folate and iron. J Womens Health Gend Based Med 2001;10:335–41.

45. Earley CJ, Allen RP, Beard JL, et al. Insight into the pathophysiology of restless legs syndrome. J Neurosci Res 2000;62:623–8.

46. Allen R. Dopamine and iron in the pathophysiology of restless legs syndrome (RLS). Sleep Med 2004;5:385–91.

47. Coccagna G, Vetrugno R, Lombardi C, et al. Restless legs syndrome: an historical note. Sleep Med 2004;5:279–83.

48. Salminen AV, Rimpilä V, Polo O. Peripheral hypoxia in restless legs syndrome (Willis-Ekbom disease). Neurology 2014;82:1856–61.

49. Minai OA, Golish JA, Yataco JC, et al. Restless legs syndrome in lung transplant recipients. J Heart Lung Transplant 2007;26:24–9.

50. Spillane JD. Restless legs syndrome in chronic pulmonary disease. Br Med J 1970;4:796–8.

51. Cavalcante AG, de Bruin PF, de Bruin VM, et al. Restless legs syndrome, sleep impairment, and fatigue in chronic obstructive pulmonary disease. Sleep Med 2012;13:842–7.

52. Winkelman JW, Shahar E, Sharief I, et al. Association of restless legs syndrome and cardiovascular disease in the Sleep Heart Health Study. Neurology 2008;70:35–42.

53. Walters AS, Rye DB. Review of the relationship of restless legs syndrome and periodic limb movements in sleep to hypertension, heart disease, and stroke. Sleep 2009;32:589–97.

54. Rajaram SS, Shanahan J, Ash C, et al. Enhanced external counter pulsation (EECP) as a novel treatment for restless legs syndrome (RLS): a preliminary test of the vascular neurologic hypothesis for RLS. Sleep Med 2005;6:101–6.

55. Hayes CA, Kingsley JR, Hamby KR, et al. The effect of endovenous laser ablation on restless legs syndrome. Phlebology 2008;23:112–7.

56. Winkelman JW, Chertow GM, Lazarus JM. Restless legs syndrome in end-stage renal disease. Am J Kidney Dis 1996;28:372–8.

57. Gigli GL, Adorati M, Dolso P, et al. Restless legs syndrome in end-stage renal disease. Sleep Med 2004;5:309–15.

58. Winkelmann J, Stautner A, Samtleben W, et al. Long-term course of restless legs syndrome in dialysis patients after kidney transplantation. Mov Disord 2002;17:1072–6.

59. Kavanagh D, Siddiqui S, Geddes CC. Restless legs syndrome in patients on dialysis. Am J Kidney Dis 2004;43:763–71.

60. Enomoto M, Inoue Y, Namba K, et al. Clinical characteristics of restless legs syndrome in end-stage renal failure and idiopathic RLS patients. Mov Disord 2008;23:811–6.

61. Pereira JC Jr, Pradella-Hallinan M, Lins Pessoa HD. Imbalance between thyroid hormones and dopaminergic system might be central to the pathophysiology of restless legs syndrome: a hypothesis. Clinics (Sao Paulo) 2010;65:547–54.

62. Fulda S, Kloiber S, Dose T, et al. Mirtazapine provokes periodic leg movements during sleep in young healthy men. Sleep 2013;36:661–9.

63. Hoque R, Chesson AL Jr. Pharmacologically induced/exacerbated restless legs syndrome, periodic limb movements of sleep, and REM behavior disorder/REM sleep without atonia: literature review, qualitative scoring, and comparative analysis. J Clin Sleep Med 2010;6:79–83.

64. Allen RP, Earley CJ. Augmentation of the restless legs syndrome with carbidopa/levodopa. Sleep 1996;19:205–13.

65. Garcia-Borreguero D, Williams AM. Dopaminergic augmentation of restless legs syndrome. Sleep Med Rev 2010;14:339–46.

66. Saper CB, Chou TC, Scammell TE. The sleep switch: hypothalamic control of sleep and wakefulness. Trends Neurosci 2001;24:726–31.

67. Lu J, Sherman D, Devor M, et al. A putative flip–flop switch for control of rem sleep. Nature 2006;441:589–94.

68. Askenasy JJ, Yahr MD. Different laws govern motor activity in sleep than in wakefulness. J Neural Transm Gen Sect 1990;79:103–11.

69. Phillips AJ, Robinson PA. A quantitative model of sleep-wake dynamics based on the physiology of the brainstem ascending arousal system. J Biol Rhythms 2007;22:167–79.

70. Rempe MJ, Best J, Terman D. A mathematical model of the sleep/wake cycle. J Math Biol 2010;60:615–44.

71. Trenkwalder C, Walters AS, Hening WA. Periodic limb movements and restless legs syndrome. Neurol Clin 1996;14:629–50.

72. Vetrugno R, Provini F, Montagna P. Restless legs syndrome and periodic limb movements. Rev Neurol Dis 2006;3:61–70.

73. Chabli A, Michaud M, Montplaisir J. Periodic arm movements in patients with the restless legs syndrome. Eur Neurol 2000;44:133–8.

74. Coleman RM, Pollak CP, Weitzman ED. Periodic movements in sleep (nocturnal myoclonus): relation to sleep disorders. Ann Neurol 1980;8:416–21.

75. Wetter TC, Collado-Seidel V, Oertel H, et al. Endocrine rhythms in patients with restless legs syndrome. J Neurol 2002;249:146–51.

76. Hornyak M, Hundemer HP, Quail D, et al. Relationship of periodic leg movements and severity of restless legs syndrome: a study in unmedicated and medicated patients. Clin Neurophysiol 2007;118:1532–7.

77. Earley CJ, Allen RP, Connor JR, et al. The dopaminergic neurons of the A11 system in RLS autopsy brains appear normal. Sleep Med 2009;10:1155–7.

78. Winkelman JW, Schoerning L, Platt S, et al. Restless legs syndrome and central nervous system gamma-aminobutyric acid: preliminary associations with periodic limb movements in sleep and restless leg syndrome symptom severity. Sleep Med 2014;15:1225–30.

79. Lerner A, Bagic A, Simmons JM, et al. Widespread abnormality of the gamma-aminobutyric acid-ergic system in Tourette syndrome. Brain 2012;135:1926–36.

80. Allen RP, Barker PB, Horská A, et al. Thalamic gluta-mate/glutamine in restless legs syndrome. Neurology 2013;80:2028–34.

81. Rizzo G, Tonon C, Testa C, et al. Abnormal medial thalamic metabolism in patients with idiopathic rest-less legs syndrome. Brain 2012;135:3712–20.

82. Cervenka S, Palhagen SE, Comley RA, et al. Sup-port for dopaminergic hypoactivity in restless legs syndrome: a PET study on D2-receptor binding. Brain 2006;129:2017–28.

83. Michaud M, Soucy JP, Chabli A, et al. SPECT imag-ing of striatal pre- and postsynaptic dopaminergic status in restless legs syndrome with periodic leg movements in sleep. J Neurol 2002;249:164–70.

84. Eisensehr I, Wetter TC, Linke R, et al. Normal IPT and IBZM SPECT in drug-naive and levodopa-treated idiopathic restless legs syndrome. Neurology 2001; 57:1307–9.

85. Trenkwalder C, Hening WA, Walters AS, et al. Circa-dian rhythm of periodic limb movements and sensory symptoms of restless legs syndrome. Mov Disord 1999;14:102–10.

86. Hening W. The clinical neurophysiology of the rest-less legs syndrome and periodic limb movements. I. Diagnosis, assessment, and characterization. Clin Neurophysiol 2004;115:1965–74.

87. Stiasny-Kolster K, Trenkwalder C, Fogel W, et al. Restless legs syndrome: new insights into clinical characteristics, pathophysiology, and treatment op-tions. J Neurol 2004;251(Suppl 6):VI/39–43.

88. Stiasny-Kolster K, Kohnen R, Carsten MJ, et al. Vali-dation of the "L-DOPA test" for diagnosis of restless legs syndrome. Mov Disord 2006;21:1333–9.

89. Comella CL. Restless legs syndrome: treatment with dopaminergic agents. Neurology 2002;58(Suppl 1): S87–92.

90. Thorpy M. New paradigms in the treatment of rest-less legs syndrome. Neurology 2005;64:S28–33.

91. Comella CL. Treatment of restless legs syndrome. Neurotherapeutics 2014;11:177–87.

Restless Legs Syndrome and Psychiatric Disorders

Susan Mackie, MD[a],*, John W. Winkelman, MD, PhD[b,c]

KEYWORDS

- Restless legs syndrome • Psychiatric disorders • Depression • Epidemiology
- Antidepressants • Psychopharmacology

KEY POINTS

- There are strong epidemiologic ties between restless legs syndrome (RLS) and a wide array of psychiatric conditions.
- Although the mechanism of this association is not fully understood, there are likely bidirectional cause-and-effect relationships.
- Appreciation of psychiatric comorbidity is an essential component of the treatment of RLS.
- Clinicians should be prepared to facilitate appropriate psychiatric treatment and consider the complex interactions between psychiatric medications, RLS medications, and the clinical course of both illnesses.

COMORBIDITY BETWEEN PSYCHIATRIC DISORDERS AND RESTLESS LEGS SYNDROME

The original description of restless legs syndrome (RLS) as *anxietas tibiarum* reflected an early understanding of the close association between RLS, psychological distress, and anxiety disorders. Recent studies of these associations estimate a lifetime prevalence of any psychiatric disorder meeting *Diagnostic and Statistical Manual of Mental Disorders* (DSM) criteria of 37% in individuals with RLS compared with 15% of persons without RLS.[1] In addition, those without threshold psychiatric conditions also frequently suffer from psychological distress and functional impairment.

The causal relationship between RLS and psychiatric disorders is likely bidirectional. Sleep disturbance, discomfort associated with leg dysesthesias, and anticipation of symptoms may all contribute to this distress and predispose patients to psychiatric disorders. Conversely, psychiatric conditions may heighten awareness of RLS symptoms and prolong waking periods at night when symptoms are prominent, and medications used to treat depression and anxiety disorders can worsen RLS.

RESTLESS LEGS SYNDROME AND SUBCLINICAL PSYCHOLOGICAL DISTRESS

Patients with RLS experience psychological distress and diminished quality of life. Epidemiologic studies indicate increased rates of self-reported social isolation, decreased libido, less frequent physical activity, and diminished self-assessment of overall mental health status.[2,3] In a recent observational study, an association with reduced quality of life was present among both treated and untreated RLS patients.[4] These investigators used the SCL-90-R Global Severity index, an indicator of generalized functional decrement, to compare RLS patients with a control sample

a Department of Internal Medicine, Brigham and Women's Hospital, Harvard Medical School, 75 Francis Street, Boston, MA 02115, USA; b Sleep Disorders Clinical Research Program, Department of Psychiatry, Massachusetts General Hospital, Harvard Medical School, 1 Bowdoin Square, 9th floor, Boston, MA 02114, USA; c Sleep Disorders Clinical Research Program, Department of Neurology, Massachusetts General Hospital, Harvard Medical School, 1 Bowdoin Square, 9th floor, Boston, MA 02114, USA
* Corresponding author.
E-mail address: semackie@partners.org

Sleep Med Clin 10 (2015) 351–357
http://dx.doi.org/10.1016/j.jsmc.2015.05.009

from the general population. The diagnosis of RLS was established by face-to-face interview. In their survey, RLS patients scored significantly worse on multiple subscales including somatization, compulsivity, depression, and anxiety. RLS severity was correlated with higher levels of psychological impairment. Although limited by its cross-sectional design, these findings suggest that the psychopathology present in RLS patients extends even to those who do not meet threshold criteria for a specific psychiatric disorder.

ANXIETY DISORDERS AND RESTLESS LEGS SYNDROME

Anxiety disorders occur at an increased prevalence among RLS patients compared with the general population. In one study by Winkelmann and colleagues,[5] 130 patients with RLS confirmed by a standardized diagnostic interview were compared with more than 2000 members of the community with other illnesses. RLS patients demonstrated a markedly increased prevalence of anxiety disorders. The strongest associations identified were between RLS and panic disorder (odds ratio [OR] = 4.7; 95% confidence interval [CI] 2.1–10.1) and generalized anxiety disorder (OR = 3.5; 95% CI 1.7–7.1).

The cause-and-effect relationship between RLS and anxiety disorders is likely complex and bidirectional, and the etiologic mechanisms are not well understood. There may be a shared neurobiological and genetic substrate that predisposes patients to both disorders, or it may be that one disorder has a causal role in precipitating the other. The aforementioned cross-sectional survey documented that patients reported that their RLS symptom onset occurred before the psychiatric disorder. Although there are other possible explanations, this suggests that the psychiatric disorder may be triggered by the RLS in at least some patients.

There are several plausible mechanisms by which RLS may precipitate or exacerbate anxiety disorders. Patients with RLS frequently experience anticipatory anxiety about the misery of their symptoms and lack of sleep, which may compound a predisposition to an anxiety disorder. In addition, RLS symptoms and the associated periodic leg movements of sleep frequently lead to inadequate total sleep time. Sleep deprivation increases sympathetic tone and increases state anxiety in normal volunteers.[6,7] Roy-Byrne and colleagues[8] have demonstrated that acute sleep deprivation is also a powerful trigger for panic attacks among patients with established panic disorder. Inadequate sleep may also play a role in

the development of panic disorder meeting DSM threshold criteria in some RLS patients who have a predisposition toward panic attacks. Also, as discussed later, medications commonly used to treat anxiety disorders may play a role in precipitating RLS.

DEPRESSION AND RESTLESS LEGS SYNDROME

Patients with RLS also have an increased risk of depressive disorders compared with the general population (for a review see Hornyak,[9] 2010). The lifetime prevalence of major depressive disorder (MDD) or dysthymia has been reported to be 36.9% in RLS patients compared with 15.2% in healthy controls, an OR of 2.9 (95% CI 1.5–4.4).[5] Similarly to anxiety disorders, most (77%) of those with comorbid MDD and RLS reported that RLS symptoms preceded depression. This directionality has been corroborated in one of the few longitudinal examinations of this issue. Using data obtained from more than 50,000 women in the Nurses' Health Study, Li and colleagues[10] found that those with RLS but no depression at baseline were more likely to develop subsequent depression at 6-year follow-up (relative risk [RR] = 1.66; 95% CI 1.18–2.35). This association remained significant after adjustment for lifestyle factors, chronic medical conditions, and sleep duration (RR = 1.5; CI: 1.1–2.1), indicating that sleep deprivation alone could not explain the association.

One of the difficulties in understanding this relationship is the diagnostic complexity attributable to the overlap in symptoms between patients with major depression and those with RLS. Patients with untreated or inadequately treated RLS are likely to report insomnia and nonrestorative sleep. This sleep disruption may also result in irritable mood, agitation, and decreased concentration. These symptoms may be mistaken for depression by the clinician not familiar with RLS symptoms. Conversely, there may be delayed recognition of MDD in patients with RLS if symptoms of depression are incorrectly attributed to the RLS. Key diagnostic indicators for the presence of depression include feelings of guilt and worthlessness, and anhedonia. These features generally should not be attributed solely to the sleep disorder. When there is diagnostic uncertainty, appropriate treatment of RLS (which usually responds rapidly to medications) should alleviate those symptoms that are secondary to the sleep disorder. In cases where symptoms persist after treatment, treatment of the psychiatric disorder is indicated.

THE IMPORTANCE OF MOOD AND ANXIETY DISORDERS IN THE TREATMENT OF RESTLESS LEGS SYNDROME

In addition to the increased risk of incident depression and anxiety disorders in RLS patients, both of these conditions have been demonstrated to predispose patients to a poor response to treatment of RLS. Godau and colleagues[11] performed a prospective observational assessment of 100 patients with idiopathic RLS, initiating guideline-based treatment for RLS in Germany.[1] The investigators found no statistically significant improvement in either International RLS (IRLS) or RLS Quality of Life (RLS-QoL) scores during the 12-month observation period. In a post hoc analysis stratifying patients according to the presence or absence of neuropsychiatric comorbidity (principally depression, anxiety, chronic pain, and somatoform disorders), those with such comorbidity (64% of the cohort) were found to have no improvement in IRLS or RLS-QoL across the study period, whereas those without neuropsychiatric conditions showed improvement according to both scales.

This study testifies to the importance of appreciating psychiatric comorbidity when treating RLS patients and when applying clinical trials data to patient care. The investigators suggest that the patients may not be able to fully separate RLS symptoms from other sources of suffering related to their psychiatric conditions, which are generally not affected by medications used to treat RLS. In addition, this frequent comorbidity may account for some of the discrepancies in outcome data between population-based studies such as this one. Whereas no improvement in RLS symptoms with treatment was found in this cohort, clinical trials, which generally exclude patients with comorbid psychiatric conditions, have demonstrated excellent efficacy of the same drugs. In clinical practice, many patients do have such comorbidity, and the clinician must be alert to the challenges of treatment in this group to serve their patients most effectively.

SCHIZOPHRENIA

There are few studies examining a possible association between untreated schizophrenia and RLS. However, the frequent use of medications with dopamine antagonist activity has led to several investigations regarding a possible increased risk of RLS among treated schizophrenia patients. In a study by Kang and colleagues,[12] 182 hospitalized schizophrenics were subjected to a structured interview for RLS.[2,3]

The observed prevalence of RLS was 21%, significantly increased in comparison with the control group ($P = .009$). The investigators performed an analysis adjusting for the presence of akathisia using an established scoring mechanism. The increased prevalence of RLS in the schizophrenia group remained significant, indicating that RLS in this group was independent of antipsychotic-induced akathisia.

In the schizophrenia study by Kang and colleagues,[12] the presence of RLS predicted more severe psychotic symptoms. However, the cumulative dose of antipsychotic medication was not associated with the presence of RLS. This finding suggests that although antipsychotics may precipitate RLS in susceptible individuals, an underlying predisposition, rather than the dose of medication, is the primary factor responsible for inducing RLS.

These findings led Jung and colleagues[13] to investigate whether there may be a genetic predisposition to antipsychotic-associated RLS.[4] These investigators compared schizophrenic patients on antipsychotic medications experiencing RLS with those without RLS, establishing the diagnosis by interview. Significant differences were found in the distribution of haplotypes in CLOCK genes between those with and without RLS. Further research is needed to determine whether genes known to have an association with primary RLS also predispose those on antipsychotics to the condition.

ATTENTION-DEFICIT/HYPERACTIVITY DISORDER

Given the shared phenotype of excessive motor activity, it is not surprising that there is evidence of misdiagnosis of RLS as attention-deficit/hyperactivity disorder (ADHD), particularly in the pediatric population.[5,14] Indeed, up to 72% of children finally diagnosed with RLS also carry a diagnosis of ADHD. Other data using more strict diagnostic criteria (Pullen criteria) found that 94 of 374 children identified with RLS also met DSM-IV criteria for ADHD.[6,7,15] Much of this overlap may be related to the diagnostic challenges of distinguishing these 2 disorders. Children may be unable to express RLS symptoms verbally, and motor hyperactivity attributable to RLS or associated sleep deprivation may be misunderstood as ADHD. It is not clear how much of the association between the 2 disorders in children is artifactual as a result of these diagnostic challenges. Although this likely explains a proportion of the overlap, shared pathophysiologic substrate may also contribute to a true association. As in the case of anxiety and mood disorders, both clinical diagnosis and interpretation of epidemiologic data should be undertaken with appreciation for these nuanced relationships.

Although ADHD is less common in adults, there are data indicating a link between RLS and adult ADHD. In one population-based study, the OR for RLS in individuals with ADHD compared with controls was 3.18 (95% CI 1.27–7.63) after adjusting for multiple confounding variables.[8,16] However, the association did not meet statistical significance after adjusting for the presence of sleep disturbance (OR = 2.02; 95% CI 0.82–4.92). This study was limited by the use of questionnaires, which may be unreliable for the diagnosis of RLS and for report of sleep time, an issue likely compounded by the aforementioned diagnostic subtleties.

PHARMACOLOGIC CONSIDERATIONS

The association between RLS and psychiatric disorders is complicated by the treatment of both with psychoactive medications (**Table 1**). Many of the agents used to treat each of these conditions have the potential to affect the other condition. This section addresses medications used to treat psychiatric disorders for which there is evidence of an exacerbating or alleviating effect on RLS symptoms, and discusses the potential psychiatric effects of various medications used to treat RLS.

Medications Used to Treat Psychiatric Conditions

Selective serotonin reuptake inhibitors (SSRIs) and serotonin norepinephrine reuptake inhibitors (SNRIs) are frequently used as first-line agents in the treatment of depression and anxiety disorders. Unfortunately, these medications have also been associated with an increased incidence of RLS. Most data on this association come from case reports, which have suggested that RLS symptoms

Table 1
The effect of psychiatric medications on RLS

Medication Class	Examples	Typical Psychiatric Indication	Likelihood of Exacerbating RLS
Selective serotonin reuptake inhibitors	Fluoxetine, citalopram, sertraline, paroxetine	Depression, anxiety	++
Serotonin norepinephrine reuptake inhibitors	Duloxetine, venlafaxine	Depression, anxiety	++
Norepinephrine dopamine reuptake inhibitor	Bupropion	Depression	–
Tricyclic antidepressants (except desipramine)	Nortriptyline, amitriptyline	Depression, anxiety	+
Tricyclic antidepressant	Desipramine	Depression, anxiety	0
Other	Trazodone	Insomnia, depression	+
Second-generation antipsychotics	Quetiapine, olazapine, risperidone	Schizophrenia, bipolar disorder	++
Second-generation antipsychotic (partial dopamine agonist)	Aripiprazole	Schizophrenia, bipolar disorder	+/–
Antihistamines	Diphenhydramine, hydroxyzine	Insomnia, anxiety	+++
Dopamine agonists	Pramipexole, ropinirole	Depression	– – –
Alkali metal	Lithium	Bipolar disorder	+/0
Benzodiazepines	Lorazepam, clonazepam, alprazolam	Anxiety disorders	–
Antiepileptics (except α2δ agents)	Topiramate, levetiracetam	Bipolar disorder	0
Antiepileptics: α2δ agents only	Gabapentin, pregabalin	Bipolar disorder	– – –

+(++), likely to cause RLS; 0, unknown or no effect; –(– –), may improve RLS.

may be triggered or exacerbated by fluoxetine, paroxetine, and venlafaxine. Ohayon and colleagues[17] found, in a population-based cross-sectional survey, that the use of an SSRI medication was a risk factor for RLS (OR = 3.11, 95% CI 1.66–5.79). However, these data were limited by their reliance on an automated telephone interview for the diagnosis of RLS. Rottach and colleagues[18] conducted a prospective study of patients initiating therapy with antidepressants including SSRIs, SNRIs, and mirtazapine (a noradrenergic and serotonergic antidepressant). In 9% of patients, RLS either emerged or worsened. Mirtazapine was associated with the highest frequency of RLS (28%). SSRI or SNRI medications were associated with a frequency ranging from 2% to 10%, with both classes averaging just below 5%. Randomized data from which to draw definitive conclusions about the association between SSRI/SNRIs and RLS are lacking, but these data and clinical experience commend awareness of this possibility and due caution when initiating these agents.

In contrast to SSRI/SNRIs, bupropion, a unique dopamine-norepinephrine reuptake inhibitor with efficacy to treat major depression, does not seem to worsen RLS and may actually be beneficial. Bayard and colleagues[19] performed a small, randomized, double-blind trial among 60 subjects with moderate to severe RLS. These investigators found a trend toward improvement in IRLS Study Group (IRLSSG) scores in the bupropion group compared with the controls, a difference that was statistically significant at 3 weeks (10.8-point improvement compared with 6.0 points in the placebo group; P = .016) but not at 6 weeks (P = .108). These data suggest that bupropion does not exacerbate RLS and may be preferable to serotonergic medications when treating depression in patients with RLS.

In addition to antidepressants, other classes of psychiatric medications also have notable effects on RLS symptoms. The atypical antipsychotics quetiapine, risperidone, and olanzapine have all been suggested as possible triggers for RLS symptoms, although most of these data are derived from uncontrolled case reports or series. On the other hand, aripiprazole, an atypical antipsychotic that has partial dopamine agonist activity, improved RLS symptoms in a few small case series.[20]

Medications Used to Treat Restless Legs Syndrome

Adverse psychiatric effects

Medications used to treat RLS also have the potential to affect primary psychiatric disorders,

and may occasionally precipitate psychiatric conditions in previously healthy individuals. Dopamine agonists, often used as first-line agents for RLS, have been associated with several psychiatric side effects. The most well-established of these is the emergence of impulse control disorders (ICD), which may include compulsive shopping, pathologic gambling, compulsive eating, hypersexuality, and punding (stereotyped repetitive actions such as sorting or manipulating objects). The estimated prevalence of ICDs among RLS patients on dopamine agonist treatment has varied from 5% to 17%.[21–24] In one of the few controlled studies on the topic, Cornelius and colleagues[21] found that RLS patients on dopaminergic treatment had a 17% prevalence of ICDs compared with 6% in a control group with obstructive sleep apnea (OSA) and 8% in a group of RLS patients not receiving dopamine agonists, a difference that was statistically significant only for the OSA control group. Factors that have been associated with increased numerical likelihood of developing ICDs on dopamine agonist include higher dose of dopamine agonist, young age at RLS onset, family history of gambling disorders, and female gender.[22] In the one controlled study mentioned, only the dose of pramipexole was statistically associated with increased ICD risk.[21] Further controlled data are needed to determine whether other predictors are valid.

Clinicians initiating treatment with dopamine agonists should warn patients (and, when feasible, their families) about the possibility of emergent ICDs. Because this complication can develop at any time during treatment, ongoing vigilance is required. Early identification of emerging compulsive habits can prompt a change in treatment and avoid potentially deleterious consequences (eg, in the case of compulsive spending/gambling).

Another risk of dopaminergic stimulation is precipitation of psychosis. Most of the research on this topic has been done in patients receiving dopamine agonists for Parkinson disease, who may have a disease-specific predisposition to psychosis. However, there is some evidence that RLS patients may also occasionally be susceptible to psychotic symptoms.[25–27] In particular, those with current psychosis should not be given a dopamine agonist, and caution should be exercised in those with a history of psychosis.

There has also been concern that dopaminergic stimulation may trigger mania in susceptible patients with clinical or subclinical bipolar disorder.[28] On the other hand, pramipexole has been used effectively for the treatment of bipolar depression in doses of 1 to 3 mg/d in at least 2 randomized controlled studies without significant increased switching.[29,30]

Regarding other drugs used to treat RLS, gabapentin and gabapentin enacarbil carry a theoretic increased risk of depression and, like other antiepileptic medications, carry a warning from the Food and Drug Administration (FDA) about suicide risk. Data on the topic are scarce, but the FDA reports 2 suicides and 3 additional cases of suicidal ideation in clinical trials with gabapentin enacarbil used for a variety of indications.[31] The FDA calculates an OR of 1.57 (95% CI 0.12–48) for the comparison of suicide risk on gabapentin versus placebo, but this CI is too wide to draw meaningful conclusions.

Possible psychiatric benefits

Despite these concerns about precipitating psychiatric disorder, dopamine agonists may also have beneficial effects on mood. Corrigan and colleagues[32] randomized 174 patients with major depression to fluoxetine, pramipexole, or placebo. Those subjects receiving pramipexole at the 1.0-mg or 5.0-mg doses had significant improvement in depression symptoms compared with the placebo group, an effect that was comparable with that of fluoxetine. The study was not powered to compare the 2 drugs statistically. It is notable that doses of pramipexole less than 1 mg, which are often used in the treatment of RLS, did not statistically improve mood.

Several studies have demonstrated improvements in depressive symptoms in patients with RLS given dopaminergic agonists. For example, Beneš and colleagues[33] found that RLS patients who also had at least mild depression showed significant improvement in depressive symptoms when ropinirole was used to treat their RLS. An investigation by Montagna and colleagues[34] evaluated a group of patients with RLS who also had mild to moderate depressive symptoms (Beck Depression Inventory [BDI] <28) and at least moderate RLS-related mood disturbance according to Item 10 of the IRLSSG scale. Patients treated with pramipexole showed a statistically significant ($P = .0199$) improvement in BDI compared with placebo. Because these study populations are similar to those frequently seen in the sleep clinic undergoing treatment of RLS, these data are encouraging, as they suggest that treatment with dopamine agonists may have benefits that go beyond the relief of restlessness.

SUMMARY

Clinicians treating RLS frequently encounter patients with comorbid psychiatric disorders. Although some forms of psychiatric pharmacotherapy may exacerbate RLS symptoms, many patients with RLS have a mental health problem that should be addressed with appropriate, directed treatment. Sleep clinicians should be comfortable screening patients for the presence of common psychiatric abnormality, initiating referral when appropriate, and collaborating with psychiatric providers to design a treatment plan that takes into account the complex interactions between RLS, psychiatric disorders, and the medications used to treat both conditions. Such complexity, when properly understood and applied, can provide substantial relief to patients suffering from the misery of both RLS and psychiatric illness.

REFERENCES

1. Lee HB, Hening WA, Allen RP, et al. Restless legs syndrome is associated with DSM-IV major depressive disorder and panic disorder in the community. J Neuropsychiatry Clin Neurosci 2008;20:101–5.
2. Ulfberg J, Nyström B, Carter N, et al. Prevalence of restless legs syndrome among men aged 18 to 64 years: an association with somatic disease and neuropsychiatric symptoms. Mov Disord 2001;16:1159–63.
3. Phillips B, Young T, Finn L, et al. Epidemiology of restless legs symptoms in adults. Arch Intern Med 2000;160:2137–41.
4. Scholz H, Beneš H, Happe S, et al. Psychological distress of patients suffering from restless legs syndrome: a cross-sectional study. Health Qual Life Outcomes 2011;9:73.
5. Winkelmann J, Prager M, Lieb R, et al. 'Anxietas tibiarum'. Depression and anxiety disorders in patients with restless legs syndrome. J Neurol 2005;252:67–71.
6. Klumpers UMH, Veltman DJ, van Tol MJ, et al. Neurophysiological effects of sleep deprivation in healthy adults, a pilot study. PLoS ONE 2015;10:e0116906.
7. Baum KT, Desai A, Field J, et al. Sleep restriction worsens mood and emotion regulation in adolescents. J Child Psychol Psychiatry 2014;55:180–90.
8. Roy-Byrne PP, Uhde TW, Post RM. Effects of one night's sleep deprivation on mood and behavior in panic disorder. Patients with panic disorder compared with depressed patients and normal controls. Arch Gen Psychiatry 1986;43:895–9.
9. Hornyak M. Depressive disorders in restless legs syndrome: epidemiology, pathophysiology and management. CNS Drugs 2010;24:89–98.
10. Li Y, Mirzaei F, O'Reilly EJ, et al. Prospective study of restless legs syndrome and risk of depression in women. Am J Epidemiol 2012;176:279–88.
11. Godau J, Spinnler N, Wevers A-K, et al. Poor effect of guideline based treatment of restless

syndrome in clinical practice. J Neurol Neurosurg Psychiatr 2010;81:1390–5.

12. Kang S-G, Lee HJ, Jung SW, et al. Characteristics and clinical correlates of restless legs syndrome in schizophrenia. Prog Neuropsychopharmacol Biol Psychiatry 2007;31:1078–83.

13. Jung J-S, Lee HJ, Cho CH, et al. Association between restless legs syndrome and CLOCK and NPAS2 gene polymorphisms in schizophrenia. Chronobiol Int 2014;31:838–44.

14. de Weerd A, Aricò I, Silvestri R. Presenting symptoms in pediatric restless legs syndrome patients. J Clin Sleep Med 2013;9:1077–80.

15. Picchietti DL, Stevens HE. Early manifestations of restless legs syndrome in childhood and adolescence. Sleep Med 2008;9:770–81.

16. Roy M, de Zwaan M, Tuin I, et al. Association between restless legs syndrome and adult ADHD in a German community-based sample. J Atten Disord 2015. http://dx.doi.org/10.1177/1087054714561291.

17. Ohayon MM, O'Hara R, Vitiello MV. Epidemiology of restless legs syndrome: a synthesis of the literature. Sleep Med Rev 2012;16:283–95.

18. Rottach KG, Schaner BM, Kirch MH, et al. Restless legs syndrome as side effect of second generation antidepressants. J Psychiatr Res 2008;43:70–5.

19. Bayard M, Bailey B, Acharya D, et al. Bupropion and restless legs syndrome: a randomized controlled trial. J Am Board Fam Med 2011;24:422–8.

20. McLean AJ. The use of the dopamine-receptor partial agonist aripiprazole in the treatment of restless legs syndrome. Sleep 2004;27:1022.

21. Cornelius JR, Tippmann-Peikert M, Slocumb NL, et al. Impulse control disorders with the use of dopaminergic agents in restless legs syndrome: a case-control study. Sleep 2010;33:81–7.

22. Voon V, Schoerling A, Wenzel S, et al. Frequency of impulse control behaviours associated with dopaminergic therapy in restless legs syndrome. BMC Neurol 2011;11:117.

23. Dang D, Cunnington D, Swieca J. The emergence of devastating impulse control disorders during dopamine agonist therapy of the restless legs syndrome. Clin Neuropharmacol 2011;34:66–70.

24. Pourcher E, Rémillard S, Cohen H. Compulsive habits in restless legs syndrome patients under dopaminergic treatment. J Neurol Sci 2010;290:52–6.

25. Signorelli MS, Battaglia E, Costanzo MC, et al. Pramipexole induced psychosis in a patient with restless legs syndrome. BMJ Case Rep 2013;2013.

26. Stoner SC, Dahmen MM, Makos M, et al. An exploratory retrospective evaluation of ropinirole-associated psychotic symptoms in an outpatient population treated for restless legs syndrome or Parkinson's disease. Ann Pharmacother 2009;43:1426–32.

27. Aiken CB. Pramipexole in psychiatry: a systematic review of the literature. J Clin Psychiatry 2007;68:1230–6.

28. Bet PM, Franken LGW, Klumpers UMH. Could pramipexole induce acute mania? A case report. Bipolar Disord 2013;15:446–8.

29. Goldberg JF, Burdick KE, Endick CJ. Preliminary randomized, double-blind, placebo-controlled trial of pramipexole added to mood stabilizers for treatment-resistant bipolar depression. Am J Psychiatry 2004;161:564–6.

30. Zarate CA, Payne JL, Singh J, et al. Pramipexole for bipolar II depression: a placebo-controlled proof of concept study. Biol Psychiatry 2004;56:54–60.

31. FDA medical review of gabapentin enacarbil. Available at: http://www.accessdata.fda.gov/drugsatfda_docs/nda/2011/022399Orig1s000MedR.pdf. Accessed June 15, 2015.

32. Corrigan MH, Denahan AQ, Wright CE, et al. Comparison of pramipexole, fluoxetine, and placebo in patients with major depression. Depress Anxiety 2000;11:58–65.

33. Beneš H, Mattern W, Peglau I, et al. Ropinirole improves depressive symptoms and restless legs syndrome severity in RLS patients: a multicentre, randomized, placebo-controlled study. J Neurol 2011;258:1046–54.

34. Montagna P, Hornyak M, Ulfberg J, et al. Randomized trial of pramipexole for patients with restless legs syndrome (RLS) and RLS-related impairment of mood. Sleep Med 2011;12:34–40.

Living with Restless Legs Syndrome/Willis-Ekbom Disease

Naoko Tachibana, MD, PhD

KEYWORDS

- Restless legs syndrome • Willis-Ekbom disease • End-stage renal disease • Hemodialysis

KEY POINTS

- Restless legs syndrome/Willis-Ekbom disease (RLS/WED) is seen in 7% to 68% of patients with end-stage renal disease (ESRD), with prevalence varying among people of differing ethnicities.
- Although RLS/WED in ESRD is classified as secondary RLS, its pathophysiology remains largely unknown, with common features with primary RLS/WED in respect to brain iron deficiency.
- Iron deficiency should be checked and corrected before starting treatment for RLS/WED in ESRD.
- Effective pharmacologic treatment includes levodopa, dopamine agonists, gamma-aminobutyric acid agonists, vitamins C and E, and intravenous iron.

THE IMPACT OF INCREASING END-STAGE RENAL DISEASE WORLDWIDE

It has been widely known that restless legs syndrome/Willis-Ekbom disease (RLS/WED) is common among patients with end-stage renal disease (ESRD). The prevalence of RLS/WED in the general population is estimated to be 5% to 15%,[1] while the prevalence in patients with ESRD is 6.6% to 68% (**Table 1**). According to the 2014 Annual Data Report from the United States Renal Data System,[2] ESRD incidence rates in 2012 varied more than 15-fold by country (25–467 new ESRD patients per million population), but in most countries, ESRD incidence rates are highest among patients aged 75 years and older, who are likely to complain about insomnia in general. Without the knowledge and awareness of RLS/WED, ESRD with RLS/WED patients might be treated as nonspecific chronic insomnia. As RLS/WED and other types of movement disorders in the elderly population were generally under-recognized,[3] many RLS/WED patients are unlikely to be properly diagnosed and treated. In particular,

RLS/WED patients with ERSD might suffer from not only from low quality of life,[4] but from also depression[5] and anxiety.[6] In addition, if RLS/WED in ERSD is untreated, it might lead to cardiovascular diseases, which are potentially lethal or cause devastating consequences to health.[7,8] Therefore, recognition and appropriate intervention for ESRD patients with RLD/ERDS are vital, and sleep specialists should provide proper information to nephrologists and ESDR patients.

EPIDEMIOLOGY OF RESTLESS LEGS SYNDROME/WILLIS-EKBOM DISEASE AMONG THE PATIENTS WITH END-STAGE RENAL DISEASE

There have been accumulating reports about the prevalence of RLS/WED in patients under hemodialysis (HD) or continuous ambulatory peritoneal dialysis (CAPD) from different countries by using either 1995 International RLS Study Group (IRLSSG) criteria[9] or 2003 National Institutes of Health (NIH) consensus criteria[10] (see **Table 1**). One may say that the prevalence of RLS/WED

Disclosure: The author has nothing to disclose.
Center for Sleep-related Disorders, Kansai Electric Power Hospital, 2-1-7 Fukushima, Fukushima, Osaka 553-0003, Japan
E-mail address: nanaosaka@aol.com

Sleep Med Clin 10 (2015) 359–367
http://dx.doi.org/10.1016/j.jsmc.2015.05.019
1556-407X/15/$ – see front matter © 2015 Elsevier Inc. All rights reserved.

Table 1
Prevalence of restless legs syndrome/Willis-Ekbom disease in end-stage renal disease patients of different countries

Country	Patients Condition	Number of Patients	Prevalence of RLS/WED (%)	Authors (References)
Brazil	HD	176	14.8	Goffredo Filho et al,[53] 2003
Brazil	HD	400	21.5	Araujo et al,[34] 2010
Canada	HD	136	26	Lee et al,[14] 2013
Germany	HD	136	23	Collado-Seidel et al,[54] 1998
Greece	HD	579	26.3	Stefanidis et al,[19] 2013
Hungary	HD	333	13.5	Mucsi et al,[4] 2005
Iran	HD	163	37.4	Rohani et al,[55] 2015
India	Chronic renal failure	121	6.6	Bhowmik et al,[56] 2004
Italy	HD	601	21.5	Gigli et al,[18] 2004
Italy	HD	100	31	La Manna et al,[7] 2011
Japan	HD	490	12.2	Takaki et al,[6] 2003
Japan	HD	228	23	Kawauchi et al,[57] 2006
Korea	HD	164	28	Kim et al,[15] 2008
Pakistan	HD	250	64.8	Haider et al,[58] 2014
Saudi Arabia	HD or CAPD	227	50.2	Al-Jahdali et al,[59] 2009
United Kingdom (Scotland)	HD	277	45.8	Siddiqui et al,[17] 2005
Taiwan	HD	1130	25.3	Lin et al,[16] 2013
Turkey	HD	81	12	Tuncel et al,[5] 2011
United States	HD	204	20	Winkelman et al,[46] 1996
United States	HD	894	32	Unruh et al,[47] 2004

among patients with ESRD is generally higher than that of general population, and the percentage of RLS/WED to the whole HD/CAPD population varies depending of the countries. This may be the reflection of the ethnic difference that has been also reported by epidemiologic studies of RLS/WED in general,[11] although little is known about the situation of the Middle East and African countries with scarce data from the general population. It has been well known that European and North American populations demonstrate higher RLS prevalence compared with Asian populations, and among European and North American populations, there is an age-related increase in the prevalence, while this is not the case among Asian populations.[11] As there have not enough data about how RLS/WED in ESRD appears in different age groups, longitudinal follow-up study about these patients will be required.

Although **Table 1** summarizes the prevalence of RLS/WSD in patients under HD or CAPD, there have been several studies showing that nondialysis-dependent chronic kidney disease (CKD) patients (estimated glomerular filtration rate <60 mL/min/1.73 m^2) also have the higher prevalence of RLS/WED compared with the general population or suffer from sleep disruption, to which RLS/WED is likely to attribute.[12–14] One should bear in mind that RLS/WED is likely when one considers the full spectrum of CKD.

ETIOLOGY OF RESTLESS LEGS SYNDROME/WILLIS-EKBOM DISEASE IN PATIENTS WITH END-STAGE RENAL DISEASE

Although RLS/WED with ESRD is classified as secondary RLS/WED, its pathophysiology is unknown. There have been a substantial number of studies investigating what factors of ESRD are involved to cause RLS/WED; however, no consistent conclusions have been made. Most studies looked into usual demographic variables such as age, sex, weight, and body mass index (BMI), but the other parameters, such as laboratory data related to ESDR severity (eg, serum blood urea nitrogen, serum hemoglobin level, ferritin) and Kt/V representing dialysis adequacy were not commonly checked.[5,15–19] Among them,

2 studies pointed out that RLS/WED risk was increased in women,[17,19] while the others not. Age did not play the role of one of the risk factors except for one study.[19] Nor did serum hemoglobin level or ferritin levels that were the common predictors of RLS in the general population increase the risk of RLS/WED.

There may be several reasons for this inconsistency about the studies looking for correlates of RLS/WED and ESRD. First, it was difficult to conform 1 dialysis program to another in all aspects. Second, as the data about blood samples and dialysis adequacy were temporal, the condition during a certain length of time might not be adequately reflected. Third, the laboratory data before the onset of RLS/WED were unavailable, and longitudinal change about the ESRD of each patient was unanalyzed.

If RLS/WED was positively related to the severity of renal failure, all the patients after renal transplantation should present complete relief from RLS/WED symptoms, but this was not the case.[20] Azar and colleagues[20] followed 28 HD patients without neuropathy who underwent renal transplantation, and found out that in 13 patients (43.3%), RLS symptoms were significantly reduced, but some still continued to have RLS with a significant association between RLS and lower serum iron and phosphorus after renal transplantation. In 1 cross-sectional survey, RLS was identified in 35 (4.5%) out of 765 post-transplant patients in 1 transplant center.[21] This prevalence was lower than that in general HD patients, but it means there were still some patients continuously suffering from RLS even after renal transplantation.

The onset of RLS/WED is probably insidious, and it has not been studied well about in what stage of renal failure RLS symptoms become full-blown. One study comparing patients under HD with and without RLS/WED found out that there was no difference between age, sex, weight, BMI, etiology of ESRD, and type of dialysis, but the period of HD dependence was significantly shorter in the group without RLS/WED.[18] Another study investigated clinical features and laboratory findings of HD patients with RLS/WED and concluded that positive family history for RLS/WEE and reduced/absent residual renal function and peripheral neuropathy were predictors of the risk for RLS/WED.[22] From these findings, and decreased prevalence of RLS/WED in post-transplant patients, one may say that once a certain group of genetically predisposed patients suffers from ESRD, these patients ultimately will have RLS/WED as their renal failure progresses, but after renal transplant, only patients with strong predisposition remain.

DIAGNOSIS OF RESTLESS LEGS SYNDROME/WILLIS-EKBOM DISEASE IN PATIENTS WITH END-STAGE RENAL DISEASE

The diagnostic procedure for RLS/WED in patients with ESRD does not differ from that for primary RLS/WED. IRLSSG consensus criteria have been recently updated,[23] and the details are described in the section concerning clinical diagnosis and diagnostic criteria. Clinical manifestation is similar between primary and secondary RLS/WED, and no specific symptoms of RLS/WED in ESRD have been described. However, as uremic neuropathy is a well-known complication of ESRD,[24] and type 2 diabetes is the most frequent cause of renal failure in the elderly population, and is often associated with diabetic neuropathy, some patients may have tingling and prickling sensation in the lower extremities with little circadian variation. Sensory disturbances caused by neuropathy often overlap RLS symptoms, so one should be careful to fail to recognize either of them.

Polysomnography (PSG) is not essential to make a diagnosis of RLS/WED in patients with ESRD, and generally there is no significant difference about sleep parameters between primary and secondary RLS/WED except for periodic leg movements while awake.[25] However, ESRD patients are also likely to have sleep apnea, which causes sleep fragmentation and results in insomnia and/or excessive daytime sleepiness in the short run.[26] In this respect, PSG is preferable to evaluate respiratory and motor events during sleep, and the sleep quality.

CONSIDERATION BEFORE STARTING TO TREAT RESTLESS LEGS SYNDROME/WILLIS-EKBOM DISEASE IN END-STAGE RENAL DISEASE

Before starting to treat RLS/WED in patients with ESRD, comorbidities and medications that exacerbate RLS/WED should be taken into consideration. Firstly, iron deficiency holds a common pivotal position in the pathogenesis of secondary RLS/WED, and evidence has been accumulated that even in primary RLS brain iron deficiency, together with abnormal dopaminergic consequences, may play the main role for its pathophysiology.[27] The criteria for defining iron deficiency has not been unambiguously determined, but in practice, ferritin level of less than 50 μg/L can be used as a rough indication.

Second, RLS/WED symptoms are distinguishable from those of polyneuropathy, but additional sensory disturbance may enhance discomfort from RLS/WED. In some cases, neurologic examinations and nerve conduction study are helpful to confirm the diagnosis of polyneuropathy.

Third, obstructive sleep apnea is the common co-morbidity of any disease in middle-aged men; however, the prevalence of obstructive sleep apnea in patients with ESRD is more than 70%,[28,29] which is much higher than the prevalence in the general population. Sleep fragmentation caused by frequent respiratory events and daytime sleepiness as a consequence usually make RLS/WED symptoms worse. To avoid the underdiagnosis, it should be borne in mind that the clinical features of sleep apnea in ESRD patients are different from with those with normal renal function in that less intense snoring and more sleep disturbance are observed.[30]

Finally, medications that can induce or exacerbate RLS/WED symptoms should be thoroughly checked. Published data are mostly case reports, and few systematic studies have been performed. They are mainly neuroleptics, tricyclics, selective serotonin reuptake inhibitors (SSRIs), and serotonin–norepinephrine reuptake inhibitors (SNRIs). Hoque and Chesson made a comprehensive review of the literature, where we can find a long list of antidepressants that induced or worsen RLS/WED as case reports. As more and more new antidepressants are going to the market, we should be cautious when prescribing a new anti-depressant for HD patients.[31,32] One case–control study of a large ESRD database showed that antidepressants, antihistamines, neuroleptics, and antiemetics are commonly used in patients with ESRD, indicating the inescapable reality that RLS/WED patients with ESRD may be prescribed one of these drugs from other sources.[33]

MANAGEMENT OF RESTLESS LEGS SYNDROME/WILLIS-EKBOM DISEASE IN END-STAGE RENAL DISEASE

ESRD patients with RLS/WED suffer from nocturnal leg discomfort associated with severe insomnia, chronic sleep deprivation, and its daytime consequences including daytime sleepiness, fatigue, poor functioning, and depression. If RLS/WED symptoms start early during the day, they may be disturbing the patient from keeping still during HD, which leads to insufficient adherence to prescribed dialysis treatment. Actually 1 Brazilian study showed 9.3% of RLS/WED patients reported RLS symptoms to be disturbing during HD.[34] Therefore, the target of management varies from one patient to another, and a tailor-made treatment strategy should be established for each individual patient. As the condition of HD is changeable according as the patient progress, fine-tune adjustment of medication for RLS/WED is also required.

PHARMACOLOGIC TREATMENT

There have not been enough data about pharmacologic treatment for RLS/WED in ESRS, mainly because systematic drug trials with large samples and longer follow-up periods usually excluded secondary RLS/WED. One systematic review trying to focus on randomized or quasi-randomized double-blind trials on treatments for uremic RLS/WED concluded that well-designed randomized controlled trials with a large sample size are needed,[35] however, it is difficult to match the HD conditions except when the study was performed in a large HD center.

Most of the available data dealt with a small number of patients, and observational periods have been from 4 weeks to 6 months (**Table 2**). In addition, most of the studies evaluated the effect of drugs by IRSSG rating scale[36] alone, and other outcomes such as sleep quality and quantity, improvement of quality of life, or comfort condition when receiving prescribed dialysis treatment were scarcely studied. The list of drugs that have been tried was similar to those recommended for primary RLS/WED, which were levodopa, dopamine agonists, gamma-aminobutyric acid (GABA) agonists, and intravenous iron. These studies showed that all of them were significantly effective for RLS/WED symptoms on a short-term basis. Although the study design was not stringent, gabapentin seemed to be superior to levodopa from 2 studies comparing these 2 drugs.[37,38] As for the time of administration, all the medications except for intravenous iron were administered at 2 hours before usual bedtime, and gabapentin was after HD session (3 times per week). So these results do not provide helpful information for the patients with RLS/WED symptoms during an extended time zone such as afternoon or early evening.

Different from these conventional medications, there was a study using antioxidant vitamin supplementation, vitamin C or vitamin E, or both of them, showing promising results.[39] This randomized, double-blind, placebo-controlled trial demonstrated that vitamins C and E, singly and in combination, improved the IRLS score by approximately 45%, 53%, and 50% respectively. These positive results could be attributable to the involvement of oxidative stress in the pathogenesis of RLS/WED,[40] and possible inflammatory/immune alteration, which can be responsible for iron deficiency. Vitamin C also increases gastrointestinal iron absorption and bioavailability of iron.[41] As there have not been enough studies about antioxidant vitamins, this field should receive special attention in the future.

Table 2
Overview of pharmacologic treatment in restless legs syndrome/Willis-Ekbom disease in patients on hemodialysis

Medication	Study Design	Daily Dose	Time of Administration	Number of Participants	Duration	Efficacy on IRLSSG Severity Scale Score	Authors (References)
Levodopa	Open-label study	125 mg/d	2 h before bedtime	15	4 wk	41% improvement in RLS severity	Micozkadioglu et al,[37] 2004
	Open randomized cross-over study	Slow-release levodopa/ carbidopa 25/100–50/ 200 mg per day	2 h before bedtime	11	14 wk	33.5% improvement in RLS severity	Pellecchia et al,[60] 2004
	Open randomized controlled study	Levodopa/carbidopa 110 mg/d	2 h before bedtime	40	4 wk	48.6% improvement in RLS severity	Razazian et al,[38] 2015
Pramipexole	Follow-up study	0.125–0.75 mg/d	2 h before bedtime	10	1 mo	70% improvement in RLS severity	Miranda et al,[61] 2004
Ropinirole	Open randomized cross-over study	0.25–2 mg/d	2 h before bedtime	11	14 wk	75% improvement in RLS severity	Pellecchia et al,[60] 2004
	Randomized, placebo-controlled study	0.25 mg/d	2 h before bedtime	7	6 mo	54% improvement in RLS severity	Giannaki et al,[43] 2013
Gabapentin	Open-label study	200–300 mg, 3 times per week	After HD session	15	4 wk	82% improvement in RLS severity	Micozkadioglu et al,[37] 2004
	Open randomized controlled study	200 mg, 3 times per week	After HD session and 2 h before bedtime	42	4 wk	72.6% improvement in RLS severity	Razazian et al,[38] 2015
Intravenous iron	Double-blind, placebo-controlled study	Iron dextran 1000 mg	N/A	11	4 wk	No data	Sloand et al,[62] 2004
Vitamin C	Randomized, double-blind, placebo-controlled study	Vitamin C (200 mg/d) and placebo	N/A	15	8 wk	45% improvement in RLS severity	Sagheb et al,[39] 2012
Vitamin E	Randomized, double-blind, placebo-controlled study	Vitamin E (400 mg/d) and placebo	N/A	15	8 wk	53% improvement in RLS severity	Sagheb et al,[39] 2012
Combination of vitamin C and vitamin E	Randomized, double-blind, placebo-controlled study	Combination of vitamin C (200 mg/d) and vitamin E (400 mg/d)	N/A	15	8 wk	50% improvement in RLS severity	Sagheb et al,[39] 2012

NONPHARMACOLOGICAL TREATMENT

Recently, 2 groups from Greece and Iran introduced intradialytic aerobic exercise training for improving RLS/WED in patients under HD.[42–45] The exercise training consisted of continuous cycling using a bedside cycle ergometer during HD 3 times a week. This kind of training had been originally used to prevent the catabolic effect and uremic myopathy and neuropathy. The trials were either 16 weeks or 6 months, and all the trials resulted in improving RLS/WED symptoms evaluated by using the IRLSSG rating scale. One randomized controlled study, in which the exercise group had readjustment of the intensity of recumbent cycle ergometers every 4 weeks and the control group continued to stick to the same intensity, demonstrated the improvement in RLS rating scale, subjective sleep quality, and Zung depression scale in the exercise group, but no significant improvement in the control group.[43] Although the mechanism of exercise-induced changes in RLS/WED severity remains unknown, the effect does not appear to due to an acute relief conferred by leg movements, but possibly systemic effect involving endogenous opiates. Another study from the same research group compared a 6-month exercise training program and a 6-month administration of 0.25 mg ropinirole, and found out that the exercise was as effective as this low-dosage dopamine agonist treatment.[44] Although supervision by exercise physiotherapists is necessary to achieve intradialytic aerobic exercise training, once the program is implemented, it may work well to prevent the onset or worsening of cardiovascular disorders. Combination of non-pharmacological and pharmacologic interventions can be a new way of treatment that is worth investigating.

RESTLESS LEGS SYNDROME/WILLIS-EKBOM DISEASE IN END-STAGE RENAL DISEASE PATIENTS AND MORTALITY

Higher short-term mortality of ESDR patients with RLS/WED compared with uremic patients who were free from RLS/WED was confirmed by several studies.[7,46] Another study focused on the severity of RLS/WED symptoms, showing that severe symptoms were significantly associated with an increased mortality.[47] La Manna and associates compared the subsets of patients with intermittent and continuous RLS/WED and found out that there were increased new cardiovascular events in patients with more severe RLS/WED characterized with persistent symptoms.[7] Regardless of comorbid RLS/WED, as cardiovascular diseases are the first cause of death in ESRD patients, it is important to decrease the risk of lethal events, and more studies will be required to know what causes increased mortality in ESRD patients with RLS/WED.

One possibility to explain this higher risk for cardiovascular diseases is that it may be more attributable to periodic leg movements during sleep (PLMS) rather than RLS/WED per se. Lindner and associates studied 100 transplanted and 50 waiting-list patients with ESRD by performing PSG, showing that an independent association between the severity of PLMS expressed by PLMS index (PLMSI) and the risk of cardiovascular and cerebrovascular disease even after adjusting for apnea-hypopnea index.[8] Another study compared the left ventricular dimensions measured by echocardiography of RLS/WED patients with PLMS group (PLMSI > 25) and non-PLMS group (PLMIS < 25) in the HD population, and speculated that a larger left ventricular morphology in PLMSI group indicated increased cardiovascular risk, although resting heart rate and blood pressure were not different between groups.[48] Other studies dealing with primary RLS/WED have also demonstrated that associated PLMS was the increased risk for the development of cardiovascular or/and cerebrovascular disease.[49–51] One should be careful about incidental PLMS with and without RLS/WED in the HD population. However, it is still the issue of controversy whether PLMS increases the risk of cardiovascular or cerebrovascular disease via sympathetic overactivity, resulting in hypertension and left ventricular hypertrophy.[52] Further interventional studies are required to see treatment of PLMS minimizes cardiovascular or/and cerebrovascular risk in ESRD patients.

REFERENCES

1. Yeh P, Walters A, Tsuang J. Restless legs syndrome: a comprehensive overview on its epidemiology, risk factors, and treatment. Sleep Breath 2012;16:987–1007.
2. United States Renal Data System. 2014 Annual data report: epidemiology of kidney disease in the United States. Bethesda (MD): National Institutes of Health, National Institute of Diabetes and Digestive and Kidney Diseases; 2014.
3. Wenning GK, Kiechl S, Seppi K, et al. Prevalence of movement disorders in men and women aged 50-89 years (Bruneck Study cohort): a population-based study. Lancet Neurol 2005;4:815–20.
4. Mucsi I, Molnar MZ, Ambrus C, et al. Restless legs syndrome, insomnia and quality of life in patients on maintenance dialysis. Nephrol Dial Transpl 2005;20:571–7.

5. Tuncel D, Orhan FO, Sayarlioglu H, et al. Restless legs syndrome in hemodialysis patients: association with depression and quality of life. Sleep Breath 2011;15:311–5.

6. Takaki J, Nishi T, Nangaku M, et al. Clinical and psychological aspects of restless legs syndrome in uremic patients on hemodialysis. Am J Kidney Dis 2003;41:833–9.

7. La Manna G, Pizza F, Persici E, et al. Restless legs syndrome enhances cardiovascular risk and mortality in patients with end-stage kidney disease undergoing long-term haemodialysis treatment. Nephrol Dial Transpl 2011;26:1976–83.

8. Lindner A, Fornadi K, Lazar AS, et al. Periodic limb movements in sleep are associated with stroke and cardiovascular risk factors in patients with renal failure. J Sleep Res 2012;21:297–307.

9. Walters AS. Toward a better definition of the restless legs syndrome. The International Restless Legs Syndrome Study Group. Mov Disord 1995; 10:634–42.

10. Allen RP, Picchietti D, Hening WA, et al. Restless legs syndrome: diagnostic criteria, special considerations, and epidemiology. A report from the restless legs syndrome diagnosis and epidemiology workshop at the National Institutes of Health. Sleep Med 2003;4:101–19.

11. Ohayon M, O'Hara R, Vitiello M. Epidemiology of restless legs syndrome: a synthesis of the literature. Sleep Med Rev 2012;16(4):283–95.

12. Merlino G, Lorenzut S, Gigli GL, et al. A case-control study on restless legs syndrome in nondialyzed patients with chronic renal failure. Mov Disord 2010;25: 1019–25.

13. Aritake-Okada S, Nakao T, Komada Y, et al. Prevalence and clinical characteristics of restless legs syndrome in chronic kidney disease patients. Sleep Med 2011;12:1031–3.

14. Lee J, Nicholl DD, Ahmed SB, et al. The prevalence of restless legs syndrome across the full spectrum of kidney disease. J Clin Sleep Med 2013;9:455–9.

15. Kim JM, Kwon HM, Lim CS, et al. Restless legs syndrome in patients on hemodialysis: symptom severity and risk factors. J Clin Neurol 2008;4:153–7.

16. Lin CH, Wu VC, Li WY, et al. Restless legs syndrome in end-stage renal disease: a multicenter study in Taiwan. Eur J Neurol 2013;20:1025–31.

17. Siddiqui S, Kavanagh D, Traynor J, et al. Risk factors for restless legs syndrome in dialysis patients. Nephron Clin Pract 2005;101:c155–60.

18. Gigli GL, Adoratib M, Dolsoa P, et al. Restless legs syndrome in end-stage renal disease. Sleep Med 2004;5:309–15.

19. Stefanidis I, Vainas A, Dardiotis E, et al. Restless legs syndrome in hemodialysis patients: an epidemiologic survey in Greece. Sleep Med 2013;14: 1381–6.

20. Azar SA, Hatefi R, Talebi M. Evaluation of effect of renal transplantation in treatment of restless legs syndrome. Transplant Proc 2007;39:1132–3.

21. Molnar MZ, Novak M, Szeifert L, et al. Restless legs syndrome, insomnia, and quality of life after renal transplantation. J Psychosom Res 2007;63: 591–7.

22. Pizza F, Persici E, La Manna G, et al. Family recurrence and oligo-anuria predict uremic restless legs syndrome. Acta Neurol Scand 2012;125:403–9.

23. Allen RP, Picchietti DL, Garcia-Borreguero D, et al. Restless legs syndrome/Willis-Ekbom disease diagnostic criteria: updated International Restless Legs Syndrome Study Group (IRLSSG) consensus criteria—history, rationale, description, and significance. Sleep Med 2014;15:860–73.

24. Krishnan AV, Kiernan MC. Uremic neuropathy: clinical features and new pathophysiological insights. Muscle Nerve 2007;35:273–90.

25. Wetter TC, Stiasny K, Kohnen R, et al. Polysomnographic sleep measures in patients with uremic and idiopathic restless legs syndrome. Mov Disord 1998;13:820–4.

26. Unruh ML, Sanders MH, Redline S, et al. Sleep apnea in patients on conventional thrice-weekly hemodialysis: comparison with matched controls from the Sleep Heart Health Study. J Am Soc Nephrol 2006; 17:3503–9.

27. Earley CJ, Connor J, Garcia-Borreguero D, et al. Altered brain iron homeostasis and dopaminergic function in Restless Legs Syndrome (Willis-Ekbom Disease). Sleep Med 2014;15:1288–301.

28. Kimmel PL, Miller G, Mendelson WB. Sleep apnea syndrome in chronic renal disease. Am J Med 1989;86:308–14.

29. Hallett M, Burden S, Stewart D, et al. Sleep apnea in end-stage renal disease patients on hemodialysis and continuous ambulatory peritoneal dialysis. ASAIO J 1995;41:M435–41.

30. Beecroft JM, Pierratos A, Hanly PJ. Clinical presentation of obstructive sleep apnea in patients with end-stage renal disease. J Clin Sleep Med 2009;5: 115–21.

31. Hoque R, Chesson AL Jr. Pharmacologically induced/exacerbated restless legs syndrome, periodic limb movements of sleep, and REM behavior disorder/rem sleep without atonia: literature review, qualitative scoring, and comparative analysis. J Clin Sleep Med 2010;6:79–83.

32. Page RL 2nd, Ruscin JM, Bainbridge JL, et al. Restless legs syndrome induced by escitalopram: case report and review of the literature. Pharmacotherapy 2008;28:271–80.

33. Bliwise DL, Zhang RH, Kutner NG. Medications associated with restless legs syndrome: a case-control study in the US Renal Data System (USRDS). Sleep Med 2014;15:1241–5.

34. Araujo S, Bruin V, Nepomuceno L, et al. Restless legs syndrome in end-stage renal disease: clinical characteristics and associated comorbidities. Sleep Med 2010;11:785–90.

35. Oliveira M, Conti C, Valbuza J, et al. The pharmacological treatment for uremic restless legs syndrome: evidence-based review. Mov Disord 2010; 25:1335–42.

36. Walters AS, LeBrocq C, Dhar A, et al. International restless legs syndrome study group. validation of the international restless legs syndrome study group rating scale for restless legs syndrome. Sleep Med 2003;4:121–32.

37. Micozkadioglu H, Ozdemir FN, Kut A, et al. Gabapentin versus levodopa for the treatment of Restless Legs Syndrome in hemodialysis patients: an openlabel study. Ren Fail 2004;26:393–7.

38. Razazian N, Azimi H, Heidarnejadian J, et al. Gabapentin versus levodopa-c for the treatment of restless legs syndrome in hemodialysis patients: a randomized clinical trial. Saudi J Kidney Dis Transpl 2015;26:271–8.

39. Sagheb M, Dormanesh B, Fallahzadeh M, et al. Efficacy of vitamins C, E, and their combination for treatment of restless legs syndrome in hemodialysis patients: a randomized, double-blind, placebocontrolled trial. Sleep Med 2012;13:542–5.

40. Cikrikcioglu MA, Hursitoglu M, Erkal H, et al. Oxidative stress and autonomic nervous system functions in restless legs syndrome. Eur J Clin Invest 2011;41: 734–42.

41. Weinstock LB, Walters AS, Paueksakon P. Restless legs syndrome -theoretical roles of inflammatory and immune mechanisms. Sleep Med Rev 2012; 16:341–54.

42. Sakkas GK, Hadjigeorgiou GM, Karatzaferi C, et al. Intradialytic aerobic exercise training ameliorates symptoms of restless legs syndrome and improves functional capacity in patients on hemodialysis: a pilot study. ASAIO J 2008;54:185–90.

43. Giannaki C, Hadjigeorgiou G, Karatzaferi C, et al. A single-blind randomized controlled trial to evaluate the effect of 6 months of progressive aerobic exercise training in patients with uraemic restless legs syndrome. Nephrol Dial Transplant 2013;28: 2834–40.

44. Giannaki C, Sakkas G, Karatzaferi C, et al. Effect of exercise training and dopamine agonists in patients with uremic restless legs syndrome: a six-month randomized, partially double-blind, placebo-controlled comparative study. BMC Nephrol 2013;14:194.

45. Mortazavi M, Vahdatpour B, Ghasempour A, et al. Aerobic exercise improves signs of restless leg syndrome in end stage renal disease patients suffering chronic hemodialysis. Scientific World J 2013;2013: 628142.

46. Winkelman JW, Chertow GM, Lazarus JM. Restless legs syndrome in end-stage renal disease. Am J Kidney Dis 1996;28:372–8.

47. Unruh ML, Levey AS, D'Ambrosio C, et al, Choices for healthy outcomes in caring for end-stage renal disease (CHOICE) study. Restless legs symptoms among incident dialysis patients: association with lower quality of life and shorter survival. Am J Kidney Dis 2004;43:900–9.

48. Giannaki CD, Zigoulis P, Karatzaferi C, et al. Periodic limb movements in sleep contribute to further cardiac structure abnormalities in hemodialysis patients with restless legs syndrome. J Clin Sleep Med 2013; 9:147–53.

49. Winkelman JW, Shahar E, Sharief I, et al. Association of restless legs syndrome and cardiovascular disease in the Sleep Heart Health Study. Neurology 2008;70:35–42.

50. Schlesinger I, Erikh I, Avizohar O, et al. Cardiovascular risk factors in restless legs syndrome. Mov Disord 2009;24:1587–92.

51. Walters AS, Rye DB. Review of the relationship of restless legs syndrome and periodic limb movements in sleep to hypertension, heart disease, and stroke. Sleep 2009;32:589–97.

52. Nannapaneni S, Ramar K. Periodic limb movements during sleep and their effect on the cardiovascular system: is there a final answer? Sleep Med 2014; 15:379–84.

53. Goffredo Filho GS, Gorini CC, Purysko AS, et al. Restless legs syndrome in patients on chronic hemodialysis in a Brazilian city: frequency, biochemical findings and comorbidities. Arq Neuropsiquiatr 2003;61(3B):723–7.

54. Collado-Seidel V, Kohnen R, Samtleben W, et al. Clinical and biochemical findings in uremic patients with and without restless legs syndrome. Am J Kidney Dis 1998;31:324–8.

55. Rohani M, Aghaei M, Jenabi A, et al. Restless legs syndrome in hemodialysis patients in Iran. Neurol Sci 2015;36:723–7.

56. Bhowmik D, Bhatia M, Tiwari S, et al. Low prevalence of restless legs syndrome in patients with advanced chronic renal failure in the Indian population: a case controlled study. Ren Fail 2004;26:69–72.

57. Kawauchi A, Inoue Y, Hashimoto T, et al. Restless legs syndrome in hemodialysis patients: health-related quality of life and laboratory data analysis. Clin Nephrol 2006;66:440–6.

58. Haider I, Anees M, Shahid SA. Restless legs syndrome in end stage renal disease patients on haemodialysis. Pak J Med Sci 2014;30:1209–12.

59. Al-Jahdali HH, Al-Qadhi WA, Khogeer HA, et al. Restless legs syndrome in patients on dialysis. Saudi J Kidney Dis Transpl 2009;20:378–85.

60. Pellecchia MT, Vitale C, Sabatini M, et al. Ropinirole as a treatment of restless legs syndrome in

patients on chronic hemodialysis: an open randomized crossover trial versus levodopa sustained release. Clin Neuropharmacol 2004;27:178–81.

61. Miranda M, Kagi M, Fabres L, et al. Pramipexole for the treatment of uremic restless legs in patients undergoing hemodialysis. Neurology 2004;62:831–2.

62. Sloand JA, Shelly MA, Feigin A, et al. A double-blind, placebo-controlled trial of intravenous iron dextran therapy in patients with ESRD and restless legs syndrome. Am J Kidney Dis 2004;43:663–70.

Restless Legs Syndrome/ Willis-Ekbom Disease Morbidity
Burden, Quality of Life, Cardiovascular Aspects, and Sleep

Mary Suzanne Stevens, MD, MS

KEYWORDS

- Restless legs syndrome/Willis-Ekbom disease (RLS/WED) • Quality of life • Burden
- Cardiovascular disease • Insomnia

KEY POINTS

- Restless legs syndrome (RLS)/Willis-Ekbom disease (WED) has a significant negative effect on quality of life. Measures show that the decreased quality of life is similar to that of other chronic diseases, such as diabetes type 2, depression, and osteoarthritis.
- RLS/WED disrupts sleep length, sleep quality, and daytime alertness. Sleep disruption can contribute to depression.
- RLS/WED has been associated with cardiovascular disease and high blood pressure, possibly because of increased sympathetic tone caused by periodic limb movements of sleep.
- RLS/WED is underdiagnosed, leading to chronic sleep disruption and daytime consequences.
- Patients with RLS/WED have decreased productivity at work, which contributes to its potentially far-reaching economic consequences.

INTRODUCTION

Restless legs syndrome (RLS)/Willis-Ekbom disease (WED) is a prevalent sensorimotor disorder that can be distressing to patients. It can result in significantly reduced quality of life (QOL), particularly through sleep deprivation resulting in daytime impairment. There has been an association between RLS/WED and cardiovascular disease (CVD), an interaction that is complex through potential mechanisms of sleep deprivation, blood pressure (BP) alterations, and inflammation. This article reviews the morbidity associated with RLS and its implications not only for QOL but for overall health and health care costs.

QUALITY OF LIFE

QOL has been shown to be significantly affected by moderate to severe RLS. In a large multinational questionnaire study, of 416 subjects with moderate to severe RLS symptoms, only 21 (5%) had been given the formal diagnosis of RLS despite 337 (81%) having discussed this with their primary care providers. Short Form-36 measures QOL across 8 domains: physical functioning, physical role functioning, bodily pain, general health perceptions, vitality, social role functioning, emotional role functioning, and mental health. Patients with RLS in the United States showed decreased scores in all domains, indicating decreased QOL,

Disclosure: The author has nothing to disclose.
Department of Neurology, University of Kansas, 3901 Rainbow Boulevard, MS 6002, Kansas City, KS 66160, USA
E-mail address: sstevens@kumc.edu

Sleep Med Clin 10 (2015) 369–373
http://dx.doi.org/10.1016/j.jsmc.2015.05.017
1556-407X/15/$ – see front matter © 2015 Elsevier Inc. All rights reserved.

to a similar degree to patients with chronic medical conditions such as type 2 diabetes mellitus, depression, and osteoarthritis.[1] Decrease in QOL across those domains has been shown in multiple studies.[2–4] Of the patients with RLS, 75% reported sleep disturbance, which is likely one of the major contributors to the impaired QOL of RLS.[1] The sleep disturbance has been shown to affect cognition during the day.[5] In one study, treatment of RLS (with dopamine agonist) not only improved polysomnographic measures of sleep after 3 months of therapy but cognitive functions improved as well, reaching the levels of healthy subjects. Parameters tested included decision making, problem solving, and categorizing abilities.[6] RLS has also been associated with depression.[7] However, prospective cohort studies show that depressive symptoms at baseline were associated with new-onset RLS over time, possibly making the relationship between depression and RLS bidirectional.[8]

Given the underdiagnosed state of RLS, high prevalence, and well-documented negative effect across all domains on QOL, the economic consequences can be far reaching. At this point in time, the full impact is unknown. Lost productivity at work, as well as the possible costs of the health care resources associated with the co-morbodities or RLS, may result in additional economic burden.[9,10] In an extensive questionnaire investigation, patients with significant RLS symptoms reported a significant productivity loss at work of 1 day per week. As RLS severity increased, there was a decrease in health status, sleep, and productivity.[2]

Longitudinally, RLS has been associated with reduced physical functioning, which is more pronounced for patients with RLS symptoms more than 15 times per month.[11] In a cross-sectional investigation, activities of daily function were impaired in patients with RLS compared with controls. Mediators were depressive symptoms and sleep disturbance.[12]

RLS in the moderate to severe range has been shown in numerous studies to decrease QOL significantly. Treatment trials have shown improvement in QOL when RLS symptoms improve. The documented underdiagnosis of RLS results in lost productivity in the workforce and unnecessarily difficult daytime consequences. Assessment of symptom severity includes not only a global measure of severity but also at least 1 other area, such as sleep quality, daytime sleepiness, daytime function, or mood. This assessment can be accomplished either with validated scales or free text.[13]

QOL plays such a large part in the disease of RLS that multiple scales to measure QOL and sleep quality have been developed and assessed specifically for RLS[14] (Box 1).

With the development of the need for evidence-based guidelines, a recent report was published discussing long-term management of RLS. The research has focused on treatment and pathophysiology, but the article notes that, "It is vital that research be performed to delineate which processes truly result in meaningful, patient-oriented improvement in outcome."[13]

CARDIOVASCULAR ASPECTS

A large cross-sectional observational study, the Sleep Heart Health Study, showed via a questionnaire that after adjusting for sex, race, body mass index (BMI), diabetes mellitus (DM), hypertension (HTN), cholesterol, and smoking history that the odds ratio for coronary artery disease or CVD were increased in the RLS population to 2.05 and 2.07 respectively.[15] In a population of elderly men, the frequency of periodic limb movements of sleep (PLMS) was associated with incident CVD.[16] However, in a prospective cohort study, Winter and colleagues[17] showed that RLS/WED was not a marker of increased CVD.

There is an association between RLS and high BP. The link might be PLMS. It is known that PLMS are present in 85% to 95% of patients with RLS, and may be the mediator between RLS and CVD or HTN.[18] PLMS have been shown to increase BP and heart rate.[19,20] More prominent BP and heart rate increases occurred when PLMS were associated with electroencephalogram (EEG) arousals. The increase in BP and heart rate may result in a higher sympathetic drive. The increased sympathetic drive that has been shown in obstructive sleep apnea (OSA) is thought to be a link to the CVD associated with OSA.[21] The PLMS that result in increases in BP and heart rate, even more so when associated with an EEG arousal, could potentially be the link between PLMS and HTN.

Box 1
Scales to assess QOL and sleep in RLS[14]

RLS QOL:

  RLS-QOL (Abetz and colleagues[3])

  RLS-QLI (RLS QOL Instrument)

  RLS-QOL (Kohnen)

Sleep questionnaires for RLS

Postsleep questionnaire for RLS

The Restless Legs Syndrome Next Day Impact questionnaire

It has been observed that, in patients who are nondippers, once the BP does not decrease at night, the patients have more CVD than the general population. Erden and colleagues[22] showed that patients with RLS have the nondipping pattern. This study used a cross-sectional method with questionnaires for RLS and ambulatory BP monitoring but no sleep monitoring, so it is unknown whether PLMS were present in these patients.

Another possible link is inflammation. C-reactive protein increases are an identified risk factor for CVD.[23] Trotti and colleagues[24] reported that patients with RLS who had PLMS had increased C-reactive protein levels. The increase also correlated with periodic limb movement frequency.

Multiple factors may contribute to the interplay between RLS and HTN/vascular disease: high BP and heart rate, high sympathetic drive, nondipping BP, sleep deprivation, and inflammation. Extensive reviews have been published on this topic[25,26] (**Box 2**).

Association does not prove causality, and the interaction may be bidirectional. Nonetheless, it is a potentially important association with significant consequences not only in QOL but in CVD prevention. Severity of RLS may be the important factor in RLS and its association with CVD.

SLEEP DISRUPTION AND RESTLESS LEGS SYNDROME

Questionnaire studies reporting sleeping disturbances show that up to 88% of patients with RLS report sleep disruption.[18,27] The sleep disturbance can encompass sleep initiation difficulties, sleep maintenance difficulties, decreased total sleep time, and daytime sleepiness, among other effects. Objective measures support the sleep disruption described with RLS.

In a cross-sectional community-based observational study, patients with RLS underwent polysomnography and showed longer adjusted mean sleep latencies than those without RLS. In addition, the more frequent the RLS symptoms, the more sleep latency increased.[28] Polysomnography in

---

Box 2
Possible interactions between RLS/PLMS and vascular disease

Insomnia

Sleep disturbances/EEG arousals

Inflammation

Nondipping BP

Sympathetic activation

Box 3
Effects of RLS on sleep

Increased sleep onset latency

Decreased total sleep time

Increased daytime sleepiness

Sleep disruption caused by discomfort associated with RLS/WED

Sleep disruption caused by arousals caused by PLMS

---

subjects with RLS and age-matched and sex-matched controls found that patients with RLS had prolonged sleep onset latency to consolidated sleep, shorter total sleep time, and higher sleep fragmentation. Both non–rapid eye movement and stage rapid eye movement (REM) were reduced[28,29] (**Box 3**). RLS is also associated with PLMS, which can further contribute to sleep fragmentation.[29]

NIGHT EATING AND SLEEP-RELATED EATING DISORDER

A cohort questionnaire study showed that 31% of patients with RLS reported episodes of night eating. Subjects with RLS with night eating had higher BMIs, reported more insomnia, and used more hypnotic and dopaminergic medications.[30] Patients with RLS were compared with patients with psychophysiologic insomnia (INS) and had statistically significantly more night eating and sleep-related eating disorder (SRED) than patients with INS. Among those with RLS, the night eating and SRED increased during treatment with sedative hypnotics and was not increased with dopaminergic therapy.[31] Night eating with RLS is categorized as a nonmotor manifestation of RLS that can have the distressing consequence of weight gain. In those patients with RLS who night eat, the compulsion to eat is categorized similarly to the compulsion to move the legs that accompanies RLS.

SUMMARY

Psychological distress is common with RLS. RLS is a chronic condition in its most severe form, interrupting any effort at resting or relaxing. It can interfere with both waking and sleep. Scholz and colleagues[32] used an observational, cross-section design and assessed psychological features of RLS. Patients with RLS had higher psychological distress overall, and subscales that were increased included compulsivity, depression, anxiety, and paranoid ideation. In general, more severe RLS correlated with greater psychological impairment. Augmentation resulted in the greatest psychological distress.

RLS is a manageable condition, although finding effective medication management can sometimes take time and creativity. Treatment may have side effects. Augmentation results in distress for the patient and more office visits. Dopaminergic medications can produce compulsive behaviors that can be costly (eg, gambling) or distressing to other people.

REFERENCES

1. Allen R, Walters A, Montplaisir J, et al. Restless legs syndrome prevalence and impact. Arch Intern Med 2005;165(11):1286.
2. Allen R, Stillman P, Myers A. Physician-diagnosed restless legs syndrome in a large sample of primary medical care patients in western Europe: prevalence and characteristics. Sleep Med 2010;11(1):31–7.
3. Abetz L, Allen R, Follet A, et al. Evaluating the quality of life of patients with restless legs syndrome. Clin Ther 2004;26(6):925–35.
4. Kushida C, Martin M, Nikam P, et al. Burden of restless legs syndrome on health-related quality of life. Qual Life Res 2007;16(4):617–24.
5. Allen RP, Abetz L, Washburn T, et al. The impact of restless legs syndrome (RLS) on sleep and cognitive function. Eur J Neurol 2002;9(Suppl 2):50.
6. Galbiati A, Marelli S, Giora E, et al. Neurocognitive function in patients with idiopathic restless legs syndrome before and after treatment with dopamine-agonist. Int J Psychophysiol 2015;95(3):304–9.
7. Lee H, Ramsey C, Spira A, et al. Comparison of cognitive functioning among individuals with treated restless legs syndrome (RLS), untreated RLS, and no RLS. J Neuropsychiatry Clin Neurosci 2014;26(1):87–91.
8. Szentkiralyi A, Völzke H, Hoffmann W, et al. The relationship between depressive symptoms and restless legs syndrome in two prospective cohort studies. Psychosom Med 2013;75(4):359–65.
9. Allen R, Bharmal M, Calloway M. Prevalence and disease burden of primary restless legs syndrome: results of a general population survey in the United States. Mov Disord 2010;26(1):114–20.
10. Salas R, Kwan A. The real burden of restless legs syndrome: clinical and economic outcomes. Am J Manag Care 2012;18(9 Supp):S207–12.
11. Zhang C, Li Y, Malhotra A, et al. Restless legs syndrome status as a predictor for lower physical function. Neurology 2014;82(14):1212–8.
12. Hanewinckel R, Maksimovic A, Verlinden V, et al. The impact of restless legs syndrome on physical functioning in a community-dwelling population of middle-aged and elderly people. Sleep Med 2015; 16(3):399–405.
13. Trotti L, Goldstein C, Harrod C, et al. Quality measures for the care of adult patients with restless legs syndrome. J Clin Sleep Med 2015;11:311–34.
14. Walters A, Frauscher B, Allen R, et al. Review of quality of life instruments for the restless legs syndrome/Willis-Ekbom disease (RLS/WED): critique and recommendations. J Clin Sleep Med 2014;10(12):1351–7.
15. Winkelman J, Shahar E, Sharief I, et al. Association of restless legs syndrome and cardiovascular disease in the Sleep Heart Health Study. Neurology 2007;70(1):35–42.
16. Koo B, Blackwell T, Ancoli-Israel S, et al. Association of incident cardiovascular disease with periodic limb movements during sleep in older men: outcomes of sleep disorders in older men (MrOS) study. Circulation 2011;124(11):1223–31.
17. Winter A, Schurks M, Glynn R, et al. Restless legs syndrome and risk of incident cardiovascular disease in women and men: prospective cohort study. BMJ Open 2012;2(2):e000866.
18. Montplaisir J, Boucher S, Poirier G, et al. Clinical, polysomnographic, and genetic characteristics of restless legs syndrome: a study of 133 patients diagnosed with new standard criteria. Mov Disord 1997;12(1):61–5.
19. Winkelman J. The evoked heart rate response to periodic leg movements of sleep. Sleep 1999;22(5):575–80.
20. Pennestri M, Montplaisir J, Fradette L, et al. Blood pressure changes associated with periodic leg movements during sleep in healthy subjects. Sleep Med 2013;14(6):555–61.
21. Somers V, Dyken M, Clary M, et al. Sympathetic neural mechanisms in obstructive sleep apnea. J Clin Invest 1995;96(4):1897–904.
22. Erden E, Erden İ, Türker Y, et al. Incremental effects of restless legs syndrome on nocturnal blood pressure in hypertensive patients and normotensive individuals. Blood Press Monit 2012;17(6):231–4.
23. Chobanian A. Seventh report of the Joint National Committee on Prevention, Detection, Evaluation, and Treatment of High Blood Pressure. Hypertension 2003;42(6):1206–52.
24. Trotti L, Rye D, Staercke C, et al. Elevated C-reactive protein is associated with severe periodic leg movements of sleep in patients with restless legs syndrome. Brain Behav Immun 2012;26(8):1239–43.
25. Innes K, Selfe T, Agarwal P. Restless legs syndrome and conditions associated with metabolic dysregulation, sympathoadrenal dysfunction, and cardiovascular disease risk: a systematic review. Sleep Med Rev 2012;16(4):309–39.
26. Ferini-Strambi L, Walters A, Sica D. The relationship among restless legs syndrome (Willis–Ekbom disease), hypertension, cardiovascular disease, and cerebrovascular disease. J Neurol 2013;261(6):1051–68.

27. Hening W. Impact, diagnosis and treatment of restless legs syndrome (RLS) in a primary care population: the REST (RLS Epidemiology, Symptoms, and Treatment) primary care study. Sleep Med 2004;5(3):237–46.

28. Winkelman J, Redline S, Baldwin C. Polysomnographic and health-related quality of life correlates of restless legs syndrome in the Sleep Heart Health Study. Sleep 2009;32(6):772–8.

29. Hornyak M, Feige B, Voderholzer U. Polysomnography findings in patients with restless legs syndrome and in healthy controls: a comparative observational study. Sleep 2007;30(7):861–5.

30. Antelmi E, Vinai P, Pizza F, et al. Nocturnal eating is part of the clinical spectrum of restless legs syndrome and an underestimated risk factor for increased body mass index. Sleep Med 2014; 15(2):168–72.

31. Howell M, Schenck C. Restless nocturnal eating: a common feature of Willis-Ekbom syndrome (RLS). J Clin Sleep Med 2012;8(4):413–9.

32. Scholz H, Benes H, Happe S, et al. Psychological distress of patients suffering from restless legs syndrome: a cross-sectional study. Health Qual Life Outcomes 2011;9(1):73.

Other Sleep Related Movement Disorders

Overview on Sleep Bruxism for Sleep Medicine Clinicians

Maria Clotilde Carra, DMD, PhD[a],*, Nelly Huynh, PhD[b],
Bernard Fleury, MD[c], Gilles Lavigne, DMD, PhD, FRCD[b]

KEYWORDS

- Sleep bruxism • Tooth grinding • Tooth clenching • Sleep arousal
- Sleep-disordered breathing • Management

KEY POINTS

- Sleep bruxism (SB) is a common sleep-related motor disorder characterized by involuntary grinding and clenching of the teeth during sleep.
- SB diagnosis relies on the awareness of tooth grinding, the presence of clinical signs and symptoms, and, when possible, on polygraphic recordings.
- Episodes of rhythmic masticatory muscle activity are more frequently observed in non–rapid eye movement sleep stages 1 and 2 and during sleep stage shifts.
- SB occurrence is related to sleep arousal–related phenomena, autonomic sympathetic cardiac activation, genetic predisposition, and psychosocial exogenous factors.
- SB treatment consists of managing tooth damage, pain, headache, and eventual comorbidities, such as sleep-disordered breathing or other movement disorders.

SLEEP BRUXISM CLINICAL CHARACTERISTICS AND DIAGNOSIS

Bruxism can be observed during wake and/or sleep. It is characterized by involuntary grinding and clenching of the teeth.[1] The wake-time habit of clenching, grinding, or gnashing the teeth can overlap in a substantial number of subjects with bruxism occurring during sleep. The prevalence of bruxism in general is estimated to be 17% in children and 8% in middle-aged adults, whereas it drops down to 3% in elderly individuals.[2,3]

SB is now classified as a sleep-related movement disorder (included in the *International Classification of Sleep Disorders,* ICSD-II, and its revised version of 2014).[4] Sleep bruxism (SB) is typically recognized during sleep by grinding sound reported by sleep partners, but such criterion is not highly reliable for current diagnosis.[3,5]

The clinical examination for SB diagnosis includes the observation of abnormal tooth wear, masticatory muscle hypertrophy, muscle tenderness, and signs and symptoms related to eventually concomitant disorders (eg, pain, headache, snoring) (**Table 1**).

Disclosure of Financial and Conflicts of Interest: G. Lavigne is a Canada Research Chair. Our group also receives—free or at reduced cost—oral appliances for research purposes (ORM-Narval, USA-Canada; Silencer, Canada; Klearway, Canada; Somnomed, USA) with no obligation attached. M.C. Carra, N. Huynh, and B. Fleury have no financial conflict of interest to disclose.
[a] Department of Periodontology, Service of Odontology, Rothschild Hospital, Assistance Publique - Hopitaux de Paris, Université Paris 7 – Denis Diderot, Unité de formation et recherche of Odontology, Paris 75006, France; [b] Faculty of Dental Medicine, Université de Montréal, CP 6128 Succursale Centre-Ville, Montreal, Quebec H3C 3J7, Canada; [c] Sleep Medicine and Respiratory Function Unit, Saint Antoine Hospital, Assistance Publique - Hopitaux de Paris, Paris 75012, France
* Corresponding author.
E-mail address: mclotildecarra@gmail.com

Sleep Med Clin 10 (2015) 375–384
http://dx.doi.org/10.1016/j.jsmc.2015.05.005
1556-407X/15/$ – see front matter © 2015 Elsevier Inc. All rights reserved.

sleep.theclinics.com

Table 1
Clinical diagnosis of sleep bruxism

Clinical Parameters	Commentary
Abnormal tooth wear, masticatory muscle hypertrophy, and morning jaw muscle tenderness	Tooth wear should be considered as an indicator of sleep bruxism (SB) because, although present in most subjects with SB, it does not confirm current tooth-grinding activity nor does it help to grade SB severity.[3,38] Other indicators include masticatory muscle (masseter and temporalis muscles) hypertrophy and jaw muscle tenderness and fatigue reported prevalently in the morning.
Report of grinding sounds during sleep	It is mandatory to ask whether a sleep partner can confirm a recent history of tooth-grinding activity (at least once a week in the recent months). However, it is not always reliable because of the SB variability over time, and the lack of perceivable grinding sounds in case of mild activity or clenching-type bruxism.[3,13,39]
Other related signs and symptoms	Presence of signs and symptoms related to concomitant pain (eg, temporomandibular pain, muscle pain, or headache), sleep-disordered breathing (eg, snoring, excessive daytime sleepiness, awareness of cessation of breathing, retrognathia, Mallampati class III and IV) and, more rarely, movement disorders (eg, tooth tapping in REM Sleep Behavior Disorder or epilepsy).[2,40,41]

For research purposes and for differential diagnosis when concomitant sleep-breathing disorders or other rare neurologic or movement disorders are suspected, it is recommended to use full polysomnography with electromyography of the masticatory muscles to score and quantify the repetitive and recurrent episodes of the activity of the masseter and temporalis muscles, called rhythmic masticatory muscle activity (RMMA) (**Table 2**).[4,6]

RMMA occurs with a frequency of 1 Hz and shows a typical cyclical occurrence pattern during sleep (**Fig. 1**).[6] RMMA episodes are observed more frequently in non–rapid eye movement (REM) sleep stages 1 and 2 (light sleep), in sleep stage shifts, and especially in the transition period from non-REM to REM sleep.[6–9] This jaw-muscle activity is observed at an index of 1 episode per hour of sleep in most people, in absence of tooth grinding; this physiologic masticatory activity is usually associated with swallowing, coughing, sleep talking, lip sucking, or other purposeless jaw movements.[10–13] In fact, SB appears to be the intensification in terms of frequency and force of a natural orofacial activity during sleep, which falls into a pathologic range of jaw-muscle activity when it is present with 2 to 4 episodes per hour of sleep in mild cases, and more than 4 episodes in severe SB cases.[14–16]

PUTATIVE EXPLANATIONS FOR SLEEP BRUXISM

The etiology and pathophysiology of SB are not based on a single explanatory mechanism and they remain largely unknown. Moreover, great between-subject variability is observed, and so far a unique and specific phenotype of the SB subject could not be extracted.[17] Putative explanations for SB occurrence include sleep arousal–related mechanisms, autonomic sympathetic cardiac activation, genetic predisposition, and psychosocial exogenous factors. When studying SB, it is important to control for age and comorbidity; the prevalence of SB is high in young subjects and drops after age 50, whereas other disorders, such as sleep-disordered breathing (SDB) and the restless legs syndrome (RLS), also known as the Willis-Ekbom disease/Wittmaack-Ekbom syndrome, increase with age (**Table 3**).[18,19] Intersecting prevalence is a challenge for family doctors who follow their patients over the years; the risk of overlapping comorbidity will arise at some time point in their life. For example, the co-occurrence of periodic limb movements during sleep, a sleep-related expression of RLS, is frequently reported with SB, but it is not obvious whether both conditions are under the same pathogenetic mechanism, and age is a critical factor to assess the independence of variance and association.[20]

Until now, the experimental and clinical evidence-based literature does suggest that SB is centrally regulated, probably in the brainstem, and its etiology is more likely multifactorial.[6,21,22] The paucity of scientific evidence to support the late 50s concept that SB is under the influence of peripheral factors, such as occlusal interferences, highlights that this hypothesis does not stand anymore.

Table 2
Polysomnographic research diagnostic criteria for sleep bruxism

Polygraphic Tools	Diagnostic Criteria
• Full-night level I polysomnography with concomitant audio and video recordings is the gold standard. Indeed, they allow achieving the highest specificity and sensitivity level in detecting and characterizing real RMMA episodes from other muscular activities occurring during sleep. However, this type of sleep recording is very sophisticated, requiring high levels of technical competence, time, and costs. • More user-friendly, level II and III polysomnographic systems with a limited number of channels and no audio-video recording also are valuable tools to assess SB activity; reliability and accuracy are ensured as long as the comparisons over time are made always with the same recording method, because an EMG overscoring of RMMA close to 25% is possible in absence of concomitant audio-video monitoring.[2,13] • Single channel level IV sleep-recording systems are good for screening purposes and large population studies owing their lower specificity to exclude atypical orofacial activities from the count of RMMA-SB episodes. • It is not wise to compare level I sleep recordings with any other type of sleep recording system (levels II, III, or IV) because, in absence of audio-video monitoring, RMMA can be overscored (lack of specificity). • Although the reported night-to-night variability, 1-night recording seems sufficient in most cases to diagnose SB.[3,42]	• Mean EMG amplitude: at least 10% of maximum voluntary clenching activity. • Types of RMMA episodes (masseter and/or temporal muscle): ○ *Phasic*: at least 3 EMG bursts lasting $\geq$0.25 s and <2 s ○ *Tonic*: 1 EMG burst lasting >2 s ○ *Mixed*: phasic and tonic bursts • EMG bursts must be separated by <2 s to be considered part of the same episode. • SB diagnosis can be made based on: ○ *The RMMA Index*: number of RMMA episodes per hour of sleep ○ *The Burst Index*: number of EMG bursts per hour of sleep ○ *The Bruxism Time Index* (%): total time spent bruxing/total sleep time × 100 ○ *Tooth-Grinding Sounds*: at least 1 RMMA episode with tooth-grinding sounds • Positive SB diagnosis (based on the frequency of EMG episodes with positive tooth-grinding history or confirmation in a sleep laboratory): ○ *Low Frequency of RMMA*: Index $\geq$2 and <4 ○ *High Frequency of RMMA*: Index is $\geq$4 and/or the Burst Index $\geq$25

Abbreviations: EMG, electromyography; RMMA, rhythmic masticatory muscle activity; SB, sleep bruxism.
Adapted from Carra MC, Huynh N, Lavigne G. Sleep bruxism: a comprehensive overview for the dental clinician interested in sleep medicine. Dent Clin North Am 2012;56:390; with permission.

Historically, the association between SB tooth grinding and sleep arousal was first observed by Reding and colleagues[23] in 1968 and by Satoh and Harada[24] in 1971. Since then, many studies have used polysomnography and electrophysiology to investigate the complex relationship between SB and sleep arousal.[7,8,14,15,22] It has been proven that most RMMA-SB episodes (close to 80%) occur in association with sleep arousals, especially in young healthy subjects, whereas this association seems lower (approximately 50%) in older patients presenting with other comorbidities.[3,7,14] Moreover, most RMMA-SB episodes occur in sleep periods that represent the so-called cyclic alternating pattern (CAP) or *phase d'activation transitoire*.[7,15,25] Precisely, most RMMA-SB episodes occur during CAP phase A, characterized by the dominance of sleep arousal activity.[6–9] Notwithstanding this strong association, sleep arousals (and CAP phase A) are more likely the "permissive window" that facilitates RMMA during sleep rather than its cause or trigger (as similarly observed for periodic limb movements).[9,15,26] New technology helped to advance the study of the association between sleep arousal and cardiac/motor activation during sleep with SB.

Reding and colleagues[23] in 1968 were also the first to show that SB was associated with a rise in heart rate activity, suggesting a role of the autonomic nervous system. Some experimental evidence further supports that RMMA onset is associated with a sequence of physiologic events that occur within a sleep arousal,[17] starting with a rise of the autonomic sympathetic cardiac activity with a concomitant withdrawal of

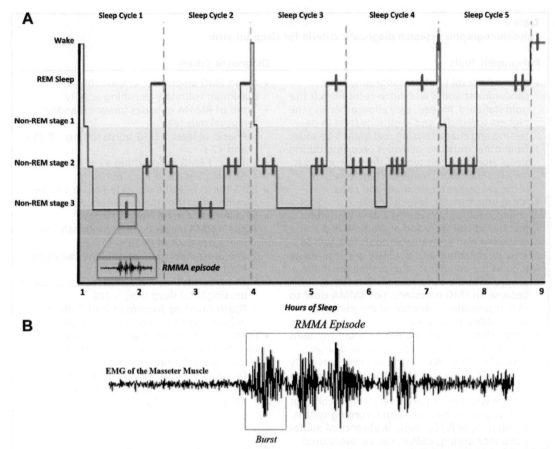

Fig. 1. Hypnogram representing the schematic distribution over the sleep cycles of RMMA episodes. (*A*) A full-night hypnogram showing the sleep stage distribution over 5 non-REM/REM sleep cycles. Green vertical lines represent episodes of RMMA. As schematically displayed, RMMA episodes are observed more frequently during non-REM sleep stages 1 and 2, sleep stage shift, and pre-REM sleep periods. (*B*) Example of an RMMA episode, defined on the masseter and/or temporalis electromyographic channels as an activity of at least 3 consecutive electromyographic bursts (frequency 1 Hz) lasting ≥0.25 second.

parasympathetic dominance[8] and culminating in the occurrence of RMMA.[2,6] A modification of the breathing patterns,[27] an increase in systolic and diastolic blood pressure,[28] and swallowing[29] also are frequently observed in close temporal association to the RMMA episode[6] (**Fig. 2**). However, such theoretic sequence of events does not explain all RMMA-SB episodes; other factors, such as hypoxia, in the presence or absence of SDB, or the level of stress and anxiety on arousal may also be considered. Fluctuation in central nervous system neurochemicals also may influence the occurrence of RMMA during sleep. As an example, a medication known to act on the noradrenergic system (eg, clonidine) was found to influence sleep architecture by altering REM sleep onset, as well as to reduce the probability of RMMA occurrence.[8,9] Similarly, an early case report of SB in a patient with Parkinson disease

treated with L-dopa was considered the first suggestion that the dopaminergic system may have a role in SB occurrence.[30] However, more recent investigations failed to confirm a dominant role of the dopaminergic axis in the genesis of RMMA-SB.[31,32]

The level of evidence supporting a genetic predisposition in SB is rather low. More recent studies suggested that 20% to 50% of subjects with SB have a direct family member who ground his or her teeth in childhood, and childhood SB persisted in adulthood in most subjects.[33] Our group found similar familial distribution.[34] The understanding of the highly variable SB phenotype probably reduces the likelihood of finding a specific set of genes that explain RMMA. Although a familial inheritance has been observed in the previously mentioned studies, this remains an open field that requires further studies able to discriminate

Table 3
Sleep bruxism and comorbidities (most are rare and information derived mainly from case report or observational comparative cohort study)

Parasomnias	• Sleep talking • Sleep walking • REM sleep behavior disorder
Other sleep-related disorders	• SDB (snoring, obstructive sleep apnea) • Sleep-related epilepsy • Periodic limb movements and restless legs syndrome
Medical and psychological conditions	• Hypertrophic tonsils and/or adenoids (suspect SDB) • Allergies • Attention-deficit hyperactivity disorder • Headaches (suspect SDB) • Orofacial pain and temporomandibular disorders • Stress and anxiety • Neurologic and psychiatric disorders (eg, dementia, depression) • Movement disorders (eg, Parkinson disease, oromandibular dystonia, tics)
Oral habits and parafunctions	• Tics • Nail biting, pen biting, etc • Wake-time tooth clenching

Abbreviations: REM, rapid eye movement; SDB, sleep-disordered breathing.

Adapted from Carra MC, Huynh N, Lavigne G. Sleep bruxism: a comprehensive overview for the dental clinician interested in sleep medicine. Dent Clin North Am 2012;56:397; with permission.

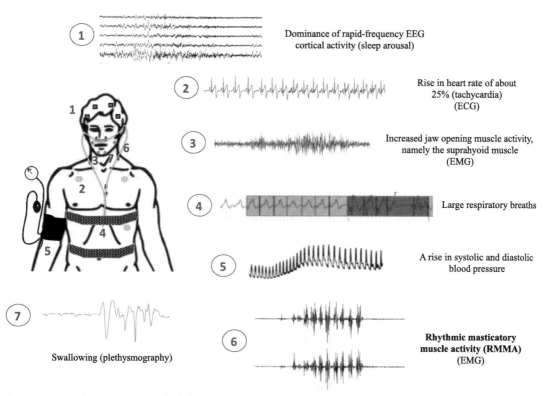

1. Dominance of rapid-frequency EEG cortical activity (sleep arousal)

2. Rise in heart rate of about 25% (tachycardia) (ECG)

3. Increased jaw opening muscle activity, namely the suprahyoid muscle (EMG)

4. Large respiratory breaths

5. A rise in systolic and diastolic blood pressure

7. Swallowing (plethysmography)

6. **Rhythmic masticatory muscle activity (RMMA)** (EMG)

Fig. 2. Genesis of an RMMA episode (schematic representation of the cascade of physiologic events that precedes RMMA onset). ECG, electrocardiogram; EEG, electroencephalogram; EMG, electromyogram. (*Data from* Refs.[8,14,22,27,28])

Table 4
Management of SB

Behavioral strategies For the majority, only empirical evidence or lack of validation[43–45]	• Avoidance of SB risk factors (eg, smoking, alcohol, caffeine, drugs) • Control of wake-time oral parafunctions • Improve sleep habits and sleep environment (sleep hygiene) • Control and reduce stress and anxiety (relaxation techniques, hypnotherapy) • Improve coping (cognitive behavioral therapy). The application of cognitive behavioral therapy was suggested but no superiority to usual dental treatment was found (ie, occlusal splint therapy).[45] • Relax muscles and reduce EMG activity during sleep (biofeedback). A newly developed biofeedback system showed some promising results but marketing such product seems to be a challenge.[44]
Pharmacotherapy For short-term treatment only. Attention to the risk/benefit ratio.	• Medications targeting the adrenergic axis acting on the autonomic nervous system and the more generally on the central nervous system were shown to reduce SB frequency in experimental trials.[6,46] However, none of these medications was submitted to effectiveness trials, assessing their safety and efficacy in real-world settings. Because most SB activity in life can be considered as transitory, pharmacologic treatments should be reserved for "acute" short-term therapy only.[6] • A placebo-controlled study found a 40% reduction of SB activity with a single dose of clonazepam (1 mg).[47] • An acute dose (0.3 mg) of the alpha₂-adrenergic agonist clonidine reduced SB by 60%.[48] What limits the use of clonidine in clinical practice is that severe morning hypotension may occur.[9,48] • Antidepressant drugs, such as low doses of amitriptyline (a tricyclic antidepressant), were shown to be ineffective for SB.[49] Serotonin selective reuptake inhibitor medications (eg, fluoxetine, sertraline, paroxetine) may increase wake time tooth grinding and clenching, whereas evidence on SB is lacking.[50] • Anecdotal reports or small sample size studies suggested a positive effect on SB of gabapentin, tiagabine, buspirone, topiramate, and botulinum toxin.[51]

Oral appliances Different designs: occlusal or stabilization splint, mandibular advancement appliances	• The most straightforward method to prevent SB-related tooth damage is the use of acrylic or rubber oral devices fitted to upper or lower jaws. Although these appliances are efficacious in protecting the teeth and attenuate the sounds of tooth grinding, there is no evidence that such devices may stop or permanently reduce SB activity; rather, their effectiveness remains unknown.[52] Most experimental or randomized trials using oral appliances for SB showed a short term/transitory reduction in the frequency of RMMA, as scored on EMG recordings.[53,54] However, some patients also may present with an exacerbation of SB activity.[54]
	• MAAs are currently used to manage snoring and mild to moderate obstructive sleep apnea. They also have been used in subjects with SB and they demonstrated to decrease RMMA-SB by close to 50% when worn in protruded positions (50%–75% of the maximal protrusion).[55] A recent controlled sleep study performed with a home-sleep monitoring system showed the beneficial effect of MAA on concomitant SB, snoring, and headache in teenagers with dentoskeletal abnormalities on a waiting list for orthodontic treatment.[56] Another study confirmed the use of MAA for managing daily idiopathic morning headaches in patients presenting with low frequency of RMMA during sleep and no SDB.[57] Although the use of an MAA for SB showed great potential, all these studies assessed the effect of MAA after short-term treatment only (2 wk on average). Their effectiveness and side effects remain to be assessed in the long term.[58,59]
	• Physicians and dentists recommending oral appliances or devices to their patients have to keep in mind that these may change their dentoskeletal morphology and dental occlusion over time. Close dental follow-ups are mandatory for all patients treated by oral appliances, and even more for patients with periodontal gum diseases.
	• Indication and safety of oral appliance use should be attentively evaluated on a patient-by-patient basis. For example, the use of single upper arch oral appliance customized for SB was shown to exacerbate obstructive respiratory events in patients with SDB (ie, rise in the apnea-hypopnea index).[60,61] In case of a patient with SB at risk of SDB (eg, obstructive sleep apnea), we recommended a mandibular occlusal splint (made for the lower jaw) or a mandibular advancement appliance.

Abbreviations: EMG, electromyography; MAA, mandibular advancement appliance; RMMA, rhythmic masticatory muscle activity; SB, sleep bruxism; SDB, sleep-disordered breathing.

the genetic component between wake-time bruxism and sleep activity, as well as to assess the role of genetics apart from the occupational and environmental influences, the impact of age, and the presence of comorbidities.[35,36]

MANAGEMENT OF SLEEP BRUXISM

It is essential to reiterate that there is no single therapy to treat or cure SB. The current medical/dental practice aims at managing and preventing the harmful consequences of SB and tooth-grinding, such as tooth damage, pain and headache, grinding sounds that have an impact on sleep partners, and eventual comorbidities, such as SDB or other movement disorders.[37] Behavioral strategies, pharmacotherapy, and oral appliance treatments are summarized in **Table 4**. It must be stressed that most management strategies are not yet fully evidence-based; most are derived from mechanistic studies, case reports, or small sample size studies assessing treatment efficacy on the short-term only.

SUMMARY

SB is a complex motor phenomenon occurring during sleep in predisposed individuals. Episodic rhythmic or sustained masticatory muscle activity may appear sporadically without significant consequences on the stomatognathic system or complaints. However, this involuntary jaw motor activity may also fall into pathologic conditions, once it is associated with comorbidities or pain symptoms. The transition from the adaptive to the maladaptive form may be determined by many factors, which remain for the most part to be identified (**Fig. 3**). Although SB is a non–life-threatening sleep-related motor disorder, it can be highly distressing because of tooth-grinding sounds that disrupt sleep partners and the potential detrimental consequences of tooth-grinding and clenching activity, including tooth damage, headaches, and orofacial pain. Sleep clinicians are responsible for detecting SB comorbidities (eg, SDB), whereas dental clinicians are primarily involved in managing and preventing the detrimental consequences of SB on patients' oral health.

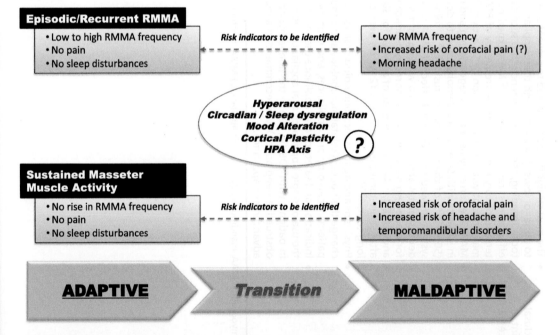

Fig. 3. Hypotheses on RMMA occurrence and genesis: "from adaptive to maladaptive Condition." RMMA, the typical electromyographic pattern of sleep bruxism, may occur as episodic rhythmic or sustained masticatory muscle activity. When occurring sporadically at low frequency and force, or without associated comorbidities, RMMA may not have significant consequences on the stomatognathic system or complaints. However, this involuntary jaw motor activity also may fall into pathologic conditions, increases in frequency and intensity of recurrent muscle contractions during sleep, and be associated with comorbidities and/or pain symptoms. The transition from the adaptive to the maladaptive form of RMMA may be determined and influenced by many factors, which remain for the most part to be identified. (*Adapted from* Riemann D, Spiegelhalder K, Feige B, et al. The hyperarousal model of insomnia: a review of the concept and its evidence. Sleep Med Rev 2010;14:21; with permission.)

REFERENCES

1. Lobbezoo F, Ahlberg J, Glaros AG, et al. Bruxism defined and graded: an international consensus. J Oral Rehabil 2013;40:2–4.

2. Carra MC, Huynh N, Lavigne G. Sleep bruxism: a comprehensive overview for the dental clinician interested in sleep medicine. Dent Clin North Am 2012;56:387–413.

3. Maluly M, Andersen ML, Dal-Fabbro C, et al. Polysomnographic study of the prevalence of sleep bruxism in a population sample. J Dent Res 2013; 92:97S–103S.

4. American Academy of Sleep Medicine, Sleep Related Bruxism, American Academy of Sleep Medicine (AASM), editors. ICSD-2 International classification of sleep disorders, 2nd edition. Diagnosis and coding manual. Westchester (IL): 2005. p. 189–92.

5. Lavigne GJ, Guitard F, Rompré PH, et al. Variability in sleep bruxism activity over time. J Sleep Res 2001;10:237–44.

6. Lavigne G, Manzini C, Huynh NT, et al. Sleep bruxism. In: Kryger MH, Roth T, Dement WC, editors. Principles and practice of sleep medicine. 5th edition. St Louis (MO): Elsevier Saunders; 2011. p. 1129–39.

7. Macaluso GM, Guerra P, Di Giovanni G, et al. Sleep bruxism is a disorder related to periodic arousals during sleep. J Dent Res 1998;77:565–73.

8. Huynh N, Kato T, Rompré PH, et al. Sleep bruxism is associated to micro-arousals and an increase in cardiac sympathetic activity. J Sleep Res 2006;15: 339–46.

9. Carra MC, Macaluso GM, Rompré PH, et al. Clonidine has a paradoxical effect on cyclic arousal and sleep bruxism during NREM sleep. Sleep 2010;33: 1711–6.

10. Dutra KM, Pereira FJ Jr, Rompré PH, et al. Oro-facial activities in sleep bruxism patients and in normal subjects: a controlled polygraphic and audio-video study. J Oral Rehabil 2009;36:86–92.

11. Lavigne GJ, Rompré PH, Montplaisir JY. Sleep bruxism: validity of clinical research diagnostic criteria in a controlled polysomnographic study. J Dent Res 1996;75:546–52.

12. Walters AS, Lavigne G, Hening W, et al. The scoring of movements in sleep. J Clin Sleep Med 2007;3: 155–67.

13. Carra MC, Huynh N, Lavigne GJ. Diagnostic accuracy of sleep bruxism scoring in absence of audio-video recording: a pilot study. Sleep Breath 2015; 19:183–90.

14. Kato T, Montplaisir J, Rompr PH, et al. Sequence of EEG and cardiac activation in relation to sleep bruxism: a controlled study. J Dent Res 2001;80: 697–6.

15. Carra MC, Rompré PH, Kato T, et al. Sleep bruxism and sleep arousal: an experimental challenge to assess the role of cyclic alternating pattern. J Oral Rehabil 2011;38:635–42.

16. Rompre PH, Daigle-Landry D, Guitard F, et al. Identification of a sleep bruxism subgroup with a higher risk of pain. J Dent Res 2007;86:837–42.

17. Lavigne GJ, Huynh N, Kato T, et al. Genesis of sleep bruxism: motor and autonomic-cardiac interactions. Arch Oral Biol 2007;52:381–4.

18. Lavigne GJ, Montplaisir JY. Restless legs syndrome and sleep bruxism: prevalence and association among Canadians. Sleep 1994;17:739–43.

19. Peppard PE, Young T, Barnet JH, et al. Increased prevalence of sleep-disordered breathing in adults. Am J Epidemiol 2013;177:1006–14.

20. van der Zaag J, Naeije M, Wicks DJ, et al. Time-linked concurrence of sleep bruxism, periodic limb movements, and EEG arousals in sleep bruxers and healthy controls. Clin Oral Investig 2014;18:507–13.

21. Lavigne GJ, Kato T, Kolta A, et al. Neurobiological mechanisms involved in sleep bruxism. Crit Rev Oral Biol Med 2003;14:30–46.

22. Kato T, Montplaisir JY, Guitard F, et al. Evidence that experimentally induced sleep bruxism is a consequence of transient arousal. J Dent Res 2003;82: 284–8.

23. Reding GR, Zepelin H, Robinson JE Jr, et al. Nocturnal teeth-grinding: all-night psychophysiologic studies. J Dent Res 1968;47:786–97.

24. Satoh T, Harada Y. Tooth-grinding during sleep as an arousal reaction. Experientia 1971;27:785–6.

25. Terzano MG, Parrino L. Origin and significance of the cyclic alternating pattern (CAP): review article. Sleep Med Rev 2000;4:101–23.

26. Fantini ML, Michaud M, Gosselin N, et al. Periodic leg movements in REM sleep behavior disorder and related autonomic and EEG activation. Neurology 2002;59:1889–94.

27. Khoury S, Rouleau GA, Rompré PH, et al. A significant increase in breathing amplitude precedes sleep bruxism. Chest 2008;134:332–7.

28. Nashed A, Lanfranchi P, Rompré P, et al. Sleep bruxism is associated with a rise in arterial blood pressure. Sleep 2012;35:529–36.

29. Miyawaki S, Lavigne GJ, Pierre M, et al. Association between sleep bruxism, swallowing-related laryngeal movement, and sleep positions. Sleep 2003; 26:461–5.

30. Magee KR. Bruxisma related to levodopa therapy. JAMA 1970;214:147.

31. Lavigne GJ, Soucy JP, Lobbezoo F, et al. Double-blind, crossover, placebo-controlled trial of bromocriptine in patients with sleep bruxism. Clin Neuropharmacol 2001;24:145–9.

32. Lobbezoo F, Soucy JP, Hartman NG, et al. Effects of the D2 receptor agonist bromocriptine on sleep

bruxism: report of two single-patient clinical trials. J Dent Res 1997;76:1610–4.

33. Hublin C, Kaprio J, Partinen M, et al. Sleep bruxism based on self-report in a nationwide twin cohort. J Sleep Res 1998;7:61–7.

34. Khoury S, Rouleau GA, Lavigne GJ. Preliminary data on the genetic of sleep bruxism. In: 30th International Symposium - GRSNC "Neurobiology & Genetics of developmental brain diseases". Montréal, Canada: Université de Montréaal; 2008.

35. Abe Y, Suganuma T, Ishii M, et al. Association of genetic, psychological and behavioral factors with sleep bruxism in a Japanese population. J Sleep Res 2012;21:289–96.

36. Lobbezoo F, Visscher CM, Ahlberg J, et al. Bruxism and genetics: a review of the literature. J Oral Rehabil 2014;41:709–14.

37. Huynh N, Manzini C, Rompré PH, et al. Weighing the potential effectiveness of various treatments for sleep bruxism. J Can Dent Assoc 2007;73:727–30.

38. Abe S, Yamaguchi T, Rompré PH, et al. Tooth wear in young subjects: a discriminator between sleep bruxers and controls? Int J Prosthodont 2009;22:342–50.

39. Kato T, Rompré P, Montplaisir JY, et al. Sleep bruxism: an oromotor activity secondary to microarousal. J Dent Res 2001;80:1940–4.

40. Abe S, Gagnon JF, Montplaisir JY, et al. Sleep bruxism and oromandibular myoclonus in rapid eye movement sleep behavior disorder: a preliminary report. Sleep Med 2013;14:1024–30.

41. Meletti S, Cantalupo G, Volpi L, et al. Rhythmic teeth grinding induced by temporal lobe seizures. Neurology 2004;62:2306–9.

42. Hasegawa Y, Lavigne G, Rompré P, et al. Is there a first night effect on sleep bruxism? A sleep laboratory study. J Clin Sleep Med 2013;9:1139–45.

43. Shulman J. Teaching patients how to stop bruxing habits. J Am Dent Assoc 2001;132:1275–7.

44. Jadidi F, Castrillon E, Svensson P, et al. Effect of conditioning electrical stimuli on temporalis electromyographic activity during sleep. J Oral Rehabil 2008;35:171–83.

45. Ommerborn MA, Schneider C, Giraki M, et al. Effects of an occlusal splint compared with cognitive-behavioral treatment on sleep bruxism activity. Eur J Oral Sci 2007;115:7–14.

46. Winocur E, Gavish A, Voikovitch M, et al. Drugs and bruxism: a critical review. J Orofac Pain 2003;17:99–111.

47. Saletu A, Parapatics S, Anderer P, et al. Controlled clinical, polysomnographic and psychometric studies on differences between sleep bruxers and controls and acute effects of clonazepam as compared with placebo. Eur Arch Psychiatry Clin Neurosci 2010;260:163–74.

48. Huynh N, Lavigne GJ, Lanfranchi PA, et al. The effect of 2 sympatholytic medications–propranolol and clonidine–on sleep bruxism: experimental randomized controlled studies. Sleep 2006;29:307–16.

49. Raigrodski AJ, Christensen LV, Mohamed SE, et al. The effect of four-week administration of amitriptyline on sleep bruxism. A double-blind crossover clinical study. Cranio 2001;19:21–5.

50. Stein DJ, Van Greunen G, Niehaus D. Can bruxism respond to serotonin reuptake inhibitors? J Clin Psychiatry 1998;59:133.

51. Lee SJ, McCall WD Jr, Kim YK, et al. Effect of botulinum toxin injection on nocturnal bruxism: a randomized controlled trial. Am J Phys Med Rehabil 2010;89:16–23.

52. Macedo CR, Silva AB, Machado MA, et al. Occlusal splints for treating sleep bruxism (tooth grinding). Cochrane Database Syst Rev 2007;(4):CD005514.

53. Harada T, Ichiki R, Tsukiyama Y, et al. The effect of oral splint devices on sleep bruxism: a 6-week observation with an ambulatory electromyographic recording device. J Oral Rehabil 2006;33:482–8.

54. Dube C, Rompré PH, Manzini C, et al. Quantitative polygraphic controlled study on efficacy and safety of oral splint devices in tooth-grinding subjects. J Dent Res 2004;83:398–403.

55. Landry-Schonbeck A, de Grandmont P, Rompré PH, et al. Effect of an adjustable mandibular advancement appliance on sleep bruxism: a crossover sleep laboratory study. Int J Prosthodont 2009;22:251–9.

56. Carra MC, Huynh NT, El-Khatib H, et al. Sleep bruxism, snoring, and headaches in adolescents: short-term effects of a mandibular advancement appliance. Sleep Med 2013;14:656–61.

57. Franco L, Rompre PH, de Grandmont P, et al. A mandibular advancement appliance reduces pain and rhythmic masticatory muscle activity in patients with morning headache. J Orofac Pain 2011;25:240–9.

58. Martinez-Gomis J, Willaert E, Nogues L, et al. Five years of sleep apnea treatment with a mandibular advancement device. Side effects and technical complications. Angle Orthod 2010;80:30–6.

59. de Almeida FR, Lowe AA, Tsuiki S, et al. Long-term compliance and side effects of oral appliances used for the treatment of snoring and obstructive sleep apnea syndrome. J Clin Sleep Med 2005;1:143–52.

60. Gagnon Y, Mayer P, Morisson F, et al. Aggravation of respiratory disturbances by the use of an occlusal splint in apneic patients: a pilot study. Int J Prosthodont 2004;17:447–53.

61. Nikolopoulou M, Ahlberg J, Visscher CM, et al. Effects of occlusal stabilization splints on obstructive sleep apnea: a randomized controlled trial. J Orofac Pain 2013;27:199–205.

Sleep-Related Leg Cramps
A Review and Suggestions for Future Research

 CrossMark

Terry M. Brown, DO

KEYWORDS

- Sleep • Leg cramps • Quinine • Continuous positive airway pressure • Statins • Elderly • Children
- Pregnancy

KEY POINTS

- Leg cramps are a common cause of sleep disruption and may be the most common sleep disorder.
- There are medications and behavioral treatments for sleep-related leg cramps, although the evidence is poor for all but quinine. Quinine is useful for leg cramps, but dangerous.
- There are numerous secondary causes of sleep-related leg cramps, although the emphasis is on idiopathic sleep-related leg cramps.
- Long-acting β-agonists may be the drug type most strongly associated with sleep-related leg cramps, with statins not being as commonly associated as some have believed.
- Because leg cramps are so common, future research into sleep-related leg cramps is important, and a standardized questionnaire would greatly facilitate this.

Sleep-related leg cramps (SRLCs), also called nocturnal leg cramps, have been insufficiently studied. The lay term is a Charley horse. However, the origin of the term remains obscure. SRLCs have also been called rest cramps in the Canadian literature.[1] In this article, the essential features of the condition, the prevalence, and the differential diagnosis are described, the primary and secondary associations and treatment effects are discussed, and opportunities for further research and education are suggested. This review is not primarily evidence based because the subject has not been well studied for a variety of reasons, and only in the cases of some treatment options are there any evidence-based data. In addition, the author has added his own anecdotal information from his patients with leg cramps, and that of his own experience with leg cramps.

The *International Classification of Sleep Disorders, Third Edition, 2014* describes 3 diagnostic criteria for SRLCs. These criteria include "a painful sensation in the leg or foot associated with sudden, involuntary muscle hardness or tightness, indicating a strong muscle contraction; the painful muscle contractions occur during the time in bed, although they may arise from either wakefulness or sleep; and third, the pain is relieved by forceful stretching of the affected muscles, thus releasing the contraction."[2] Often, the coping strategy involves getting out of bed to put weight on the afflicted limb.[3] Nocturnal cramps are generally in the calf or muscles in the foot and rarely include the thigh muscles. The cramp is sometimes preceded by an early warning tightening sensation and sometimes can be prevented by dorsiflexing the foot, according to the author's patients. The other essential feature of SRLCs is that they disturbs sleep. Some individuals have multiple leg cramps nightly, whereas others have only the occasional SRLC. If cramps are severe, there

Disclosure: the author has nothing to disclose.
Sleep Medicine Associates, LLC, Sleep Disorders Center, St. Joseph Memorial Hospital, 2 South Hospital Drive, Murphysboro, IL 62966, USA
E-mail address: terry.brown@sih.net

Sleep Med Clin 10 (2015) 385–392
http://dx.doi.org/10.1016/j.jsmc.2015.05.002
1556-407X/15/$ – see front matter © 2015 Elsevier Inc. All rights reserved.

may be residual tenderness and soreness in the muscle for 1 to 2 days. In addition to the obvious diurnal variation, there is some evidence of a seasonal variation, with more quinine being prescribed for leg cramps in the midsummer as opposed to midwinter in a Canadian study.[4]

SRLCs may be idiopathic or secondary to metabolic or other medical disorders. The most common type is probably idiopathic or this may reflect our incomplete knowledge of etiopathology. Secondary associations have included pregnancy,[5] peripheral vascular disease,[6] hypokalemia,[1] hypocalcemia,[7] hypomagnesemia,[8] spinal stenosis[9] dialysis,[10] dehydration and other electrolyte disturbances,[11] other metabolic disorders including metabolic syndrome,[12] and diabetes mellitus, although 1 study[6] suggested no correlation between diabetes and leg cramps. Various drugs have also been associated with the condition (to be discussed later). In addition, prolonged standing has been associated with both nocturnal leg cramps and varicose veins.[13]

PREVALENCE

The prevalence is unclear, but it is clear that SRLCs are common. Some studies have suggested that 50% to 60% of the adult population[6,14] may experience SRLCs and some children also experience them.[15] In general, SRLCs are increasingly common with advancing age, although they have been reported in another study in children as young as age 8 years.[15] That study showed a 7% prevalence in children 8 years or older although the frequency of cramps was low by adult standards. It is not clear that there is a gender predominance, although some studies have suggested a greater prevalence in females.[14] The frequency of this disorder within individuals varies considerably. In the author's opinion, leg cramps are rarely the primary reason for a sleep medicine referral or self-referral. The perception of many patients seems to be that SRLCs are just an unpleasant part of getting older and many may not recognize that treatments are available. This attitude of the patient may also be another reason why SRLCs have not been thoroughly studied. There is no clear evidence of familial pattern thus far. Pregnant women may be more likely to have SRLCs, which normally resolve after delivery. Estimates are that between 30% and 45% of pregnant women have SRLCs.[5,16]

The author's own unpublished data from his busy sleep medicine practice show that only 2.3% of patients interviewed for the first time reported a problem with leg cramps. This finding included 75 patients of 3257 patients who had been interviewed and examined between January,

2011 and December, 2014. Clearly, this is not a measure of prevalence but may suggest certain things about patients' willingness to bring up the problem voluntarily. Another factor is that patients often come to see the sleep specialist for a more severe sleep disorder, and there may not be time to investigate SRLCs from both the clinician's and the patient's viewpoint.

DIFFERENTIAL DIAGNOSIS

In discussing leg cramps with patients, it seems that some do not differentiate well the distinctions between restless legs syndrome (RLS) and SRLCs; however, the determination should be easy for the clinician if one keeps in mind the sudden nature of SRLCs versus the gradual and persistent effect of RLS. In general, the patient with SRLC describes a tightened or cramped muscle, which the pure RLS case does not describe. Dystonias can be confused with SRLCs but involve agonist versus antagonist simultaneous muscle activation. RLS is difficult for the patient to describe, whereas SRLCs are specifically described. Also, leg cramps are not expected to be alleviated with dopaminergic agonists. Dystonias generally are not relieved by stretching or standing on the affected limb, as are SRLCs. In general, the phenomenologies are distinct. It may be that RLS and SRLCs cluster together in the same individuals, and that may be 1 reason why the patient seems to often confuse these 2 conditions. Growing pains in children can be differentiated by their lack of sudden onset. Secondary causes of leg cramps are probably rarer than idiopathic. The primary focus of this review is the idiopathic leg cramp.

Muscular pain fasciculation syndrome has been described and involves muscular aching, fasciculations, fatigue, and paresthesias.[17] It is not more or less prominent during sleep and does seem to be a rare disorder. Like SRLCs, it is worsened by exercise, but unlike SRLCs, the symptoms subside at rest generally. Various myelopathies may mimic the condition, but once again, these are more likely to occur with muscular effort and not at rest, as do leg cramps generally. A similar disorder was described[18] called cramp fasciculation syndrome, which seems to be a peripheral nerve disorder. Fibromyalgia has been believed to be associated with both leg cramps and RLS in the literature,[19] but clearly, more study is needed to determine degree of overlap.

Secondary Sleep-Related Leg Cramps

Leg cramps while awake during the day may have the same etiopathology as SRLCs, but this has not been confirmed. However, because the literature on waking leg cramps is likely relevant, it is reviewed here as well. Athletes have been known to report leg cramps in the course of exercise and often warm up with stretching exercises to decrease the odds of these. The assumption has been that dehydration and electrolyte disturbances may lead to leg cramps in athletes, but some studies[11] have suggested that electrolyte changes may have nothing to do with the cramps of athletes that are exercise induced. Electrolyte disturbance in various medical conditions that may lead to leg cramps has been reported anecdotally in much of the literature, although the author is not aware of any systematic analyses of this in nonathletes. Other associations with leg cramps in the literature concern various drugs, including oral contraceptives,[20] intravenous iron sucrose (Venofer),[21] raloxifene (Evista),[22] teriparatide (Forteo),[23] pyrazinamide,[24] long-acting β-agonists,[1] and statins.[1] Garrison and colleagues[1] have studied in patients aged 50 years and older the frequency of quinine (Qualaquin) usage for leg cramps and looked at what prescriptions have preceded the prescription of quinine for leg cramps in a large Canadian database. These investigators also compared the frequency of quinine use in those not receiving one of the index drug classes of diuretics, statins, and long-acting β₂-agonists. Quinine was still being used to treat leg cramps in Canada at the time of the study.[1] The investigators found that medications that are most associated with quinine treatment of cramps were long-acting β-agonists, potassium-sparing diuretics, and thiazidelike diuretics. If, as some think, hypokalemia is a putative cause of leg cramps, it is interesting that Garrison and colleagues[1] found that there was a stronger association of prescribing quinine after the addition of the potassium-sparing diuretics than there was with prescribing of quinine after addition of the potassium-depleting diuretics. A further interesting finding was that statins were not highly associated with quinine use. It may be that statins have obtained this leg cramp reputation association because they cause myopathies, but it is certainly not clear that they cause leg cramps. The main limitation of the study other than being retrospective was not having a direct measure for leg cramp frequency, but quinine use, at least until recently, does seem to be a good surrogate indicator for presence of leg cramps in Canada. Other drugs have not been systematically studied and most of the evidence is anecdotal.

Other secondary causes of leg cramps or SRLCs include peripheral neuropathies caused by cancer treatment or metastasis,[25,26] cardiovascular disease,[6] cirrhosis,[27] venous insufficiency,[13] osteoarthritis (largely anecdotal), Parkinson disease,[28] multiple sclerosis,[29] and gout (largely anecdotal).

PATHOPHYSIOLOGY

Little is known about the pathophysiology, because the spontaneous nature of the leg cramps makes observing them challenging. Experimental electrical and magnetic stimulations have been performed, and there seems to be a rapid firing of the anterior horn neurons. Patients with a history of leg cramps require a lower-frequency (15 Hz) signal to elicit the cramp in the flexor hallucis brevis muscle than do patients without such a history.[30] It is not known if this characteristic is inherited or acquired, but it is a useful research finding. Why the motor cells fire in spontaneous cases of leg cramp is not clear. Afferent pathways from the muscle may elicit the motor neuron firing and possibly help to end it as well. However, the central versus peripheral origin of the leg cramp has not been fully elucidated.[31]

TREATMENTS

A wide variety of pharmacologic and some behavioral treatments have been used. In the United Kingdom and in Canada, it seem that quinine is used a great deal still to treat SRLCs. In 2012, the US Food and Drug Administration (FDA) put out a memo stating that quinine was approved for malaria and was not safe for treatment or prevention of leg cramps. Although off-label prescribing has been tolerated by the FDA for most drugs, this was a rare time that they stated that it was not safe. Among the side effects cited were thrombocytopenia, hypersensitivity reactions, and QT prolongation.[32]

However, the evidence for the efficacy of quinine to treat SRLCs is good.[33,34] For this reason, and because the drug is no longer used for treatment of leg cramps in the United States, the subject of the efficacy of quinine is left as a given, in the interests of brevity.

Magnesium salts have been tried in several groups of elderly patients with leg cramp, with primarily negative results. In 1995, Frusso and colleagues[35] published a double-blind, placebo-controlled trial in 93 patients with 900 mg of magnesium citrate twice a day. There was no significant difference in outcome measures between the magnesium condition versus the placebo condition. In 2002, Roffe and colleagues[36] performed a randomized placebo-controlled crossover study of 46 persons of mixed gender using 300 mg (12 mmol) per day of oral magnesium citrate. There was no significant difference between the placebo versus magnesium condition, but patients reported that their leg cramps were perceived as improved after magnesium treatment, even although frequency of cramps was not significantly different. This result occurred even although the study was double blinded.[36] Garrison and colleagues,[37] 2011, performed a double-blind placebo-controlled trial of intravenous magnesium (2011) in 46 elderly patients (69 ± 7.7 years) and found no difference between placebo infusion and magnesium infusion. In this study, serum magnesium levels were normal. Of course, in all of these studies, the preparations were different salts of magnesium, and elemental magnesium dosage varied.

Magnesium for the treatment of leg cramps in pregnancy has also been studied. Dahle and colleagues[8] in 1995 studied 73 pregnant patients in a randomized double-blind trial of oral magnesium (5 mmol per day of a combined citrate and lactate preparation). Serum magnesium in all patients was low to low normal, but therapy did not significantly increase serum magnesium levels. However, there was an overall significant effect of magnesium over placebo in terms of leg cramp frequency. Nygaard and colleagues[38] performed a double-blind placebo-controlled study of 38 women using 360 mg per day of oral magnesium citrate or lactate, believed to be 5 mmol, versus placebo. Both serum magnesium and urinary excretion of magnesium were measured but were not significantly different between the 2 groups before or after the intervention. There was also no significant difference in leg cramp frequency between the treated group and the placebo group. Supakatisant and Phupong[39] performed a randomized, double-blind, placebo-controlled study of 86 women using 300 mg bisglycinate chelate per day oral magnesium versus placebo. Leg cramp frequency in the treated group was significantly lower than it was in the placebo group after treatment.

A Cochrane database study was performed by Sebo and colleagues,[40] who reviewed 7 randomized controlled studies that met their criteria and concluded that magnesium had no effect in nonpregnant adults but may have a slight positive effect on pregnant women with leg cramps. These investigators suggested that we needed more studies in pregnant patients. It may be that the studies of nonpregnant adults were not positive because of normal baseline serum magnesium levels, if this had been measured. Clearly, all of the studies, both in the nonpregnant and the pregnant, should have had preserum and postserum magnesium levels to help tease out the

magnesium deficiency issue. Maybe some pregnant patients respond to magnesium because of magnesium deficiency, which the nonpregnant adult patients might not have.

Other medications and supplements have been tried in the treatment of leg cramps, but most of the evidence is weak. These treatments include diltiazem (Cardizem), verapamil (Calan; Isoptin) (open-label small study),[41] gabapentin (Neurontin),[42] orphenadrine (Norflex),[43] carisoprodol (Soma),[44] B complex vitamins,[45] and vitamin E.[46] The quality of evidence on all of these treatments is low, and some of it is just anecdotal. However, there was 1 letter to the editor by Wen-Chol Voon[47] in 2001 describing a double-blind crossover study of diltiazem versus placebo in 13 patients. Diltiazem was found to be safe and efficacious. Vitamin E was compared with quinine in 29 hemodialysis patients in the study by Roca and colleagues[46] in 1992. Similar efficacy between 325 mg of quinine and 400 EU of vitamin E at bedtime was shown, but, although the study was blinded and randomized and there was a placebo washout, there was no placebo group. However, this finding may suggest some efficacy for vitamin E in this patient group. However, Connolly[48] performed a placebo-controlled crossover study of 27 male veterans not on dialysis comparing all 3 conditions and showed that quinine, but not vitamin E, was effective compared with placebo. More studies are needed before any of these secondary agents can be recommended.

Behavioral Treatments

Leg stretching has been recommended as a treatment of SRLCs, because stretching before practice seems to help athletes avoid exercise-induced cramps. However, the data are confusing. Hallegraeff and colleagues[49] found that nightly stretching of the calves and hamstrings in 80 adults older than 55 years decreased the severity and frequency of leg cramps compared with a control group who did nothing. Random assignment occurred, but of course, this study could not be blinded. The study shows photographs of the type of stretching exercises that were performed, which should aid in standardization if other studies like this are performed. If plantar flexion of the foot is the main elicitor of SRLCs, it is difficult to understand how stretching exercises would prevent the cramps. It may be that the muscles need to be tense at baseline for the plantar flexion to elicit the cramps. Although stretching is recommended, there have been dissenters regarding methodological issues in the Hallegraeff study.[50] Other types of treatments such as avoiding heavy bed covers, heating pads, and so forth have not been systematically studied. Getting out of bed and walking seems to help according to a survey study,[3] but whether walking during the day would help prevent leg cramps at night is not known.

Continuous positive airway pressure (CPAP) has been suggested to be therapeutic for leg cramps in patients with obstructive sleep apnea in 1 study.[51] It is a case study of 4 individuals, 3 of whom had complete resolution of SLRCs after starting CPAP, and the fourth had a near complete resolution after starting CPAP. These patients did not have periodic limb movements or RLS. More research in this area would be interesting.

FUTURE DIRECTIONS FOR RESEARCH

SRLCs in the author's opinion may be the most common sleep disorder. Because SRLCs are so prevalent, it would be good if we had more effective treatments for the condition. Quinine works well; however, the risks of quinine use may be too great, in any population, but especially, in the population that is likely to have the most frequent leg cramp complaints. Behavioral treatments may be effective in some persons.

Another issue is that it is not certain if SRLCs share the same pathophysiology as waking daytime cramps, although the phenomenology seems similar. We need to know more about the pathophysiology, why there is such rapid firing of motor neurons, and whether muscle afferent receptors are involved in starting the rapid firing of the motor neurons. The author was once giving a lecture to a group of elderly laypersons who asked about leg cramp treatment. The author demonstrated the plantar flexion motion as an elicitor of leg cramps and proceeded to have a cramp there in front of the audience. It was relieved quickly by stomping the affected foot on the floor and putting weight on it, which is the opposite of the plantar flexion that normally occurs when the cramps start. Although this incident was not sleep related, it had the same phenomenology as that of sleep-related cramps. Anecdotally, heavy bed covers have also been associated with plantar flexion and leg cramps in the author's experience and that of his patients. Sleeping prone may elicit these too if a significant plantar flexion of the feet occurs.

If various vitamin or nutritional substances are continued to be studied as possible treatments, it would be important to know the preintervention and postintervention blood levels of these nutritional substances in these clinical trials. It is regrettable that we do not have a safe drug treatment of SRLCs, but do we need a drug treatment is still another question. If a behavioral intervention would work, this would be preferable. If plantar flexion instigates the cramp, which certainly seems to be the case from the survey literature[3] and the author's viewpoint of having had these cramps, both sleep related and during the day with similar phenomenology, then maybe we should be telling patients with leg cramp to avoid heavy bed covers on the feet, because these might promote plantar flexion. Perhaps even a therapeutic bootie could be designed that keeps the foot dorsiflexed to some degree while sleeping. Many patients report the cramps while lying supine, where the bed covers may be more likely to plantar flex the feet. Also many of the author's patients have reported that when they first wake in the morning, they tend to stretch their legs in bed, and with this to plantar flex their feet, eliciting the cramp. The author has educated some patients not to plantar flex their feet while they are stretching in bed, with beneficial results, although no systematic study has been performed regarding any of this.

Another area that is intriguing is whether CPAP therapy in those patients with obstructive sleep apnea can improve SRLCs. A more extensive prospective study should be performed to determine if the leg cramps improve in most persons receiving CPAP. Anecdotally, it is said that sometimes RLS improves with CPAP therapy. The extent to which SRLCs overlap in individuals with RLS and other sleep disorders would be a useful thing to know as well.

A standardized leg cramp rating instrument would help us perform research related to SRLCs. Such questionnaires should explore the age of onset of the cramps, the frequency, a quantification of the severity of the pain, and the location of the pains, as well as how much the condition disturbs sleep. To tease out daytime versus night cramps, the questionnaire should ask about both and the environmental circumstances preceding each type of cramp. Of course, what the patient does to alleviate the pain, behavioral as well as over-the-counter remedies, should be explored along with inquiries to health care professionals about possible treatment. Medical conditions known to be associated with secondary SRLCs would be important to cover, as well as whether cramps occurred during pregnancy. Blyton and colleagues'[3] survey of patients with the condition and what treatments they found effective may represent the beginnings of such a questionnaire research instrument, and the author would like to praise and encourage such efforts. Medication lists to obtain a better idea of the type of medications associated with SRLCs would also be a useful part of the rating instrument.

Another issue is that there are contradictory data about the role of hypokalemia in leg cramps. The study by Garrison and collegaues[1] suggested that potassium-sparing diuretics are more likely to produce leg cramps than potassium-depleting diuretics and that seems to be inconsistent with standard anecdotal connections between hypokalemia and leg cramps. But Garrison and colleagues[1] note that hyperkalemia is more neurostimulating than hypokalemia would be based on what we know about the nerve cell mechanism of excitability. Garrison and colleagues,[1] of course, admit the limitations of their quinine prescribing data, so more studies are clearly needed to determine if hypokalemia is or is not a common cause of SRLCs. The author once admitted a 35-year-old woman to a psychiatric facility, and in the routine laboratory tests, we discovered that potassium levels were low. The patient was complaining of leg cramps, which piqued this author's interest. The potassium level when she first came in was 3.3 meq/L. The author then started giving her KCL at recommended doses of 20 meq per day. By the time of discharge 5 days later, her leg cramps had gone and her potassium level was now 3.8. She was taking no medications other than an antidepressant and had no medical problems other than generalized anxiety disorder. After discharge, she was to follow up with the author, but did not for an entire year. When the author saw her in the office a year later, she was also complaining of leg cramps. The author checked her potassium level again and it was 3.4. Once again, he gave her 20 meq per day of KCL for a week and her cramps disappeared, and the blood level of potassium was 3.7. This was unpublished data with only 1 patient, but it did make this author curious about how frequent hypokalemia could be a cause of SLRCs. The seasonal variation that Garrison and colleagues[4] describe could suggest that because the prescribing of quinine was more frequent in the summer, the summer shows a higher frequency of leg cramps, and this might fit with the hypokalemia issue, through more sweating in the summer months. However, this study was carried out in Canada, where the summers are milder than in the United States, and thus, the connection with hypokalemia may not be supported by this 1 Canadian study. Also, in Canada, it may be that patients have heavy bed covers on their feet throughout the year, and these could instigate plantar flexion at any time of year. Clearly, more research is needed on the seasonality of leg cramps, but they may be more frequent in the summer for whatever reason(s).

PATIENT EDUCATION AND CLINICIAN EDUCATION

It may be that a lot of primary care doctors are unaware of leg cramps, or just do not ask about them after the FDA put out the warning on using quinine for treatment of SRLCs. Dr Richard Allen and Dr K. Kirby in their review of leg cramps in the journal *American Family Practice*[52] have begun this education mission already.

Patient education may be slower to progress, because patients do not seem to realize that SRLCs are something to talk about with their doctor (or at least their sleep specialist), do not seem to realize it is a sleep disorder, and are unaware of treatments generally. The fact that few of the author's patients (2.3%) even mentioned SRLCs to the sleep specialist may reflect these concerns. Since December, 2014, the author has been trying to systematically ask the patients who come in for any sleep disorder if they have SRLCs. Traditional sleep questionnaires have often not addressed leg cramps. Once again, a standardized questionnaire might assist with clinical treatment as well as with research agendas.

However, there are other patient educational problems, in that many over-the-counter leg cramp remedies are sold over the Internet. One site that this author looked at in preparing this review was a remedy described by its proponents as an old remedy. It consists of apple cider vinegar, ginger plant juice, and garlic juice. Claims are that it prevents or stops cramps of any kind but also specifically treats nocturnal leg cramps, in 1 to 2 minutes. One can swallow the liquid remedy, or just rub it on one's affected area(s). The mechanism of action is not specified. It occurs to the author that SRLCs often resolve in 1 to 2 minutes with no treatment other than getting out of bed and standing up. Several remedies described on the Internet contain quinine in homeopathic doses from the *Chinchona officinalis* plant or quinine bark. The safety or efficacy of such a homeopathic remedy is difficult to evaluate, and we may need to caution our patients about use of such over-the-counter remedies.

SRLCs are the probably the most frequent sleep disorder. They are easy to diagnose, but difficult to treat. Known effective medication treatments are dangerous. Behavioral treatments may be effective. Future research is needed into cause and treatments. Future research could be facilitated by a standardized questionnaire. Patients may underreport SRLCs to their doctors, and thus, more education is needed.

REFERENCES

1. Garrison SR, Dormuth RL, Morrow RL, et al. Nocturnal leg cramps and prescription use that precedes them: a sequence symmetry analysis. JAMA Intern Med 2012;172(2):120–6.

2. American Academy of Sleep Medicine. International classification of sleep disorders. 3rd edition. Darien (IL): American Academy of Sleep Medicine; 2014. p. 299.

3. Blyton F, Chuter V, Burns J. Unknotting night-time muscle cramps: a survey of patient experience, help-seeking behaviour and perceived treatment effectiveness. J Foot Ankle Res 2012;5:7.

4. Garrison SR, Dormuth CR, Morrow RL, et al. Seasonal effects on the occurrence of nocturnal leg cramps: a prospective cohort study. CMAJ 2015; 187:1–6.

5. Hensley JG. Leg cramps and restless legs syndrome during pregnancy. J Midwifery Womens Health 2009;54(3):211–8.

6. Oboler SK, Prochazka AV, Meyer TJ. Leg symptoms in outpatient veterans. West J Med 1991;155:256–9.

7. Palal B, Sinsakul M, Reutrakul S. Case report: life-threatening hypocalcemia following subtotal parathyroidectomy in a patient with renal failure and previous Roux-en-Y gastric bypass surgery. Case Rep Endocrinol 2011;2011:1–6.

8. Dahle LO, Berg G, Hammar M, et al. The effect of oral magnesium substitution on pregnancy-induced leg cramps. Am J Obstet Gynecol 1995;173(1): 175–80.

9. Matsumoto M, Watanabe K, Tsuji T, et al. Nocturnal leg cramps: a common complaint in patients with lumbar spinal canal stenosis. Spine (Phila Pa 1976) 2009;34(5):E189–94.

10. Raymond CR, Wazney LD. Treatment of leg cramps in patients with chronic kidney disease receiving hemodialysis. CANNT J 2011;21(3):19–23.

11. Schwellnus MP, Nicol J, Laubscher R, et al. Serum electrolyte concentrations and hydration status are not associated with exercise associated muscle cramping (EAMC) in distance runners. Br J Sports Med 2004;38(4):488–92.

12. Mania MN. Leg cramps in relation to metabolic syndrome. Georgian Med News 2009;1(166):51–3 [English translation].

13. Bahk JW, Kim H, Jung-Choi K, et al. Relationship between prolonged standing and symptoms of varicose veins and nocturnal leg cramps among women and men. Ergonomics 2012;52(2):133–9.

14. Abdulla AJ, Jones PW, Pearce VR. Leg cramps in the elderly: prevalence, drug and disease associations. Int J Clin Pract 1999;53(7):494–6.

15. Leung AK, Wong BE, Chan PY, et al. Nocturnal leg cramps in children: incidence and clinical characteristics. J Natl Med Assoc 1999;91(6):329–32.

16. Valbø A, Bøhmer T. Leg cramps in pregnancy: how common are they? [Abstract in English]. Tidsskr Nor Laegeforen 1999;119(11):1589–90 [Article in Norwegian].

17. Hudson AJ, Brown WF, Gilbert JJ. The muscular pain-fasciculation syndrome. Neurology 1978; 28(11):1105–9.

18. Tahmoush AJ, Alonso RJ, Tahmoush GP, et al. Cramp-fasciculation syndrome: a treatable hyperexcitable peripheral nerve disorder. Neurology 1991; 41(7):1021–4.

19. Yunus MB, Aldaq JC. Restless legs syndrome and leg cramps in fibromyalgia syndrome: a controlled study. BMJ 1996;312(7042):1339.

20. Grant EC. Venous effects of oral contraceptives. Br Med J 1969;4(5675):73–7.

21. Physicians' desk reference. Venofer. 2015. Available at: http://www.pdr.net/drug-summary/venofer?druglabelid=805. Accessed January 16, 2015.

22. Mok CC, Ying KY, To CH, et al. Raloxifene for prevention of glucocorticoid-induced bone loss: a 12-month randomized double-blinded placebo-controlled trial. Ann Rheum Dis 2011;70(5):778–84.

23. Stroup J, Kane MP, Abu-Baker AM. Teriparatide in the treatment of osteoporosis. Am J Health Syst Pharm 2008;65(6):532–9.

24. Gupta S, Gupta V, Kapoor B, et al. Pyrazinamide induced hyperuricaemia presenting as severe bilateral leg cramps. J Indian Med Assoc 2007;105(6): 341–2.

25. Steiner I, Sieqal T. Muscle cramps in cancer patients. Cancer 1999;63(3):574–7.

26. Jhawer M, Mani S, Lefkopoulou M, et al. Phase II study of mitomycin-C, adriamycin, cisplatin (MAP) and bleomycin-CCNU in patients with advanced cancer of the anal canal: an Eastern Cooperative Oncology Group study E7282. Invest New Drugs 2006;24(5):447–54.

27. Hidaka H, Nakazawa T, Kutsukake S, et al. The efficacy of nocturnal administration of branched-chain amino acid granules to improve quality of life in patients with cirrhosis. J Gastroenterol 2013;48(2):269–76.

28. Barone P, Amboni M, Vitale C, et al. Treatment of nocturnal disturbance and excessive daytime sleepiness in Parkinson's disease. Neurology 2004;63(8 Suppl 3):S35–8.

29. Mueller ME, Gruenthal M, Olson WL, et al. Gabapentin for relief of upper motor neuron symptoms in multiple sclerosis. Arch Phys Med Rehabil 1997;78(5): 521–4.

30. Miller KC, Knight KL. Electrical stimulation cramp threshold frequency correlates well with the occurrence of skeletal muscle cramps. Muscle Nerve 2009;39:364Y8.

31. Minetto MA, Botter A. Elicitability of muscle cramps in different leg and foot muscles. Muscle Nerve 2009;40(4):535–44.

32. Derbis, J. Serious risks associated with using quinine to prevent or treat nocturnal leg cramps. 2012. Retrieved from: memo to physicians (public domain). Available at: http://www.fda.gov/ForHealthProfessionals/ArticlesofInterest/ucm317811.htm. Accessed January 16, 2015.

33. Man-Son-Hing M, Wells G. Meta-analysis of efficacy of quinine for treatment of nocturnal leg cramps in elderly people. BMJ 1995;310(6971):13–7.

34. Young G. Leg cramps. BMJ Clin Evid 2009;2009. pii: 1113.

35. Frusso R, Zarate M, Augustovski F, et al. Magnesium for the treatment of nocturnal leg cramps: a crossover randomized trial. J Fam Pract 1999;48(11): 868–71.

36. Roffe C, Sills S, Crome P, et al. Randomized, crossover, placebo controlled trial of magnesium citrate in the treatment of chronic persistent leg cramps. Med Sci Monit 2002;8(5):CR326–30.

37. Garrison SR, Birmingham CL, Koehler BE, et al. The effect of magnesium infusion on rest cramps: randomized controlled trial. J Gerontol A Biol Med Sci 2011;66(6):661–6.

38. Nygaard IH, Valbo A, Pethick SV, et al. Does oral magnesium substitution relieve pregnancy-induced leg cramps? Eur J Obstet Gynecol Reprod Biol 2008;141(1):23–6.

39. Supakatisant C, Phupong V. Oral magnesium for relief in pregnancy-induced leg cramps: a randomized controlled trial. Matern Child Nutr 2015;11:139–45. Available at: http://onlinelibrary.wiley.com/doi/10.1111/j.1740-8709.2012.00440.x/abstract.

40. Sebo P, Cerutti B, Haller DM. Effect of magnesium therapy on nocturnal leg cramps: a systematic review of randomized controlled trials with meta-analysis using simulations. Fam Pract 2014;31(1): 7–19.

41. Baltodano N, Gallo BV, Weidler DJ. Verapamil vs quinine in recumbent nocturnal leg cramps in the elderly. Arch Intern Med 1988;148(9):1969–70.

42. Serrao M, Rossi P, Cardinali P, et al. Gabapentin treatment for muscle cramps: an open-label trial. Clin Neuropharmacol 2000;23(1):45–9.

43. Popkin RJ. Orphenadrine citrate (Norflex) for the treatment of "restless legs" and related syndromes. J Am Geriatr Soc 1971;19(1):76–9.

44. Chesrow EJ, Kaplitz SE, Breme JT, et al. Use of carisoprodol (soma) for treatment of leg cramps associated with vascular, neurologic or arthritic disease. J Am Geriatr Soc 1963;11:1014–6.

45. Chan P, Huang TY, Chen YJ, et al. Randomized, double-blind, placebo-controlled study of the safety and efficacy of vitamin B complex in the treatment of nocturnal leg cramps in elderly patients with hypertension. J Clin Pharmacol 1998;38(12):1151–4.

46. Roca AO, Jarijoura D, Blend D, et al. Dialysis leg cramps: efficiency of quinine versus vitamin E. ASAIO J 1992;38(3):M481–5.

47. Voon W, Sheu S. Letter to the Editor. Age Aging 2001;30(1):91–2.

48. Connolly PS, Shirley EA, Wasson JH, et al. Treatment of nocturnal leg cramps: a crossover trial of quinine vs vitamin E. Arch Intern Med 1992;152:1877–80.

49. Hallegraeff JM, Van Der Schans C, De Ruiter R, et al. Stretching before sleep reduces the frequency and severity of nocturnal leg cramps in older adults: a randomized trial. J Physiother 2012;58(1):17–22.

50. Garrison SR. Prophylactic stretching is unlikely to prevent nocturnal leg cramps. J Physiother 2014; 60(3):174.

51. Westwood AJ, Spector AR, Auerbach SH, et al. CPAP treats muscle cramps in patients with obstructive sleep apnea. J Clin Sleep Med 2014;10(6):691–2.

52. Allen RP, Kirby KA. Nocturnal leg cramps. Am Fam Physician 2012;86(4):350–5.

Hypnic Jerks
A Scoping Literature Review

Norma G. Cuellar, PhD, RN*,
Debra Whisenant, PhD, MSPH, RN, Marietta P. Stanton, PhD, RN

KEYWORDS

- Parasomnia • Sleep start • Polysomnography • Scoping framework

KEY POINTS

- Although there is a common perception that hypnic jerks are benign, studies suggest that they may be a characteristic of certain illness, are more prevalent with chronic health conditions that interrupt sleep, and may be mimicked by other movement disorders.
- It is important to identify differential diagnosis, including nocturnal seizures, nonepileptic seizures, other parasomnias, hyperekplexia, restless legs syndrome (RLS), periodic limb movements in sleep (PLMS), excessive fragmentary myoclonus, and psychiatric diagnosis.
- Lifestyle (caffeine, smoking, anxiety) and hereditary contributions may be responsible for hypnic jerks and should be included in sleep education.
- The diagnostic value of hypnic jerks may be overlooked, specifically in patients with Parkinson disease.
- Pediatric health care providers should ask about sleep problems in children, specifically if they have hypnic jerks, as this may identify other childhood issues.

Case study

Mrs Smith is a 66-year-old woman who was seen in the clinic for routine checkup and to renew medications. She states she has been experiencing "a startle" or a "jerking awake" when she nods off to sleep in her chair at night. She remembers little as she nods off but suddenly she jerks awake and is simultaneously "propelled forward" or "falls forward". She said that this had happened in the past sporadically but that it appears to be happening more frequently and she is concerned she will fall and injure herself. She states this sleep event happens at work especially after lunch when working at the computer. She takes regular breaks when working on the computer to stay awake. When she nods off, she invariably "jerks" awake as she is in the process of falling forward. She has hit her face on her keyboard and computer screen. She states that she is not experiencing any other distress, is taking her medications as prescribed, and continues to work full-time. She has no history of sleep disorders but has never been evaluated.

INTRODUCTION

Parasomnias are abnormal events during sleep, including arousal disorders, sleep-wake transition disorders (SWTDs), events associated with rapid eye movement sleep, and other parasomnias.

Hypnic jerks (aka hypnogogic jerks, sleep start, sleep twitch, night starts, hypnic myoclonia, nocturnal myoclonus, or sleep jerks) are included in the SWTD. For the purpose of this article, the term hypnic jerks is used to include the various terms in the literature. At the moment of sleep

---

Capstone College of Nursing, University of Alabama, 650 University Boulevard, Tuscaloosa, AL 35401, USA
* Corresponding author.
E-mail address: ncuellar@ua.edu

Sleep Med Clin 10 (2015) 393–401
http://dx.doi.org/10.1016/j.jsmc.2015.05.010
1556-407X/15/$ – see front matter

onset, the physiologic phenomena of hypnic jerks cause a sudden start of the motor centers resulting in a startling awakening. Hypnic jerks may occur intermittently in 70% of the population, with 10% of this group having daily symptoms.[1] In most cases, hypnic jerks are considered a normal common variant and a benign disorder without sequelae.

Pathophysiology

SWTDs are due to modulatory systems in the brainstem and forebrain.[1] Hypnic jerks involve a major portion of the brain and occur quickly during sleep onset. Hypnic jerks presumably arise from sudden descending volleys that originate in the brainstem reticular formation and are activated by the instability of the system at the transition between sleep and wake.[2]

Diagnosis

Diagnoses of the parasomnias are based on clinical information through an interview (or sleep history) plus nocturnal polysomnography (PSG). The International Classification of Sleep Disorders-2 identifies hypnic jerks as sudden, brief jerks at sleep onset, mainly affecting the legs or arms, associated with at least 1 description of a feeling of falling, a sensory flash, or a hypnagogic dream, and must not be better explained by another disorder, medication, or substance use disorder. Unfortunately, these diagnostic criteria have not been established for interrater reliability. In a study to determine the interrater reliability of the parasomnias using the minimal diagnostic criteria, hypnic jerks showed only moderate interobserver reliability for diagnosis.[3]

A thorough sleep history should help identify concerns for the patient who may report feeling fearful and not knowing what has happened when awakened by a hypnic jerk. As hypnic jerks are intensified, sleep may be disturbed, resulting in insomnia. This condition in turn may worsen the occurrence of hypnic jerks. Hypnic jerks may be exacerbated during stressful conditions occurring during a normal part of sleep onset.[4] These stressful conditions that may cause hypnic jerks include fatigue, stress, sleep deprivation, vigorous exercise, and stimulants like caffeine and nicotine. The bed partner may also be bothered with the jerks, resulting in sleep problems for the partner as well.

At sleep onset, there are gradual changes in muscle tone on the electroencephalography (EEG). During a hypnic jerk, changes in PSG have been recorded during quiet wakefulness, drowsiness, or N1 sleep stage.[1] The jerks consist of non-periodic myoclonic movements occurring at sleep

onset with K-complexes or an EEG arousal. With each jerk, an autonomic activation occurs, resulting in tachycardia, tachypnea, and sudomotor activity described as a shock or falling feeling. The jerks are immediately followed by alpha activity on the EEG. If not carefully observed, the hypnic jerks mimic epileptic myoclonic seizures, especially in children.

Treatment

If a person feels the hypnic jerks may be a risk to themselves or someone else, if sleep is impaired as a result of the hypnic jerks, and if the frequency or intensity of the hypnic jerks increase, treatment such as self-management, sleep hygiene, or pharmacologic interventions may be considered. Self-management includes health promotion activities, that is, stress reduction, exercise, and dietary management. Good sleep hygiene should be followed, that is, avoiding caffeine and alcohol, ensuring the environment is conducive to sleep, having a good mattress, and practicing bedtime rituals. Clonozapam (Klonopin) has been helpful for treatment, but there have been no major studies examining benefits of pharmacologic agents to help with hypnic jerks.[1] It is important to reassure patients that this phenomenon is considered benign.

The ultimate aim of a scoping article is to perform a systematic review if there are enough data in the literature to support this. It is not the intent of this scoping review to describe research findings in detail but to map the fields of study in this area. Therefore, this article (1) conducts a scoping review of the literature to determine the extent, range, and nature of the research activity related to hypnic jerks and (2) identifies research gaps in the existing literature.

METHODS

This scoping review explored the current literature to identify the extent, range, and nature of the literature on hypnic jerks. Following the framework by Arksey and O'Malley,[5] a scoping review is an approach to identify or map the extent of key concepts and main sources and types of evidence available where an area may be comprehensive.[5] Unlike a systematic review, a scoping article (1) addresses broader topics whereby many different designs may be included, (2) is less likely to seek to address specific research questions, and (3) does not assess the quality of the studies included in the review. See **Box 1** for the stages of the scoping framework. The reporting of findings follows the Stages of the Scoping Framework methodology.

Stage 1: Identifying the Research Question

The research question identified for this scoping study was "What is known from the existing research literature about hypnic jerks?" The authors purposely kept the question broad to increase the amount of coverage for the review.

Stage 2: Identifying Relevant Studies

A comprehensive review was done to include research articles, case studies, and abstracts. A scoping study team, the authors, identified articles for breadth and comprehensiveness. The search was conducted in December of 2014 and again in February of 2015 to yield articles about hypnic jerks and other terms synonymously used with hypnic jerks, including hypnogogic jerks, sleep start, sleep twitch, night starts, hypnic myoclonia, nocturnal myoclonus, or sleep jerks. The electronic search was conducted in Medline, PubMed, CINAHL, psyINFO, and Google Scholar. Abstracts were searched for the last 5 years from the Annual Meetings of Associated Professional Sleep Societies. Articles were reviewed in all languages and were reviewed if the abstracts were written in English. Reference lists were reviewed to determine other articles relevant to the review. See **Fig. 1** for the flow diagram used by Preferred Reporting Items for Systematic Reviews and Meta-Analyses (PRISMA).

Stage 3: Selecting the Studies

The search was conducted by all 3 authors. The studies were then compared and combined to review. The first author read each article in its entirety. The 3 authors met at the beginning,

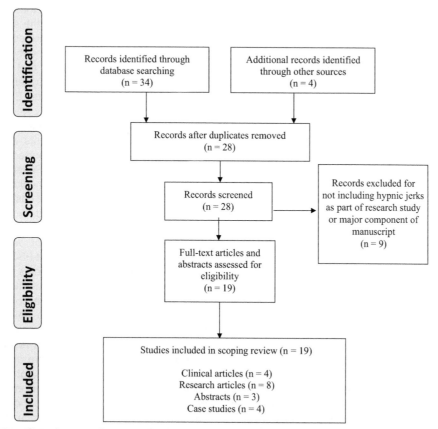

Fig. 1. PRISMA flow diagram. (*From* Moher D, Liberati A, Tetzlaff J, Altman DG, The PRISMA Group. Preferred reporting items for systematic reviews and meta-analyses: the PRISMA statement. PLoS Med 2009;6(6):e1000097.)

midpoint, and final stages of the literature review to discuss challenges or uncertainties related to study selection and refine the search as needed. Inclusion criteria were determined based on consensus of the team. Articles included in the review were categorized by research articles that identified hypnic jerks somewhere in the paper, abstracts from the APSS, case studies, and clinical articles. Inclusion criteria included any article that identified hypnic jerks as findings or as primary outcomes. There was no exclusion based on age or gender.

Stage 4: Charting the Data

Findings from the scoping review included 11 research articles/abstracts, 4 case studies, and 4 clinical articles. The research articles (n = 8) and abstracts (n = 3) are presented in **Table 1**. The case studies are described in a narrative; the clinical articles were used to write the introduction and background of the article.

Stage 5: Collating, Summarizing, and Reporting the Results

Research articles and abstracts

Of the research articles (n = 8) and abstracts (n = 3), the sample consisted of pediatric, obstetric, psychiatric, and adult populations from 7 different countries, including Finland, Germany, India (n = 2), Italy, Singapore, Turkey, and the United States (n = 4). Only 2 of the studies were specific to hypnic jerks as an outcome. Most of the articles just mentioned hypnic jerks as a finding but did not specifically address the issues of hypnic jerks or measure hypnic jerks, or it was not a major outcome of the study.

The methodologies used in these studies included subjective and objective measures of sleep. Self-reported data and/or historical data gathered through questionnaires or interviews were reported. Of the 11 studies, 6 used objective measures of sleep, including PSG, EEG, or video-EEG. The sample sizes varied from 10 to 4972 patients. Of the 11 studies, 4 focused on children's sleep disorders. Of the 11 studies, 3 included patients with paroxysmal nonepileptic events or seizures (PNEs) as their sample.

Research gaps in the literature were identified. All of the studies were descriptive in design; none addressed treatment options or improving outcomes or consequences of hypnic jerks over time. There were no intervention studies. No studies on the long-term consequences of hypnic jerks have been reported. With the startle effect of hypnic jerks and the autonomic nervous system

response, implications to chronic health conditions have not been identified.

From the scoping review, it is frequently reported that hypnic jerks are prevalent in the population and do not represent any significant pathology. They are seen across the life span and are not associated with seizure activity. Hypnic jerks may be associated with sleep disorders such as obstructive sleep apnea (OSA) and insomnia. They may be related to symptoms associated with Parkinson disease and to a bouncing walk seen with falls in the elderly.

Case studies

The case studies are presented as a descriptive analytical methodology within a narrative approach. The authors reviewed 4 published articles that presented case studies. Each case was uniquely different in description of sleep jerks, in concurrent medical diagnosis, and in medical history. The case studies provide an in-depth description about hypnic jerks.

In the first article, 2 cases involving a 42-year-old woman and a 29-year-old woman were published in 1998. Both patients reported several years of transient body jerks at sleep onset and also during daytime drowsiness. Increased stress and sleep deficiency increased the episodes. No sleep cycle disorders were reported, and sleep was undisturbed. One patient underwent electrocardiography, brain MRI, EEGs, and PSG testing with normal results. The second patient underwent a brain MRI with normal results. Both patients were considered to have sensory sleep jerks with no specific treatment recommended.[6]

In the second article, 5 patients with different symptoms and histories were reported to have significant sleep start episodes. Patients' medical histories consisted of hypothyroidism, ocular myopathy, and hepatitis C, and 2 cases had medical history. Each patient reported involuntary jerks at sleep onset, with 2 patients also reporting jerks during nocturnal arousals and on waking in the morning. Each patient underwent PSG with varied results. In an effort to evoke the jerks patients also experienced sensory and mental stimulus. Each case was determined to have a correlation between sleep jerks and the sleep-wake transition. Sleep jerks were noted only in the relaxation phase before sleep occurred. The jerks resolved in the earliest stages of sleep and were absent during all sleep cycles. One patient was noted to experience jerks during nocturnal awakening and on morning awakening. When sensory or mental exercises were instituted during relaxation before sleep, the jerks as well as the EEG alpha activity were not present. Each patient experienced

Table 1
Research articles and abstracts on hypnic jerks

Title, Year, Study Location	Study Population	Aims of the Study	Methodology	Outcome Measures	Important Results
Sleep motor activity in parkinsonism at disease onset: a possible marker for differential diagnosis (2012), Italy[10]	23 patients with Parkinson disease (PD)	To describe the possible diagnostic value of videopolysomnographic (VPSG) motor findings in patients with recent-onset parkinsonism	Descriptive, comparative	VPSG	Half of patients diagnosed with PD displayed more than 1 hypnic jerk during VPSG
Intensified hypnic jerks: a polysomnographic and polymyograhic analysis (2013), USA[11]	10 patients with repeated jerking movements at sleep onset	To analyze the nature and propagation of muscle bursts in patients presenting with intensified hypnic jerks and sleep-onset insomnia	Descriptive	Polysomnography (PSG)	There may be several physiologic subtypes of hypnic jerks Hypnic jerks involve generalized body and limb jerks and, occasionally, head jerks bilaterally
Sleep problems and daytime somnolence in a German population-based sample of snoring school-aged children (2007), Germany[12]	1144 snoring school-aged children; 114 in follow-up 1 y later	To assess associations between habitual snoring and sleep problems in primary school children	Exploratory survey population-based cross-sectional study with a nested cohort	Self-report questionnaire	Long-term habitual snorers were at risk for SWTD including hypnic jerks

(continued on next page)

Table 1
(continued)

Title, Year, Study Location	Study Population	Aims of the Study	Methodology	Outcome Measures	Important Results
Parasomnias decline during pregnancy (2002), Finland[13]	325 pregnant women in various stages of pregnancy across time	To determine the frequency of parasomnias during pregnancy by using patients' self-reports	Descriptive, comparative over time	Self-report questionnaire	Reported sleep starts decreased during pregnancy and 3 mo after, more in primiparas than multiparas
Sleep-disordered breathing in Dombivli and Mumbai (India): interesting observations (2014), India[14]	133 patients with habitual snoring	Not reported	Descriptive study	PSG, clinical evaluation	9.7% of habitual snorers in this study had hypnic jerks
Paroxysmal nonepileptic events in children and adolescents (2002), USA[15]	134 patients with paroxysmal nonepileptic events (PNEs)	To examine the relative frequency of different PNE disorders encountered during a 6-y period	6-y longitudinal study, descriptive, comparative	Prolonged video-EEG monitoring	91% of patients with hypnic jerks had a diagnosis of epilepsy, developmental delay, and attention-deficit disorder
Survey of sleep problems amongst Singapore children in a psychiatric setting (2006), Singapore[16]	490 children in a psychiatric setting	To estimate the prevalence of sleep problems in children and adolescents attending psychiatric services and to identify the correlates of sleep problems in this population	Descriptive study	Self-report questionnaire	Approximately 21% of the sample had symptoms of sleep starts; 5% had previous history of sleep starts

Study	Sample	Aim	Study type	Method	Results
Frequency of parasomnias in patients with non-epileptic seizures (2011), USA[17]	9 patients with parasomnic nonepileptic seizure (PNES)	Not reported	Descriptive, comparative	Video-EEG recordings, self-report questionnaire	PNES had a higher frequency of nonrapid eye movement parasomnias with then 77.8% of PNES having hypnic jerks
Violent behavior during sleep (1997), USA[18]	4972 of a representative sample	To examine the frequency of violent or injurious behavior during sleep and associated psychiatric risk factors	Descriptive, comparative study	Telephone interviews	Of the 2% of the sample who reported violent behavior during sleep (VBS), 62.5% reported hypnic jerks. Of the 98% of the sample who reported non-VBS, 33.8% reported hypnic jerks
Sleep paralysis and sleep starts (1962), India[19]	792 students	Not reported	Descriptive, questionnaire distributed to college students	Self-report questionnaire	47% of the sample experienced independent sleep jerks; in 11%, hypnic jerks were associated with sleep hallucinations
Childhood paroxysmal nonepileptic events (2013), Turkey[20]	95 children with PNEs	To evaluate the demographic features of children with PNEs and the nature, relative frequency, and clinical manifestations of the events documented and to determine whether these differ in children with PNEs that originated from organic or physiologic and psychogenic causes	13-y study, descriptive	Long-term video-EEG monitoring	6.3% of children with PNE had hypnic jerks

altered sleep activity with reports of insomnia. No causative effect could be found for the sleep jerks, and no correlation to concurrent medical diagnosis was noted.[7]

In 2008, a case report of a 64-year-old woman was reported with presenting complaints of "cracking" sounds on transitioning to sleep and then waking with jerking present in all 4 limbs. She could experience this up to 15 times each night while attempting to sleep. The patients' medical history consisted of pulmonary and extrapulmonary sarcoidosis. Treatment had been effective, with no sequela noted. She reported sleep issues beginning with current diagnosis 12 years earlier. Treatment of sleep issues was unsuccessful until bromazepam was instituted. MRI revealed T2-hyperintense pontomesencephalic lesion with a normal neurologic examination. The location of the lesion indicated that it could affect sleep, but it was determined that the patient's sarcoidosis was the greater cause. No specific therapy was recommended.[8]

The most recent case study described a patient with a current history of hypnic jerks preventing sleep onset. The 35-year-old patient reported insomnia due to involuntary jerks of the trunk and limbs and a feeling of "petrified head". He underwent a PSG study resulting in the observation of 5 spontaneous jerks and 2 jerks evoked by an acoustic stimulus. His hypnic jerks were random, not associated with body position, and occurred only in the sleep-wake transition period. The patient received a diagnosis of intensified hypnic jerks. He was treated with clonazepam and reported an improvement of his insomnia and hypnic jerks.[9]

Case study: Mrs Smith Mrs Smith may have hypnic jerks that could be ignored in the health assessment; however, she brings up major concerns of her risk of falling and her sleep fragmentation. It is important to examine her sleep history, as improving her sleep may in fact improve her other health conditions and decrease her hypnic jerks. Falling asleep during the day is not normal, and further evaluation of her health status is needed, particularly other sleep disorders that may be causing poor sleep, such as OSA. She also is in need of sleep hygiene instruction to help promote restorative sleep. Hypnic jerks have been associated with falls in older adults, and therefore, fall prevention should be discussed in her plan of care.

SUMMARY

Although there is a common perception that hypnic jerks are benign, recent studies suggest

that hypnic jerks may be a characteristic of certain illness, are more prevalent with chronic health conditions that interrupt sleep, and may be mimicked by other movement disorders. It is important to identify differential diagnosis, including nocturnal seizures, nonepileptic seizures, other parasomnias, hyperekplexia, RLS, PLMS, excessive fragmentary myoclonus, and psychiatric diagnosis. Lifestyle (caffeine, smoking, anxiety) and hereditary contributions may be responsible for hypnic jerks and should be included in sleep education.

The diagnostic value of hypnic jerks may be overlooked, specifically in patients with Parkinson disease. The long-term effects of hypnic jerks and the impact on children has not been addressed. Persons with sleep-disordered breathing witness hypnic jerks that may affect sleep/health outcomes. Pediatric health care providers should ask about sleep problems in children, specifically if they have hypnic jerks, as this may identify other childhood issues. This scoping study identifies that there is a lack of research in the area of hypnic jerks with gaps in the literature. Owing to the lack of clinical trials in the area, there are not enough research studies to conduct a systematic review or meta-analysis.

REFERENCES

1. Vetrugno R, Montagna P. Sleep-to-wake transition movement disorders. Sleep Med 2011;12(Suppl 2): S11–6.
2. Walters AS. Clinical identification of the simple sleep-related movement disorders. Chest 2007; 131(4):1260–6.
3. Vignatelli L, Bisulli F, Zaniboni A, et al. Interobserver reliability of ICSD-R minimal diagnostic criteria for the parasomnias. J Neurol 2005;252(6):712–7.
4. Lozsadi D. Myoclonus: a pragmatic approach. Pract Neurol 2012;12(4):215–24.
5. Arksey H, O'Malley L. Scoping studies: towards a methodological framework. Int J Soc Res Methodol 2005;8(1):19–32.
6. Sander HW, Geisse H, Quinto C, et al. Sensory sleep starts. J Neurol Neurosurg Psychiatr 1998; 64(5):690.
7. Vetrugno R, Provini F, Meletti S, et al. Propriospinal myoclonus at the sleep-wake transition: a new type of parasomnia. Sleep 2001;24(7):835–43.
8. Salih F, Klingebiel R, Zschenderlein R, et al. Acoustic sleep starts with sleep-onset insomnia related to a brainstem lesion. Neurology 2008;70(20):1935–7.
9. Calandra-Buonaura G, Alessandria M, Liguori R, et al. Hypnic jerks: neurophysiological characterization of a new motor pattern. Sleep Med 2014;15(6): 725–7.

10. Alessandria M, Calandra-Buonaura G, Sambati L, et al. Sleep motor activity in Parkinsonism at disease onset: a possible marker for differential diagnosis. Sleep 2012;35 [Abstract Supplement].

11. Chokroverty S, Bhat S, Gupta D. Intensified hypnic jerks: a polysomnographic and polymyographic analysis. J Clin Neurophysiol 2013;30(4):403–10.

12. Eitner S, Urschitz MS, Guenther A, et al. Sleep problems and daytime somnolence in a German population-based sample of snoring school-aged children. J Sleep Res 2007;16(1):96–101.

13. Hedman C, Pohjasvaara T, Tolonen U, et al. Parasomnias decline during pregnancy. Acta Neurol Scand 2002;105(3):209–14.

14. Iyer S, Iyer R. Sleep disordered breathing in Dombivli and Mumbai (India): interesting observations. Sleep 2014;37 [Abstract Supplement].

15. Kotagal P, Costa M, Wyllie E, et al. Paroxysmal non-epileptic events in children and adolescents. Pediatrics 2002;110(4):e46.

16. Mahendran R, Subramaniam M, Cai Y, et al. Survey of sleep problems amongst Singapore children in a psychiatric setting. Soc Psychiatry Psychiatr Epidemiol 2006;41(8):669–73.

17. Miglis M, Rodriguez A. Frequency of parasomnias in patients with non-epileptic seizures. Sleep 2011;34 [Abstract Supplement].

18. Ohayon MM, Caulet M, Priest RG. Violent behavior during sleep. J Clin Psychiatry 1997;58(8):369–76.

19. Rao VR, Rindani TH. Sleep paralysis and sleep starts. J Postgrad Med 1963;9:50–6.

20. Yilmaz U, Serdaroglu A, Gurkas E, et al. Childhood paroxysmal nonepileptic events. Epilepsy Behav 2013;27(1):124–9.

Moving?

Make sure your subscription moves with you!

To notify us of your new address, find your **Clinics Account Number** (located on your mailing label above your name), and contact customer service at:

Email: journalscustomerservice-usa@elsevier.com

800-654-2452 (subscribers in the U.S. & Canada)
314-447-8871 (subscribers outside of the U.S. & Canada)

Fax number: 314-447-8029

Elsevier Health Sciences Division
Subscription Customer Service
3251 Riverport Lane
Maryland Heights, MO 63043

*To ensure uninterrupted delivery of your subscription, please notify us at least 4 weeks in advance of move.

ELSEVIER

Printed and bound by CPI Group (UK) Ltd, Croydon, CR0 4YY

03/10/2024

01040375-0003